Erectile Disorders

ERECTILE DISORDERS

Assessment and Treatment

Edited by
RAYMOND C. ROSEN
SANDRA R. LEIBLUM
University of Medicine and Dentistry of New Jersey
Robert Wood Johnson Medical School

FOREWORD BY JOHN BANCROFT

Medical Consultant: R. Taylor Segraves

THE GUILFORD PRESS
New York   London

This book is dedicated to our cherished
friends and colleagues in the field.

© 1992 The Guilford Press
A Division of Guilford Publications, Inc.
72 Spring Street, New York, NY 10012

Printed in the United States of America

This book is printed on acid-free paper.

Last digit is print number: 9 8 7 6 5 4 3 2 1

Library of Congress Cataloging-in-Publication Data
Erectile disorders: assessment and treatment / edited by Raymond C.
  Rosen and Sandra R. Leiblum.
      p.   cm.
  Includes bibliographical references and index.
  ISBN 0-89862-792-3
    1. Impotence. I. Rosen, Raymond, 1946-   . II. Leiblum, Sandra
Risa.
    [DNLM: 1. Penile Disorders—diagnosis. 2. Penile Disorders—
therapy. 3. Penile Erection.   WJ 790 E67]
RC889.E74   1992
616.6'92—dc20
DNLM/DLC
Library of Congress   91-38062
                                                                 CIP

Contributors

STANLEY E. ALTHOF, Ph.D., Department of Psychiatry, Case Western Reserve University School of Medicine, Cleveland, Ohio; Male Sexual Health Center, University Hospitals of Cleveland, Cleveland, Ohio

JULIAN M. DAVIDSON, Ph.D., Department of Molecular and Cellular Physiology, Stanford University School of Medicine, Stanford, California

SANDRA R. LEIBLUM, Ph.D., Department of Psychiatry and Sexual Counseling Service, University of Medicine and Dentistry of New Jersey, Robert Wood Johnson Medical School, Piscataway, New Jersey

STEPHEN B. LEVINE, M.D., Department of Psychiatry, Case Western Reserve University School of Medicine, Cleveland, Ohio; Center for Human Sexuality, University Hospitals of Cleveland, Cleveland, Ohio

JOSEPH LOPICCOLO, Ph.D., Department of Psychology, University of Missouri-Columbia, Columbia, Missouri

BARRY W. MCCARTHY, Ph.D., Washington Psychological Center/Department of Psychology, American University, Washington, D.C.

ARNOLD MELMAN, M.D., Department of Urology and Center for Male Sexuality, Montefiore Medical Center and Albert Einstein College of Medicine, Bronx, New York

RAYMOND C. ROSEN, Ph.D., Department of Psychiatry and Sexual Counseling Service, University of Medicine and Dentistry of New Jersey, Robert Wood Johnson Medical School, Piscataway, New Jersey

RAUL C. SCHIAVI, M.D., Department of Psychiatry, Mount Sinai School of Medicine, New York, New York

LESLIE R. SCHOVER, Ph.D., Center for Sexual Function, The Cleveland Clinic Foundation, Cleveland, Ohio

KATHLEEN B. SEGRAVES, Ph.D., Department of Psychiatry, MetroHealth Medical Center, Cleveland, Ohio; Department of Psychiatry, Case Western Reserve University School of Medicine, Cleveland, Ohio

R. TAYLOR SEGRAVES, M.D., Ph.D., Department of Psychiatry, Case Western Reserve University School of Medicine, Cleveland, Ohio; Department of Psychiatry, Cleveland Metropolitan General Hospital, Cleveland, Ohio

LEONORE TIEFER, Ph.D., Department of Urology and Psychiatry, Montefiore Medical Center and Albert Einstein College of Medicine, Bronx, New York

LOUISA A. TURNER, Ph.D., Department of Psychiatry, Case Western Reserve University School of Medicine, Cleveland, Ohio; Private Practice, Cleveland, Ohio

BERNIE ZILBERGELD, Ph.D., Private Practice, Oakland, California

Foreword

When I first entered the field of sex therapy in the 1960s, it was widely assumed that erectile dysfunction was a psychogenic problem in at least 90% of cases. Not only was there no evidence to support such an assumption, there was also no understanding of how psychological processes might result in erectile failure. Anxiety and anger were regarded as of central importance by therapists of both psychoanalytic and behavioral persuasions. There were naive explanations based on a dichotomous concept of the autonomic nervous system, with the parasympathetic system underlying positive, "desirable" responses such as relaxation and erection, and the sympathetic system mediating the effects of anxiety or anger in inhibiting such "positive" responses. With the entry of Masters and Johnson into this therapeutic field in 1970, the role of performance anxiety and the negative impact of being a "spectator" rather than a "participant" were given particular emphasis. There followed a substantial increase in both therapeutic activity and optimism among psychologically oriented therapists. Their results were encouraging to the extent that a fair proportion of cases of erectile failure benefited. But there remained an equally impressive proportion who failed to respond, and for those who did respond, the reasons for the success remained somewhat obscure.

Over the past 15 years or so, and somewhat in parallel to the developments in sex therapy, we have also seen a dramatic change in the medical (or perhaps more correctly, surgical) approach to erectile dysfunction. This has in part reflected the changing pattern of health care and the need for prestigious, highly paid specialties to diversify their role. Thus we see the conventional work of urologists and, to a lesser extent, vascular surgeons shrinking as health patterns change and surgical management gives way to medical. Both of these professional groups, but especially the urologists, have moved into the field of male sexual dysfunction.

In contrast to the earlier, ill-founded assumption that the large majority of erectile problems were psychogenic in origin, we increasingly hear the counterclaim that nearly all cases of impotence are organic in nature. Again, this assertion is based on no valid evidence. But this time, in addition, we are told that nearly all such cases are treatable. The breakthrough has arrived; men should no longer suffer this tribulation. A veritable industry has evolved within the private sector of medicine, exhorting men with erectile problems to seek the medical and surgical treatments that are currently available.

This process has colluded with certain prevailing social attitudes—in particular, the equation of male sexuality with power, inherent in the term "potency." Thus a man's erectile function tends to be central to his self-esteem. The term "impotent" captures the sense of "loss of power" which has significance well beyond the individual's capacity for sexual pleasure. The female counterpart is "frigid," a term that emphasizes the effect of the woman's response or lack of response on the man. She is cold; to whom is she cold? The man. Both terms are pejorative. Interestingly, for that reason, the term "frigid" has largely disappeared from use. By contrast, there has been an exponential growth in the use of the term "impotent" and hardly any attempt to drop its use despite its pejorative, stigmatizing connotations. It is encouraging to see that in this book the term is largely missing.

Looking at sexual attitudes more closely, at an individual level, we see a further sex difference. For men—and this is not the case for women—a physical explanation is preferable to a psychological one, and physical treatment is more acceptable than psychological, regardless of the fact that the psychogenic problem has a much greater chance of satisfactory resolution.

We see these attitudes reflected in official policy. Recently, when colleagues of mine in the United States sought official approval for the investigation of a new drug in the treatment of sexual problems of women, they were told that what a sexually troubled woman required was not a drug, but a new or better sexual partner. Elsewhere, we are told that what the sexually troubled, impotent man requires is not a new partner, but a new or more effective penis, kicked into action by its injection with drugs, or reinforced with plastic rods. From this viewpoint, male sexuality is the key to human sexuality. The crucial issue is to get that right; female sexuality will then follow.

We can therefore, with some confidence, conclude that the "medicalization" of sexuality that we have been observing in recent years is in the *male* and not the *female* domain.

In addition to the dubious claims of therapeutic breakthrough, there is another aspect to this medicalization process. It is acknowledged that some cases of erectile dysfunction can be psychogenic and responsive to psychological treatment. Hence, it is important to investigate such cases, and demonstrate that organic causation exists before advocating surgical treatment. So another parallel industry has emerged: the diagnostic investigation of impotence, using just about every available form of modern diagnostic technology and, of course, involving the impotent man in a considerable amount of extra expense.

   This diagnostic revolution has, in fact, been of considerable interest. It has provided us with a wealth of information about the pathophysiology of erectile response. However, as a diagnostic approach, its use has, with a few exceptions, been seriously and significantly flawed. These tests are based on the assumption that the erectile machinery and its associated vasculature can be tested and evaluated in isolation from the man and his psychological nature. Let me examine this assertion in more detail. In doing so, I have relied heavily on the invaluable literature review by Jacques Buvat and his colleagues (Buvat, Buvat-Herbaut, Lemaire, Marcolin, & Quittelier, 1990).

   These diagnostic procedures are of two types. The first aims to assess the man's capacity for erectile response, aiming to distinguish between so-called "organic" and "nonorganic" (psychogenic) causation, without attempting to identify the specific organic process involved. Thus we see measurement of nocturnal penile tumescence (NPT), of erectile response to visual erotic stimuli, and of response to intracavernosal injections of smooth-muscle-relaxing drugs such as papaverine or prostaglandin E_1. Secondly, we have tests aimed at specific etiologies, in particular, vascular and neurological abnormalities.

   The investigation of the arterial factor has progressed from the early and comparatively primitive measurement of the penile blood pressure index (PBPI) to the use of modern, highly sophisticated ultrasonographic techniques, which have so far reached their acme with color Doppler, which distinguishes, by color, arteries from veins. Duplex ultrasonography is perhaps the most widely used of these modern techniques, and we are investigating this in our clinic in Edinburgh. This procedure combines the imaging capacity of ultrasound, and the resulting ability to locate arteries in the penis, with the computer-directed application of Doppler to measure pulsatile flow in these arteries. It is generally accepted that such assessment should be carried out both before and after intracavernosal injection of smooth-muscle-relaxant drugs such as papaverine. Various techniques are used to investigate so-called "venous incompetence."

   While many of the above techniques are sophisticated and informative, their value diagnostically is based on the assumption that they will evaluate erectile mechanisms, uninfluenced by psychological factors. However, increasingly the evidence is showing such an assumption to be suspect. The mind–body dichotomy is once again being challenged.

   NPT is suppressed in depressive illness (Thase et al., 1987). It is no longer possible to assume that impaired NPT indicates solely organic disease affecting the peripheral erectile mechanisms. The response to intracavernosal drugs varies considerably from one occasion to another. It is now evident that such response may be impaired in psychogenic cases, presumably as a result of some psychological mechanism (Buvat et al., 1990). Response to visual erotic stimuli may be augmented by intracavernosal drugs. In other words, there is an interaction between the peripheral drug effects within the erectile tissues and the psychically mediated influences (Bancroft, Smith, Munoz, & Ronald, in press). Some men with demonstrable obstructions in their penile arteries have been cured with psychological treatment (Buvat-Herbaut, Lemaire, & Buvat, 1984). Increasingly, it is becoming evident that measures of penile blood flow after intracavernosal injections reflect the functional response of the penis to the injection and not the structural condition of the penile vasculature (Buvat et al., 1990).

The inevitable conclusion, therefore, is that most of these diagnostic procedures require, for their interpretation, an understanding of the psychosomatic process. We can assert that the penis cannot be meaningfully separated from the man. Even the effects of drugs injected directly into the erectile tissues appear to be modified by higher influences. However, the mechanisms by which the "man" influences or overrides such local effects remain of crucial importance and have been almost totally ignored.

The key question that therefore emerges is, "How are psychological influences on erectile response physiologically mediated?" The neglect of this question is perhaps not surprising. The complexities of mind–body interaction are welcomed neither by the patient, who often feels most comfortable with a physical explanation; nor by the sex therapist, who is unable to assess physiological parameters; nor by the surgeon, who prefers a body–mind distinction that will justify the reliance on physical methods of management and the relative neglect of the psychological component.

But the question remains of fundamental importance. It goes to the heart of the clinical problem of psychogenic erectile failure. To what extent has it been pursued by psychologists or psychophysiologists? We do have an elegant series of laboratory-based experiments in which the role of cognitive and affective factors on erectile response have been investigated. These studies have mostly been carried out by Barlow and his associates, and are well reviewed by Cranston-Cuebas and Barlow (1990). The common assumption that sexual dysfunction is a consequence of either anxiety or anger, and the more recent emphasis given by Masters and Johnson on the importance of the "spectator role," have been further shown to be misleading oversimplifications. In this series of experiments it has been demonstrated that:

1. Experimental induction of anxiety often facilitates sexual response, though this is more likely to occur in men who are not already experiencing sexual difficulties.

2. Performance demand, induced in the experimental situation, again distinguishes "functional" from "dysfunctional" men, apparently facilitating response in the former and hindering it in the latter.

3. Heightened arousal, induced by whatever means, appears to accentuate the typical pattern. Thus in functional men, who tend to focus on erotic cues in the experimental setting, this focus is enhanced and the sexual

response facilitated. Dysfunctional men, who characteristically focus on nonerotic cues, in these circumstances, are even more likely to do so. In other words, the arousal strengthens the response, erotic in the functional group, nonerotic in the dysfunctionals.

4. Distraction (i.e., being asked to listen to a nonerotic cue while attending to an erotic stimulus) substantially reduces the erotic response in functional men. In dysfunctional men it either makes little difference or even increases the response. The assumed explanation for this difference is that the dysfunctional men are already attending to nonerotic cues, which may be even more countererotic than the distracting cue.

5. When asked to report on their level of genital response to erotic stimuli, functionals tend to report accurately or to overreport their response. Dysfunctionals tend to underreport.

We can conclude from this evidence that affective states and specific cognitive processes do not have consistent effects on sexual response. We find functional and dysfunctional men reacting to these states and processes differently. But we do not know whether that difference is a cause of the dysfunction, representing some characteristic that *precedes* the dysfunction, or is a consequence of dysfunction, so that once men regard themselves as dysfunctional, for whatever reason, they react differently, possibly accentuating the problem in the process.

Let us consider the situation in terms of information processing, with the functionals and dysfunctionals processing in a different way. A crucial question is whether such differences, even if they are causal, are a *sufficient* explanation for the sexual dysfunction. In my opinion, that is doubtful. Such factors may represent aggravating influences, or they may serve to initiate some other type of mechanism. But I find it difficult to believe that disturbances in information processing alone could account for the total failure of response, both psychically and reflexively (e.g., in response to appropriate tactile stimulation), that can occur in cases of psychogenic erectile failure.

For a sufficient explanation, some form of neuropsychological inhibition is required, specifically inhibiting the erectile response in the presence of appropriate sexual stimuli. It is widespread, if not universal, within the central nervous system, for function to depend on a balance between excitation and inhibition. We see the effects on erection of reducing such inhibition in some men with spinal cord injury, whose threshold for reflexive erection is markedly reduced. Is it possible that those same inhibitory mechanisms can be invoked to account for the occurrence of erectile failure in many psychogenic cases?

When we consider such fundamental explanations for human function such as this, we tend to look for comparable animal models. Barry Everitt and I have recently explored the animal evidence, particularly that relating to rodents, for such leads (Everitt & Bancroft, in press). Two types of systems that might be inhibited need to be considered, namely, sexual motivation ("appetitive" behavior) and initiation of sexual activity ("consummatory" behavior).

So far, while the role of androgens in the *excitation* of appetitive behavior is clear, at least for the males of most species, mechanisms producing active *inhibition* of such behavior have not yet been identified. Our current difficulties in understanding and managing the common problem of so-called "inhibited sexual desire" emphasize the importance of this unresolved issue.

For consummatory behavior there are some potentially interesting leads. Perhaps the most interesting is the role of the medial preoptic area (MPOA) of the hypothalamus. We know from implanted electrode stimulation studies in mobile rhesus monkeys, that stimulation of this area leads to sexual mounting but not to the point of ejaculation (Perachio, Marr, & Alexander, 1979). Lesions of the MPOA, in virtually all species studied, result in marked impairment of sexual behavior (Hart & Leedy, 1985). However, this impairment does not involve sexual motivation as such. Such animals will continue to work for access to a receptive female, whereas a castrated animal, whose androgen-dependent motivation is reduced, will not (Everitt, 1990). Nor do MPOA lesions reduce the frequency of autosexual activity; monkeys continue to masturbate as before. Put with a receptive female, however, they will be unable to copulate (Slimp, Hart, & Goy, 1978). Is this an animal model for erectile dysfunction? Before seeking an answer to such a question, it is important to consider that the behavioral manifestations of such a specific mechanism, as is located and disrupted by MPOA lesions, are likely to vary from species to species, even if the central mechanism is basically similar.

More recent evidence from Herbert's group in Cambridge has shown that infusion of β-endorphin into the MPOA of rats produces a similar deficit to the lesion. However, they were able to show a much more subtle impairment, which raises some fascinating questions of relevance to the human (Stavy & Herbert, 1989). If the animal had already mounted and intromitted the female, infusion of the β-endorphin would have no effect on subsequent mounting and copulation *with that same female*. But if after the infusion the original female was replaced with a different one, then sexual activity with that female would fail. Clearly, to account for this phenomenon, some kind of information processing is involved. These workers concluded that the MPOA is involved in the matching of incentive stimuli to specific behavioral responses, perhaps an interface between information processing and the appropriate physiological–behavioral response. The effect of β-endorphin as described can be seen to disrupt this interface, resulting in the effective inhibition of the physiological–behavioral response. Is this comparable to the inhibition of erection in the man with psychogenic erectile failure? Everitt and Bancroft (in press) speculated that, if so, the principal difference be-

Masters, W. H., & Johnson, V. E. (1970). *Human sexual inadequacy.* Boston: Little, Brown.

Perachio, A. A., Marr, L. D., & Alexander, M. (1979). Sexual behavior in male rhesus monkeys elicited by electrical stimulation of preoptic and hypothalamic areas. *Brain Research, 177,* 127–144.

Slimp, J. C., Hart, B. L., & Goy, R. W. (1978). Heterosexual, autosexual and social behavior of adult male rhesus monkeys with medial preoptic–anterior hypothalamic lesions. *Brain Research, 142,* 105–122.

Stavy, M., & Herbert, J. (1989). Differential effects of β-endorphin infused into the hypothalamic preoptic area at various phases of the male rat's sexual behavior. *Neuroscience, 30,* 433–442.

Thase, M. E., Reynolds, C. F., Glanz, L. M., Jennings, J. R., Sewitch, D. E., Kupfer, D. J., & Frank, E. (1987). Nocturnal penile tumescence in depressed men. *American Journal of Psychiatry, 144,* 89–92.

Wagner, G., Gerstenberg, T., & Levin, R. J. (1989). Electrical activity of corpus cavernosum during flaccidity and erection in the human penis; a new diagnostic method? *Journal of Urology, 142,* 723–725.

Preface

The past decade has witnessed a rapid evolution in our conceptual understanding of male erectile disorders. Major changes have occurred in the diagnostic terminology, laboratory assessment methodology, and treatment modalities for male disorders. Surgical implants in a wide range of models and types, intracorporal injection therapy, vacuum pump devices, oral medications, laser-based venous ligation procedures, and other technologically sophisticated procedures have all attained prominence in recent years. Not surprisingly, the number of professional and scientific publications on erectile disorders has grown exponentially, as have the clinics and treatment centers specializing in male sexual problems. In this volume, the latest biomedical and laboratory-based approaches to assessment and treatment are reviewed by a distinguished group of experts, including Arnold Melman, Raul Schiavi, and Julian Davidson.

Compared to developments in medicine and surgery, psychological approaches to erectile disorders have been relatively neglected overall. With the increasing "medicalization" of the field, less attention has been paid to the psychological or interpersonal underpinnings of the problem. Yet psychological issues are fundamental to sexual response, as recent research by David Barlow, Gayle Beck, and others has demonstrated. In the first two chapters of the present volume, social and psychological dimensions of erectile failure are explored in depth. Several chapters, particularly those by Bernie Zilbergeld, Joseph LoPiccolo, Stephen Levine, and ourselves, address the essentially dyadic nature of erectile disorders, and the crucial importance of involving the sexual partner in all phases of assessment and treatment.

Not only has our understanding of anatomical mechanisms and psychophysiological processes evolved in recent years, but major changes have taken place in the official nomenclature for erectile difficulties. Our terminology in this regard has evolved from the original classifications—primary and secondary impotence—as used by Masters and Johnson (1970), to the currently preferred "male erectile disorder" (DSM-III-R; American Psychiatric Association, 1987). Despite the pressure for change in the official nomenclature, most physicians and laypersons continue to make widespread use of the term "impotence" in referring to the man with erectile difficulties.

Although we strongly prefer the terms "erectile disorder" or "erectile dysfunction," we have opted, after considerable discussion and debate, to grant each author editorial discretion and freedom of choice in this regard.

In the second edition of *Principles and Practice of Sex Therapy* (Leiblum & Rosen, 1989), we predicted that a focus on erectile disorders was likely to dominate sex therapy attention in the 1990s. This has clearly occurred, and with this trend in mind, we have sought to update readers on the latest conceptual and technological advances in the field. Our contributors represent a nationally known and highly regarded group of researchers and practitioners, each of whom has a distinctive orientation and therapeutic style. We have emphasized both biomedical and psychological perspectives throughout the book, as we have sought to provide a more balanced and holistic view of the field. As in our previous volumes, contributors were asked to discuss both theoretical and clinical aspects, and to illustrate critical points with case examples wherever possible.

As in any work of this nature, many friends and colleagues have guided our thinking and encouraged our efforts. In particular, we acknowledge the invaluable contributions of R. Taylor Segraves, M.D., Ph.D., who served as medical consultant for this volume. Not only did he provide a painstaking review of the medical and psychiatric aspects of each chapter, but he has given unstintingly of his friendship and support throughout. Valuable comments and suggestions on specific chapters were also provided by Daniel Goldberg, Ph.D., and Placido Grino, M.D. Many others have contributed ideas and encouragement, including John Bancroft, Raul Schiavi, Patricia Schreiner-Engel, Kathleen Segraves, Harold Lief, Julian Davidson, Leonore Tiefer, David McWhirter, Julia Heiman, and John Gagnon. We deeply appreciate their contributions.

Special thanks are due to our publisher and friend, Seymour Weingarten, for his unswerving support of our writing projects over the past decade. Judith Grauman, our editor at The Guilford Press, also provided many valuable comments and suggestions. And finally, to our secretary and long-time friend, Agnes Bertelsen, our heartfelt thanks!

RAYMOND C. ROSEN
SANDRA R. LEIBLUM

REFERENCES

American Psychiatric Association. (1987). *Diagnostic and statistical manual of mental disorders* (3rd ed., rev.). Washington, DC: Author.

Masters, W. H., & Johnson, V. E. (1970). *Human sexual inadequacy*. Boston: Little, Brown.

Leiblum, S. R., & Rosen, R. C. (1989). *Principles and practice of sex therapy* (2nd ed.): Update for the 1990s. New York. Guilford Press.

Contents

Introduction
and Overview

I

Erectile Disorders: An Overview of Historical Trends and Clinical Perspectives

RAYMOND C. ROSEN AND SANDRA R. LEIBLUM

Throughout recorded history, male erectile disorders have rarely been perceived with equanimity or detachment. Rather, an endless succession of potions and prescriptions, drugs and devices has been advocated for overcoming the problem. Both men and their partners have displayed a considerable investment in maintaining a "working penis," and descriptions of treatments for combating erectile problems have long been a focus of literature and mythology. As long ago as 2000 B.C., Egyptian papyri contained specific recipes for curing impotence, and the mandrake root has been extensively used throughout Africa as a tribal cure for male erectile problems. We begin this chapter with a brief historical journey through the various commentaries on and approaches to erectile disorders.

ERECTILE DISORDERS FROM ANCIENT TIMES TO THE 19TH CENTURY

Biblical references to erectile failure describe it as a form of punishment for adultery. A well-known passage in Genesis, for example, describes how Abimelech was punished by God with impotence for considering having sexual relations with Abraham's wife: "Behold thou art but a dead man, for the woman which thou has taken; for she is another man's wife" (Genesis 20:3). The use of the word "dead" to refer to erectile failure is clearly extreme, although it is a common reflection of how many men feel when unable to develop an erection. Apparently, the equation of adequate erections with vitality and life is several thousand years old!

It was in Greek mythology that psychological causes for erectile dysfunction first came to be recognized. According to Greek legend, Iphiclus, son of King Phylacus, as a young boy, saw his father coming toward him with a blood-stained gelding knife and became terrified that his father would use the knife on him. Iphiclus subsequently developed chronic erectile failure, and the legend may represent the earliest historical account of castration anxiety. The Greeks may also be credited with recognizing the therapeutic value of systematic desensitization. Iphiclus was subsequently cured by his physician, Melampus, with gradual exposure to the dried blood and rust on the gelding knife (Johnson, 1968).

Church authorities in the Middle Ages attributed erectile failure to the effects of demoniacal possession or witchcraft. In the 12th century, for example, the practice of "ligature" became widespread for inflicting impotence on unsuspecting victims. A ligature was a type of sexual hex, in which a series of knots was tied in a cord or strip of leather, which was then hidden in a secret place. Depending upon the number and configuration of knots, the victim could be rendered partially impotent, totally impotent, or sterile. The stage of "ligature" was recognized as valid grounds for dissolution of a marriage, and was referred to by no less an authority than Thomas Aquinas: "The Catholic faith teaches both that there are demons and that by their doings, they can inflict injury on men and prevent carnal copulation" (cited in Johnson, 1968, p. 5).

The potential role of underlying physical determinants of erectile failure was identified during the Age of Enlightenment. Perhaps the most famous case of the period was that of Louis XVI, king of France from 1774 to 1789. Louis was 16 years old at the time of his marriage to Marie Antoinette, and he was unable to consummate the marriage for at least 7 years because of his condition of "total impotence" (Hastings, 1963). News of Louis's problem traveled throughout the courts and palaces of Europe. After consultation with many authorities, the cause of his problem was finally determined to be an excessively tight foreskin, and Louis was subsequently circumcised. According to one source (Johnson, 1968), Marie Antoinette wrote several letters afterwards detailing her satisfaction with the results of surgery! This historical episode illustrates the emerging concept of erectile failure as a medical (as opposed to a psychological or spiritual) problem, and may represent the first attempt to employ a surgical intervention to effect a cure for impotence.

The role of genetic or hormonal factors was first recognized in the 19th century. Napoleon Bonaparte, in particular, was reputed to have suffered from an unidentified endocrine disorder, which resulted in erectile failure in middle age. In the postmortem report by his personal physician, Napoleon's genitals were described as follows: "He had granules in his prostate, the penis and testicles were very small, and the whole genital system seemed to exhibit a physical cause for the absence of sexual desire and the chastity which has been stated to have characterized the deceased" (cited in Johnson, 1968, p. 7). Recent developments in the hormonal evaluation and treatment of erectile disorders are reviewed in Chapter 4 of this volume by Davidson and Rosen.

MODERN APPROACHES
TO ERECTILE DISORDERS

In the 20th century, two major themes have emerged in the discussion of erectile disorders. First, psychological factors have been identified as both major causes and consequences of erectile dysfunction. In particular, Freud, Stekel, and other early psychoanalysts emphasized the contribution of psychogenic factors in their psychodynamic formulations of the disorder. The role of anxiety, in particular, has been widely discussed by both analytical and behavioral theorists. Second, there has been a growing emphasis, particularly in the recent past, on the potential etiological role of organic factors in erectile dysfunction (Krane, Goldstein, & Saenz de Tejada, 1989; Morley, 1986). Currently, the professional literature on the topic is dominated by discussion of the role of physical factors in both the assessment and treatment of erectile disorders.

Although psychoanalytic theorists have emphasized the importance of resolving unconscious conflicts that may inhibit erectile function, there has also been a growing recognition that reliance on "uncovering" therapy is not always successful in reversing erectile disorders. Nevertheless, the traditional psychoanalytic position has viewed psychogenic factors as the primary causative agent in erectile failure. Freud commented, for example, "We are accustomed confidently to promise recovery to psychically impotent patients who come to us for treatment, but we ought to be more guarded in making this prognosis so long as the dynamics of the disturbance are unknown to us" (Freud, 1919/1955, p. 197). The suggestion is that if treatment is not successful, it is because the "true" unconscious conflicts interfering with erectile response have not been resolved.

Among the early analysts, it was Stekel (1927) who first realized that organic factors were important as well, and recommended the observation of sleep erections as a means for distinguishing between psychogenic and organic erectile disorders:

> It is a frequent, one might say an almost universal, observation that these ostensibly impotent men still have more or less strong erections in the morning, during a dream, or on awakening. Mistakenly, these erections are considered to be due to an accumulation of urine in the bladder and are attributed to the reflex action of a distended bladder. There is no greater

physiological absurdity. As a matter of fact, a morning erection is the most reliable indication that impotence is psychic and ensures a more favorable prognosis with psychotherapy. (Stekel, 1927, p. 187)

The early behavior therapists are credited, however, with the development of modern treatment approaches to erectile disorders. Wolpe (1958) and Lazarus (1965), in particular, recommended the use of systematic desensitization as a means of overcoming anxiety, and thereby improving erectile function. Before Masters and Johnson, Joseph Wolpe had emphasized the importance of eliminating performance anxiety, with instructions *not* to attempt intercourse: "The patient is told that he must on no account perform sexually unless he has an unmistakable positive desire to do so, for otherwise he may consolidate or even extend his inhibitions" (1958, p. 194). The sensate focus approach developed by Masters and Johnson (1970) and widely utilized in the treatment of all sexual dysfunctions has been interpreted as a form of *in vivo* desensitization of sexual anxiety (O'Leary & Wilson, 1987). Systematic desensitization was a staple of the early behavioral approaches to the treatment of erectile failure, as well as the specific use of guided imagery rehearsal.

More recently, Bancroft (1989) has suggested that it may be the "threat" of negative consequences, rather than anxiety per se, that causes erectile failure. Recent research by Barlow and his associates has strongly suggested that anxiety can have mixed effects on arousal and erectile responses to erotic stimuli, depending upon the level of cognitive distraction involved (Barlow, Sakheim, & Beck, 1983). In other words, it is not anxiety specifically that causes erectile failure, but the cognitive interference that accompanies it. These authors suggest that men with psychogenic erectile failure have the capacity to function sexually, but that they have difficulties in performance because their cognitive focus is inappropriately directed toward thoughts that are not sexually arousing.

Cognitive distraction as a cause of erectile problems has received considerable recent attention in the psychological and behavioral literature (Rosen & Beck, 1988). In a study by Cohen, Rosen, and Goldstein (1985), for example, a pattern of right temporal lobe activation was observed to accompany maximum erection responses in responsive, nondysfunctional men during visual erotic presentations. In contrast, the men with erectile failure showed significant activation in the right temporal and occipital sites during erotic audiotapes, but not during video presentations. Cohen et al. suggested that these patterns of hemispheric asymmetry may indicate increased cognitive activity, concurrent with negative affective responses in men with erectile dysfunction.

The results of this and similar studies suggest that it is not the peripheral, autonomic, or skeletal dimension, but possibly the central-attentional dimension of performance anxiety that is most relevant in understanding the psychogenic mechanisms of erectile dysfunction. In Barlow's (1986) terminology, this is the "cognitive distraction" process that is so important in the genesis of erectile disorders.

Among sex therapists, Kaplan (1974) was the first to attempt a more integrated biological, behavioral, and systemic formulation of erectile dysfunction. She described performance anxiety as the immediate cause of most sexual dysfunctions, including erectile disorders, and unconscious conflicts and developmental inhibitions as the remote causes. Investigation of the latter must occur only if the elimination of the debilitating performance anxiety is not accomplished. Like Masters and Johnson (1970), Kaplan asserts that sexual performance is essentially reflexive or "natural," and will occur without difficulty if performance anxiety and unconscious conflicts do not interfere.

Recently, sex therapists have focused also on the systemic or interactional nature of many erectile disorders. Couples dynamics are strongly emphasized nowadays in both assessment and treatment of erectile disorders, as we discuss in Chapter 9 of this volume.

Despite this recognition of the role of psychological and interpersonal factors, much of the current emphasis in the medical and sex therapy literature has been on the role of organic factors as either primary or secondary determinants of erectile dysfunction. Whereas 25 years ago it was widely believed that most cases of erectile dysfunction were attributable solely to psychogenic causes, nowadays it is often stated that physical factors are responsible for the problem in more than 50% of cases (e.g., Morley, 1986). As we (and our contributors) have emphasized repeatedly, the attempt to differentiate erectile problems on the basis of psychogenic versus organogenic etiology alone is misguided and incorrect. The issue is particularly addressed by Joseph LoPiccolo in Chapter 7 of this volume. Simple dichotomies are seldom demonstrated in real life, and this is certainly no exception.

PROBLEMS OF DEFINITION AND DIAGNOSIS

Historically, the term "impotence" has been applied to a wide array of male sexual dysfunctions. Past usages, in fact, often included premature ejaculation, ejaculatory incompetence, and sexual aversions, as well as erectile dysfunction per se. Numerous authors have commented also on the potentially pejorative and stigmatizing connotations of the term "impotence," which nonetheless continues to enjoy widespread popular and professional usage today.

Major arguments against the use of the term "impotence" include the lack of diagnostic specificity, as well as the implied personality characteristics of the so-called "impotent male." Moreover, Tiefer (1986) has related the increased use of the stigmatizing and stress-inducing lable of "impotence" to the increasing "medicalization" of male sexuality. She argues that economic interests among physician/providers and medical technology manufacturers lie in expanding the range of services offered to increasing numbers of patients. Impotence is therefore labeled as a biomedical disorder, which is "common in men of all ages, best served by thorough evaluation and appropriate medical treatment when any evidence of organic disorder is identified" (Tiefer, 1986, p. 594). Continued use of the term "impotence" by the biomedical community clearly serves these needs.

Some authors have also suggested that reverse sexism may be operative in the whole-hearted professional rejection of the term "frigidity," while "impotence" continues to be widely used in the professional literature (Elliott, 1985). In fact, Alfred Kinsey and colleagues may have unwittingly sparked this trend by using the term "impotence" uncritically and often in the 1948 volume on males, while commenting strongly on the pejorative connotations of "frigidity" in the volume on females: "We dislike the term ["frigidity"], for it has come to connote either the unwillingness or incapacity to function sexually. In most circumstances neither of these implications is correct" (Kinsey, Pomeroy, Martin, & Gebhard, 1953, p. 354). This trend was continued by Masters and Johnson (1970). Whereas female problems were classified by Masters and Johnson as "disorders of penetration" (vaginismus and dyspareunia) and "orgasmic dysfunctions," male problems were characterized as either "ejaculatory problems" (premature ejaculation and ejaculatory incompetence) or "impotence" (primary and secondary impotence). Desire disorders in men were included with secondary impotence.

Both the terms "impotence" and "frigidity" were used in the first *Diagnostic and Statistical Manual of Mental Disorders* (DSM-I; American Psychiatric Association, 1952). In the 1968 version of the manual (DSM-II), however, only impotence was retained in the category of "urogenital dysfunction." By the time DSM-III appeared in 1980, "impotence" had been removed in favor of "male inhibited sexual excitement." Despite this advance in the psychiatric nomenclature, little change has been apparent in the overall usage of the term (Elliott, 1985; Tiefer, 1986). In the latest revision of the American Psychiatric Association's diagnostic manual (DSM-III-R), "male erectile disorder" is defined as follows:

(1) persistent or recurrent partial or complete failure in a male to attain or maintain erection until completion of the sexual activity [or]
(2) persistent or recurrent lack of a subjective sense of sexual excitement and pleasure in a male during sexual activity
(American Psychiatric Association, 1987, p. 294)

It is noteworthy that erectile dysfunction has come to be defined *independently* of the ability to obtain or sustain erections adequate for intercourse. This definition includes reference not only to the physiological achievement of erection, but also to the subjective sense of sexual excitement and pleasure that is experienced during sexual activity. The DSM-III-R definition acknowledges that some men are able to achieve erections without experiencing pleasure or a feeling of sexual arousal, and that this lack of subjective arousal may be problematic in some instances. The definition is also very broad in referring to "sexual activity," which can include masturbation, oral stimulation, or anal stimulation in addition to vaginal intercourse.

Although "impotence" continues to be widely used in the medical and psychiatric literature, sex therapists have repeatedly urged replacing this term with "erectile dysfunction," "erectile failure," or "erectile disorders." Vasculogenic impotence is also frequently referred to as "erectile insufficiency" or "erectile incompetence." These latter diagnoses may also be viewed as having pejorative connotations.

Many attempts have been made to classify erectile disorders on the basis of etiology (psychogenic vs. biogenic), as well as on other dimensions. The extent and duration of the disorder have also been viewed as key factors. For example, as noted above, Masters and Johnson (1970) distinguished between primary and secondary impotence. "Primary" impotence refers to a clinical situation in which successful intercourse has *never* been achieved with a partner of either sex. It is noteworthy that Masters and Johnson defined primary impotence as a male's never having been "able to achieve and/or maintain an erection sufficient to accomplish successful coital connection" (1970, p. 137). Masters and Johnson considered erection sufficient for intercourse to be a *sine qua non* of the "cultural demand for effectiveness of sexual performance" (1970, p. 159), implying an association between masculinity and the ability to achieve erections sufficient for intercourse.

"Secondary" or "situational" erectile failure, as the name implies, refers to an inability to perform adequately with certain partners or in particular situations or activities. Male patients with a "madonna–whore" syndrome, for example, may function well only in extramarital sexual situations (see Chapter 7 by LoPiccolo). Diagnostic distinctions have also been made among "chronic," "acute," and "global" erectile dysfunction (Rosen, 1983).

In summary, although some progress has been made toward a more refined and less ambiguous diagnostic terminology, there remains a clear lack of consensus in the field. We would anticipate that a current poll of urologists and other physicians would show widespread endorsement of the term "impotence," whereas sex therapists and mental health clinicians are increasingly inclined to use "erectile disorder" or "erectile dysfunction" in diagnosing the problem. Certainly, the term "impotence" remains highly controversial, although it appears unlikely to be replaced in the immediate future.

INCIDENCE AND PREVALENCE

A cursory reading of the popular literature would suggest that problems of erectile inadequacy are rampant among men of all ages. Has there been an increase in the actual incidence of the disorder? Or is the increased attention paid to erectile problems an artifact of the increased availability of new medical and surgical treatments, a greater tendency to identify and treat sexual problems generally among couples of all ages, or greater sophistication in sexual inquiry among both physicians and mental health clinicians?

Estimates regarding the prevalence of erectile dysfunction tend to vary greatly, depending on individuals' age, health status, medication history, and alcohol and drug use, as well as the definition of erectile dysfunction used in the particular study (Morley, 1986). In one study (Slag, Morley, Elson, & Trence, 1983), a large sample of middle-aged men ($n = 1,180$) in a medical outpatient clinic were screened for the presence or absence of erectile dysfunction. A substantial number (34%) of patients complained of erectile difficulties. Subsequent medical evaluation revealed a wide range of causal factors, including medication effects (25%), primary or secondary hypogonadism (19%), diabetes (9%), and psychogenic factors (14%). It is highly likely that psychogenic factors were underestimated because of the type of clinical setting involved and lack of in-depth interviewing in the study.

Several studies have implicated age as a major determinant of the prevalence of erectile dysfunction. As discussed by Segraves and Segraves (Chapter 5, this volume), there is a gradual decrease in penile sensitivity with aging, as well as declining plasma testosterone levels and sexual desire after age 60. There is some disagreement, however, as to the specific etiological role played by declining testosterone levels in the increased prevalence of erectile dysfunction in older men (Schiavi, 1990). Nocturnal penile tumescence (NPT) has also been shown to decline steadily after age 60, although some men continue to maintain adequate daytime function. This observation needs to be considered when performing diagnostic studies in older men.

How common are erectile difficulties in the general population? In the often-quoted study of self-reported "happily married," nonclinical couples by Frank, Anderson, and Rubinstein (1978), inability to achieve an erection was reported by 7% of the sample, while 9% indicated difficulties in maintaining erections. In their recent review of results from several community surveys and prevalence studies, Spector and Carey (1990) reported an average incidence of 4–9% for erectile disorders. These authors also concluded that erectile failure is presently the leading complaint among males attending sex therapy clinics.

Several studies have indicated that erectile disorders account for a large and possibly growing proportion of the total number of sex therapy cases in treatment. For example, two early studies reported that approximately 35–40% of male partners in sex therapy had erectile failure as their primary complaint (Frank, Anderson, & Kupfer, 1976; Bancroft & Coles, 1976). Other authors have suggested that the proportion may be increasing, as Hawton (1982) reported erectile dysfunction in 53% of his sample, and our own clinic data have similarly shown that more than 50% of males currently seeking services complain of erectile difficulties (Rosen, Leiblum, & Hall, 1987). As noted by Wincze and Carey (1991), these incidence data have been obtained from psychosocially oriented sex therapy clinics, and the number of males presenting with erectile disorders would certainly be much higher in sexual dysfunction programs located within urology departments or other medical services.

The incidence of erectile failure also varies considerably, depending upon the diagnosis or type of dysfunction under consideration. For example, primary erectile dysfunction is far less common that secondary erectile dysfunction (Masters & Johnson, 1970). As noted above, primary erectile dysfunction is generally viewed as psychogenic in origin, although medical conditions such as hypogonadism can result in primary erectile failure. Renshaw (1988) reported that 3.5% of men seeking treatment for erectile disorders received a diagnosis of "primary" erectile dysfunction, compared to the 48% of the sample who received a "secondary" diagnosis. Similarly, in the original Masters and Johnson (1979) report, 50% of men requesting treatment experienced "secondary impotence," while only 8% were diagnosed with "primary impotence."

Obviously, unbiased estimates of the incidence and prevalence of erectile failure are difficult to come by. As Tiefer and Melman (1989) point out, several factors have fueled increased awareness and concern about the problem in recent years: (1) the importance accorded to sexual function in personal life generally; (2) the relatively new expectation that sexual function is a lifelong capacity; (3) women's increased expectations for ongoing sexual gratification; (4) the increasing trend for physicians and other health care providers to advertise their services in the popular media; and (5) the disproportionate amount of attention paid to erectile difficulties, as opposed to other sexual problems, in the professional literature (Elliott, 1985).

ASSESSMENT AND FORMULATION

Diagnostic procedures for the assessment of erectile disorders have proliferated in recent years, leading to a broad array of available methods for evaluating vascular, hormonal, and neurogenic factors (e.g., Buvat, Buvat-

Herbaut, Lemaire, Marcolin, & Quittelier, 1990; Krane et al., 1989). Along with the use of new diagnostic procedures, increasingly complex and sophisticated decision-making models have appeared in the past decade. Vascular assessment procedures, ranging from duplex ultrasonography to angiographic studies of venous and arterial function, are advocated in many centers, as well as NPT testing and intracorporal injection studies. A lesser effort overall has been directed toward assessment of psychological or interpersonal functioning (Mohr & Beutler, 1990), and the major emphasis of current diagnostic approaches is clearly medical. Whereas organic factors were identified in only 5% or fewer of Masters and Johnson's (1970) cases, recent clinical reports have suggested that these factors may be present in up to 50% of patients presenting with complaints about erectile function (Melman, Tiefer, & Pedersen, 1988).

In a review of alternative models for diagnostic decision making, some general trends are apparent. To begin with, most authors recommend an initial physical examination and psychosexual history, prior to laboratory screening and more direct measures of erectile function. Hormonal evaluation is increasingly emphasized in most centers (see Davidson & Rosen, Chapter 4). Specialized vascular testing and neurogenic testing are also widely utilized, although these procedures are typically reserved for the latter stages of assessment. Patients without specific organic involvement are typically referred for sexual counseling evaluation and/or treatment. In our own center, a stepwise, multidisciplinary approach that includes interactive and concurrent evaluation of urological, endocrinological, and psychological factors has evolved. This model is illustrated in Figure 1.1 and is summarized briefly as follows.

The process of assessment typically begins with a review of the patient's medical, sexual, and psychological history. A detailed relationship history, as we described in Chapter 9 of this volume, is also obtained in most cases. Unless the problem is clearly situational (i.e., it only occurs with specific activities or partners, and especially if the man continues to masturbate with firm and lasting erections), a physical examination is recommended. Patients over 60 are routinely referred for medical examinations.

Although the physical examination is seldom sufficient in itself for establishing a diagnosis, certain conditions, such as Peyronie's disease or testicular atrophy, are easily detected during a routine office examination and should be eliminated at the outset. The physical examination also provides an important opportunity to assuage any of the patient's worries concerning penis size or function. Along with the physical examination, most patients are also required to provide blood and urine samples for laboratory screening. We have previously recommended fasting blood sugar, serum testosterone, and prolactin studies for selected patients (Fracher,

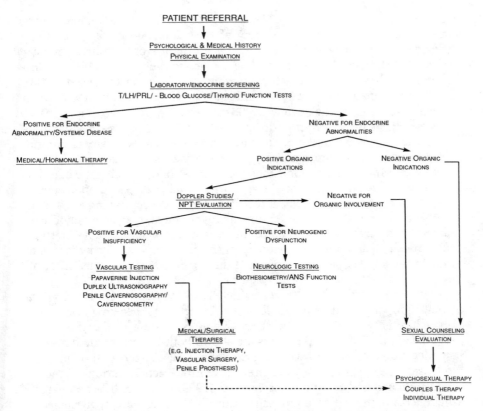

FIGURE 1.1. A flow-chart model for diagnosis and treatment of erectile dysfunction. T, serum testosterone; LH, luteinizing hormone; PRL, prolactin; NPT, nocturnal penile tumescence; ANS, autonomic nervous system.

Leiblum, & Rosen, 1981), but have recently begun to include thyroid function and glucose challenge tests as well.

Others (e.g., Kaplan, 1990) recommend a more complete blood and hormone screening for all patients, including plasma testosterone, luteinizing hormone, follicle-stimulating hormone, prolactin, estrogen, thyroid studies, lipids, glycohemoglobin, and acid phosphatase. These latter two tests are useful for assessing symptoms of diabetes and prostatic cancer, respectively, which may not have been evaluated by the referring physician. Obviously, cost-benefit considerations will come into play in this decision-making process, depending upon the type of patient being evaluated and the nature of the clinical practice setting (Tiefer, 1986).

Several criteria are used to determine the need for additional testing at this point. First, the medical history of the patient needs to be carefully considered. This may include coronary heart disease or peripheral vascular disease, neurological symptoms, drug or alcohol abuse, or other medical conditions that generally affect erectile function (Schover & Jensen, 1988). The current medication status of the patient is particularly important to assess, as noted in the review by Segraves and Segraves (Chapter 5) of adverse effects of prescription drugs. Psychosocial history is equally important, because erectile dysfunction is frequently seen as secondary to chronic depression, relationship conflicts, or disorders of sexual desire (Rosen & Leiblum, 1987). In general, only those patients without significant medical or psychiatric histories, and/or those with documented situational erectile disorders, are referred directly at this stage for sexual counseling evaluation.

For patients with suspected organic involvement, erectile function may be directly assessed in at least one of three ways: (1) by means of NPT testing; (2) through visual stimulation studies; or (3) pharmacologically, by means of intracorporal injection studies. Each of these methods is presented in detail by Schiavi in Chapter 6 of this volume.

It is noteworthy that the *least* widely used method by far is the visual stimulation approach. As described by Tiefer and Melman (1989), this procedure is performed in the sleep laboratory on one of the two nights scheduled for NPT testing. Patients are shown both X-rated erotic films and an educational video with scenes of explicit sexual activity, with permission to masturbate if desired. Any occurrences of firm erection during the procedure are noted and quantified. As Bancroft (1989) observes, "It is an interesting reflection on medical attitudes to sexuality that there are many surgeons who do not hesitate to elicit an erection by injecting a drug into the penis, but who would be very reluctant to elicit an erection with the use of erotic stimuli" (p. 427).

Vascular studies for erectile dysfunction are typically initiated with the monitoring of penile arterial function in the flaccid penis by means of a Doppler ultrasound probe or penile plethysmography (Krane et al., 1989). A small pressure cuff is placed around the penis, and systolic blood pressures are assessed by means of a Doppler ultrasound recorder. Pressure and pulse amplitude can be evaluated separately (Bancroft, 1989). Although the Doppler procedure is relatively brief, is simple to perform, and is very widely used, it may be grossly lacking in sensitivity. Mellinger, Vaughan, Thompson, and Goldstein (1987), for example, reported that Doppler studies failed to identify 54% of men suffering from vasculogenic erectile disorders. Other limitations of the procedure are discussed by Schiavi in Chapter 6.

Additional vascular assessment methods are available if either the NPT or Doppler studies are positive for vasculogenic impairment. Duplex ultrasonography, for example, involves the combination of high-frequency ultrasonography with pulsed Doppler analysis, and the test may be used along with intracavernosal injection. As noted by Schiavi (Chapter 6), this test requires considerable experience to administer and interpret, and is not widely used at present.

More invasive testing is generally reserved for those cases in which erectile function is severely compromised, and vascular bypass or venous ligation surgery is being considered. Venous insufficiency problems, for example, are now accessible to study by means of radiographic techniques such as *penile cavernosography*. The goal is to assess venous outflow resistances, and the procedure requires infusion of X-ray contrast medium into the corpora cavernosa, followed by radiographic visualization of venous leakage sites. Penile cavernosometry involves infusion of saline into the penile corpora and monitoring of perfusion rates required to obtain or maintain an artificial erection. These procedures are costly, invasive, and potentially risky; moreover, there is currently little agreement concerning the clinical relevance of specific test findings from either one

Neurological studies are less frequently employed, in part because of the lack of specific tests or procedures for assessment of penile innervation. In particular, no tests are currently available to evaluate the efferent autonomic nerve supply to the penile corpora (Krane et al., 1989). Some authors have recommended the use of penile biothesiometry for measurement of afferent conduction in the dorsal nerve of the penis. The technique involves measuring the threshold of vibratory stimulation in the glans and penile shaft by means of an electormagnetic vibration device. Neurological tests of other parasympathetic functions, such as the cystemetrogram test of bladder function, may be of some value in determining the effects of peripheral neuropathy in some patients. Neurological examination is also obviously important when erectile failure is associated with head injury or spinal cord damage.

Although our current diagnostic model presents vascular and neurological testing as relatively independent assessment options, in clinical practice the two areas are often concurrently evaluated. For example, patients with a history of chronic diabetes frequently show signs of vascular insufficiency, in addition to peripheral autonomic neuropathy. In such instances, a combination of vascular and neurological testing may be indicated. The separation of medical and psychosocial components of the evaluation is also somewhat artificial, as both areas are typically assessed simultaneously.

Several authors have sought alternative conceptualizations of the organic–psychogenic dichotomy that pervades much of the clinical literature in the area. In fact, *both* organic and psychogenic factors are encountered in many cases, and LoPiccolo (Chapter 7) argues that psychogenic and organic factors should be represented as two separate and independently varying dimensions, as Sandra Bem (1974) has proposed for masculinity and femininity. According to this approach, the degree of organic and psychogenic involvement should be separately quantified in each specific case. Mohr and Beutler (1990) have also argued that diagnostic assessment should be targeted toward treatment decisions and prognostic outcomes, rather than emphasizing etiological determinants exclusively.

For some patients, the assessment process has come to resemble a bewildering "smorgasbord" of testing options and diagnostic possibilities. One patient complained, "I don't know which way to turn. I've seen three urologists so far, and each one has recommended a completely different approach. How does one decide which direction to go in?" Particularly for older patients, or those with a history of systemic illnesses, hormonal deficits, or alcohol and drug abuse, the range of diagnostic tests to be considered is potentially overwhelming. Moreover, there is little consistency or standardization of procedures from one clinic to another. In some centers, NPT continues to function as the "gold standard" of diagnostic testing for impotence (Mohr & Beutler, 1990) and is a central feature in most research studies. In other centers, intracorporal injections are widely used as a "first-step" diagnostic tool (Lue, Hricak, Schmidt, & Tanagho, 1986; Buvat et al., 1990). Still others, such as Melman and Tiefer (1989), have emphasized the value of the visual stimulation method. Given the confusing array of diagnostic options, it is essential for clinicians to guide both patients and their partners through the diagnostic decision-making process, helping them to respond emotionally as well as intellectually at each stage of the evaluation process.

Case Vignette

J. H. was a 68-year-old Danish accountant referred to our Sexual Counseling Service for evaluation of chronic erectile dysfunction. Mr. H. complained of progressive deterioration of erectile functioning during the past 10 years, culminating in his being unable to achieve or sustain erection sufficient for intercourse. Three years earlier he had undergone a transurethral prostatectomy, following which he had begun to experience "dry orgasms." He also complained of an occasional lack of sensation and a feeling of "numbness" in the penis during partner stimulation.

Psychosocial evaluation revealed that the patient had recently entered a new relationship after the loss of his wife 4 years earlier to cancer. His current partner was a 51-year-old bookstore owner, who had been divorced 8 years previously. He described her as a "strong-minded" woman, who frequently expressed her frustration at the lack of intercourse and other deficiencies in the relationship. However, he found her attractive and desirable, and had recently proposed marriage. The patient's current erectile difficulties had begun during the last 2 years of his wife's illness, at which time he experienced a loss of libido and increasing difficulty in maintaining erection during intercourse.

Laboratory screening was negative for endocrine or blood glucose abnormalities. Penile Doppler testing was similarly negative (penile-brachial index = 0.92). Two nights of NPT testing, however, showed a mild to moderate degree of erectile impairment. Maximum circumference changes equaled 14 mm at base and 8 mm at tip, with an absence of firm erection on either night. Normal pulsations were observed on both nights.

Intracorporal injection testing was undertaken next, on the advice of the patient's urologist. In keeping with the NPT results, the patient failed to achieve satisfactory erection during three successive administrations of papaverine and phentolamine. At this point it was concluded that vasculogenic factors were involved, in addition to performance anxiety and relationship conflicts. Several sessions were scheduled to discuss the patient's growing interest in a surgical implant, and to address the sexual demands experienced from his partner.

NEW TREATMENTS, NEW DILEMMAS

Along with the proliferation of assessment techniques, numerous treatment options are currently available for assisting men (and their partners) with erectile dysfunction. Psychotherapy and couples therapy, oral medications and intracorporal injections, vacuum pump devices and constriction rings, vascular surgery, and a variety of new surgical prostheses are all widely recommended. How does one decide which treatment to recommend for any particular man? What are the costs and benefits for each, and which criteria should be applied in selecting a specific treatment option for a given individual? What are the contraindications and long-term risks? Who is most likely to benefit from each of the various approaches? These and other questions regarding the efficacy and outcome of treatment remain to be addressed.

Surgical Techniques

From the perspective of technological innovation, perhaps the most significant advances have taken place in the area of penile prosthesis surgery. Surgical implantation of a penile prosthesis dates back to 1936, when a piece of human rib was first used for this purpose. In the past decade, at least six new types of surgical implant procedures have been developed and are currently available. Each of these methods is described and evaluated by Melman and Tiefer in Chapter 10 of this volume. Penile prosthesis surgery continues to be the mainstay of surgical treatment for erectile failure, in large part because of the allure of permanent freedom from concern about erectile functioning (Tiefer, 1986), as well as the enthusiastic recommendations for such devices by both urologists and manufacturers.

Although the exact number of penile prostheses implanted each year is difficult to estimate, Collins and Kinder (1984) reported that between 1974 and 1980, over 400 Scott-Bradley inflatable penile prostheses were implanted at the Mayo Clinic alone. These numbers have undoubtedly skyrocketed in the last decade. It has recently been estimated, for example, that approximately 25,000 prostheses are implanted annually (Krane et al., 1989), although this may represent a conservative estimate.

How effective is the surgical implant in restoring sexual function for the male and his partner? Although overall success rates tend to be quite high, several factors may influence the outcome in individual cases. According to Collins and Kinder (1984), at least two-thirds of implant recipients tended to be reasonably satisfied with the results, with similar levels of satisfaction reported by partners. However, they noted that when patients were interviewed separately, lower levels of satisfaction were reported. Postoperative intercourse frequencies tended to be higher than in the preoperative period. Middle-aged patients were more satisfied overall than either younger or older men, and the least satisfaction was observed in couples with severe relationship conflicts or lack of sexual desire. Schover and von Eschenbach (1985) have reported that surgical implants may be less successful in cases where a concomitant female sexual dysfunction exists; where the man has unrealistic or inaccurate expectations regarding the prosthesis; where the female partner is opposed to surgery (or, conversely, where she is pressuring her partner to undergo surgery); and where the couple has abandoned all sexual intimacy because of an inability to achieve penile-vaginal intercourse.

Although semirigid prostheses continue to be widely recommended as less costly and more reliable, satisfaction rates tend to be higher with the inflatable implants. For example, Beutler, Scott, Karacan, Baer, and Morris (1984) reported satisfaction ratings in 49 women whose sexual partners had received either inflatable or noninflatable penile prostheses. These authors found that women in the inflatable prosthesis group were significantly more satisfied with the overall quality of their sexual relations and with their partners' prostheses than were women in the noninflatable prosthesis group. Women reported that their husbands, too, were more satisfied with the inflatable prostheses.

Other surgical procedures for erectile dysfunction include arterial reconstructive (bypass) surgery and venous ligation. As discussed by Melman and Tiefer (Chapter 10), the success rates associated with these techniques are extremely variable, ranging from 20% to 80%. The absence of long-term outcome data for these procedures is also problematic. Although vascular surgery techniques are not widely used at present, we anticipate that technological advances in the next decade will lead to an increasing emphasis on both arterial and venous surgeries for erectile failure.

Nonsurgical Approaches to Treatment

Despite the obvious appeal, surgery continues to be a relatively costly and irreversible treatment approach. Given the current trend in medicine toward less costly and invasive treatments generally, sex therapists nowadays are likely to recommend alternative treatment approaches—for example, intracorporal injections, constriction rings, or vacuum pump devices—before advocating a surgical implant for patients with organogenic dysfunction. Although the long-term risks of these latter treatments are relatively unknown, at least the need for irreversible surgery is forestalled.

Intracavernosal injection of smooth muscle relaxants, such as papaverine and phentolamine, has been used with increasing frequency since the mid-1980s for treatment of erectile dysfunction (Brindley, 1986; Virag, Frydman, Legman, & Virag, 1984; Zorgniotti & Lefleur, 1985). As discussed by Althof and Turner in Chapter 11 of this volume, there are several major risks and advantages associated with this approach. Specifically, Althof and Turner report that injection therapy is accepted by only 40–50% of men who are referred for this treatment. Many men are extremely uncomfortable with the notion of self-injection, and such individuals are obviously poor candidates for this form of treatment. The cost of injection therapy is also considerable (approximately $75 or more per month). Various side effects have been reported, ranging from fibrotic nodules, scarring, and liver problems to occasional instances of priapism. Moreover, information is not yet available on long-term use (i.e., 5 years or more) of injection therapy.

For men who tolerate the procedure well, a major advantage of injection therapy appears to be that it is less intrusive than vacuum pumps or constriction rings, and is therefore attractive to single men or those who feel uncomfortable in advertising their erectile difficulties to their partners. Moreover, injection therapy can be combined with traditional sex therapy techniques in the treatment of selected patients with psychogenic dysfunctions (Kaplan, 1990).

Vacuum pump devices, such as the "ErecAid" system, offer certain advantages over injection therapy, according to Althof and Turner (Chapter 11). These devices are generally well tolerated by most patients, and can be used with a wide variety of neurogenic, vasculogenic, and psychogenic problems. Side effects appear to be minimal. Although these devices require an initial outlay of $200–400, the expense is well justified if they are used regularly. Reznichek, Price, Reznichek, and Blackwell (1991) have suggested that these devices are particularly appealing to men with mechanical aptitude, some of whom can be found in their workshops tinkering with ways of improving the device! If a man is in a comfortable, long-standing, and supportive relationship, the vacuum pump approach offers a cost-effective and relatively safe form of treatment.

Althof and Turner also suggest that some men with psychogenic erectile failure may benefit from vacuum pump therapy. Patient acceptance of external pump devices appears to be very high (i.e., 80–90%, unlike that of self-injection treatment. Less costly, and occasionally helpful as well, is the use of constricting bands or so-called "performance rings." These metal or plastic rings are placed around the base of the penis, and help to maintain erections in men who are able to attain a satisfactory erection but are unable to sustain the erection during intercourse.

Case Vignette

Mr. S., a 62-year-old widower, married a 41-year-old divorcee less than 1 year after the unexpected and tragic death of his first wife. From the start of his dating relationship, he experienced severe erectile difficulties with his new partner. He consulted a urologist, who suggested that the patient's hypertensive medication might be the source of his problem. After changing medications and ultimately discontinuing medication altogether, without any noticeable impact on his erectile function, Mr. S. reluctantly accepted referral to our Sexual Counseling Service.

Laboratory evaluation was negative for endocrine or other systemic disorders. Furthermore, two nights of NPT testing indicated relatively intact erectile function in this patient. In treatment, it became clear that Mr. S. had not resolved his grief over the loss of his first wife. In addition, he appeared to have significant regrets over his hasty commitment to a woman with three children from a previous marriage. Conflicts with his stepchildren, the silent accusations from his own son because of his second marriage, and his own misgivings about his choice of marital partner all appeared to contribute to his difficulty in sustaining erections. Mr. S. minimized discussion of these issues and kept insisting that his penis could and should work. "After all," he protested, "I have great erections when I get up in the morning!"

In order to facilitate treatment, a trial of vacuum pump therapy was recommended in addition to conjoint couples therapy. The procedure was carefully explained by a consulting urologist, and the couple were able to incorporate the pump with relatively little difficulty into their lovemaking script. Over a period of several months, Mr. S. began to experience increasing erections without the aid of the pump, at which point termination was recommended.

Psychological Approaches to Treatment

Individual and couples therapy approaches for erectile dysfunction have evolved considerably since the early sensate focus and guided intercourse approach of Masters and Johnson (1970). As noted by LoPiccolo (Chapter 7), the notion of forbidding intercourse and directing the male and his partner to nondemand body caressing can be traced back to the writings of an 18th-century British physician, Sir John Hunter. The Masters and Johnson treatment for erectile failure is also similar in concept to the *in vivo* desensitization approach of the early behaviorists, as described above.

Although the sensate focus and guided intercourse techniques continue to be widely used, significant advances have recently been made in the cognitive–behavioral and systemic approaches to erectile disorders. Beginning with the early work of Albert Ellis (1980), the use of rational–emotive and other cognitive interventions has been increasingly utilized in altering pervasive irrational and self-defeating expectations. In Chapter 2 of this volume, for example, Zilbergeld discusses a number of fundamental and widely held beliefs about male sexuality. Other cognitive–behavioral approaches are detailed by LoPiccolo in Chapter 7.

Couples issues are clearly pivotal in many cases of erectile failure, and we have increasingly emphasized the role of couples therapy approaches in the treatment of erectile disorders. In our experience, couples dynamics are perhaps the single most important determinant of treatment prognosis, as couples with strong, committed, and supportive relationships appear to develop effective coping strategies even in the face of the most severe sexual dysfunctions. Core areas for treatment intervention are status and dominance issues, intimacy and trust, lack of desire, and script discrepancies. We discuss each of these areas in detail in Chapter 9.

Single men with erectile difficulties present a special challenge for the sex therapist. In some instances, these men may lack the social skills or willingness to develop or maintain an intimate relationship. In other instances, fears of rejection or excessive performance anxiety can lead to a complete avoidance of sexual intimacy. Treatment of erectile difficulties in such cases requires a strong emphasis on relationship factors, in addition to the often unrealistic expectations that many single males present with. These and other treatment issues are discussed in Chapter 12 of this volume by McCarthy.

Although less has been published about the incidence, prevalence, and treatment of erectile difficulties among gay men, homosexual males are hardly exempt from concerns about erectile performance. The current human immunodeficiency virus (HIV) and acquired immune deficiency syndrome (AIDS) epidemic has certainly affected the sexual behavior of homosexual men (Coleman & Reece, 1988), and has increased the risks and anxieties attendant on sexual exchange in general. Many gay men have responded to the AIDS epidemic with an initial period of sexual withdrawal or abstinence. Fear, anxiety, somatic symptoms, insomnia, increased use of alcohol and drugs, and sometimes a period of social isolation are not uncommon (McWhirter & Mattison, personal communication, 1990). At times, this is followed by denial and an increase in high-risk sexual behavior; for some men, sexual dysfunction ensues.

According to one large-scale study of the incidence of sexual dysfunctions in 500 gay men seeking treatment, Paff (1985) reported that approximately 50% of this sample complained of arousal phase disorders. In a more in-depth study of 22 gay male couples, it was found that 45% complained of erectile dysfunction, which was the most common sexual problem overall. Interestingly, primary erectile problems were almost nonexistent among these men. Rather, situational erectile problems were commonplace and tended to occur more frequently among intimates than in situations of anonymous sexual encounters. The changing sexual climate has undoubtedly caused important and necessary changes in the sexual scripts of gay men, and it seems likely that anonymous sex is accompanied by greater anxiety nowadays.

Unlike their heterosexual counterparts, gay men are less likely to enter treatment with erectile failure as the "ticket of admission" for psychotherapy or sex therapy (McWhirter, personal communication 1990). Rather, as one gay therapist noted:

> The sexual practices of gay men these days in my practice are focused rather on transmission, how to negotiate and implement safer sex, how to form relationships with HIV infection as a factor, loss of sexual desire related to HIV disease, guilt regarding homosexuality, sex associated with illness and death, etc. (McWhirter, personal communication, 1990)

Probably few clinicians would disagree with the statement that all men experiencing erectile failure attributable to psychogenic factors could benefit from some form of individual or conjoint counseling. However, psychotherapy is clearly not equally beneficial for all patients. Men with little interest in, or capacity for, self-reflection or self-examination are less likely to benefit from solely psychological interventions. Often these men are unwilling or unable to understand how relationship conflicts interfere with sexual desire or performance, or how their early experiences of abuse, shame, guilt, fear, and the like may be subverting their current sexual functioning. Rather, they come for therapy requesting an immediate "fix" for their flagging penises. These attitudes and expectations are explored in depth by Zilbergeld in Chapter 2 of this volume.

The last decade has witnessed a remarkable upsurge in the use of technological interventions for assessing and treating erectile failure. In addition to a variety of surgical interventions, the use of physician- or self-administered intracavernosal injections has gained widespread acceptance. What is particularly noteworthy is the willingness of many clinicians to prescribe these treatments for men with psychogenic erectile failure. In the past, such medical or surgical interventions were generally reserved for men with clear-cut organic impotence. Nowadays, there is a greater willingness to treat long-standing and refractory "psychogenic" dysfunction with medical or surgical means.

Implications of the New Technologies

The current proliferation of technological solutions for erectile dysfunction can be seen as strong testimony to the seriousness of the problem for male patients and their partners. In many instances, erectile failure continues to be viewed as a debilitating and potentially emasculating condition. Despite the current rhetoric in the field about sex and intimacy's involving more than penile–vaginal intercourse, the quest for a rigid erection appears to dominate both popular and professional interest. Moreover, it seems likely that our diligence in finding new ways for overcoming erectile difficulties serves unwittingly to reinforce the male myth that rock-hard, ever-available phalluses are a necessary component of male identity. This is indeed a dilemma.

How can we as sex therapists challenge the "myth of the perfect penis," as Tiefer (1986) describes it, while we assiduously look for new and better ways of insuring erections? It may be time for us to re-examine our initial assumptions, and to practice what we preach about the importance of relationships, intimacy, nongenital touching, and affection as the basic ingredients in a rewarding sexual life.

REFERENCES

American Psychiatric Association. (1952). *Diagnostic and statistical manual of mental disorders* (1st ed.). Washington, DC: Author.

American Psychiatric Association. (1968). *Diagnostic and statistical manual of mental disorders* (2nd ed.). Washington, DC: Author.

American Psychiatric Association. (1980). *Diagnostic and statistical manual of mental disorders* (3rd ed.). Washington, DC: Author.

American Psychiatric Association. (1987). *Diagnostic and statistical manual of mental disorders* (3rd ed., rev.). Washington, DC: Author.

Bancroft, J. (1989). *Human sexuality and its problems.* New York: Churchill Livingstone.

Bancroft, J., & Coles, L. (1976). Three years' experience in a sexual problems clinic. *British Medical Journal, i,* 1575–1577.

Barlow, D. H. (1986). Causes of sexual dysfunction: The role of anxiety and cognitive interference. *Journal of Consulting and Clinical Psychology, 54,* 140–157.

Barlow, D. H., Sakheim, D. K., & Beck, J. G. (1983). Anxiety increases sexual arousal. *Journal of Abnormal Psychology, 92,* 49–54.

Bem, S. (1974). The measurement of psychological androgyny. *Journal of Consulting and Clinical Psychology, 42,* 155–162.

Beutler, L. E., Scott, F. B., Karacan, I., Baer, P. E., & Morris, J. (1984). Women's satisfaction with partners' penile implant. *Urology*, *24*, 552-558.

Brindley, G. S. (1986). Maintenance treatment of erectile impotence by cavernosal unstriated muscle relaxant injection. *British Journal of Psychiatry*, *149*, 210-215.

Buvat, J., Buvat-Herbaut, M., Lemaire, A., Marcolin, G., & Quittelier, E. (1990). Recent developments in the clinical assessment and diagnosis of erectile dysfunction. *Annual Review of Sex Research*, *1*, 265-308.

Cohen, A. S., Rosen, R. C., & Goldstein, L. (1985). EEG hemispheric asymmetry during sexual arousal: Psychophysiological patterns in responsive, unresponsive, and dysfuntional males. *Journal of Abnormal Psychology*, *94*, 580-590.

Coleman, E., & Reece, R. (1988). Treating low sexual desire among gay men. In S. R. Leiblum & R. C. Rosen (Eds.), *Sexual desire disorders* (pp. 413-445). New York: Guilford Press.

Collins, G. F., & Kinder, B. N. (1984). Adjustment following surgical implantation of a penile prosthesis: A critical overview. *Journal of Sex and Marital Therapy*, *10*, 255-271.

Elliott, M. L. (1985). The use of "impotence" and "frigidity": Why has "impotence" survived? *Journal of Sex and Marital Therapy*, *11*, 51-56.

Ellis, A. (1980). Treatment of erectile dysfunction. In S. R. Leiblum & L. A. Pervin (Eds.), *Principles and practice of sex therapy* (pp. 235-261). New York: Guilford Press.

Fracher, J. C., Leiblum, S. R., & Rosen, R. C. (1981). Recent advances in the comprehensive evaluation of erectile dysfunction. *International Journal of Mental Health*, *10*, 110-121.

Frank, E., Anderson, C., & Kupfer, D. J. (1976). Profiles of couples seeking sex therapy and marital therapy. *American Journal of Psychiatry*, *133*, 559-562.

Frank, E., Anderson, C., & Rubinstein, D. (1978). Frequency of sexual dysfunction in "normal" couples. *New England Journal of Medicine*, *299*, 111-115.

Freud, S. (1955). 'A child is being beaten': A contribution to the study of the origin of sexual perversions. In J. Strachey (Ed. and Trans.), *The standard edition of the complete psychological works of Sigmund Freud* (Vol. 17, pp. 175-204). London: Hogarth Press. (Original work published 1919)

Hastings, D. W. (1963). *Impotence and frigidity*. Boston: Little, Brown.

Hawton, K. (1982). The behavioral treatment of sexual dysfunction. *British Journal of Psychiatry*, *140*, 94-101.

Johnson, J. (1968). *Disorders of sexual potency in the male*. Elmsford, NY: Pergamon Press.

Kaplan, H. S. (1974). *The new sex therapy*, New York: Brunner/Mazel.

Kaplan, H. S. (1990). The combined use of sex therapy and intrapenile injections in the treatment of impotence. *Journal of Sex and Marital Therapy*, *16*, 195-207.

Kinsey, A. C., Pomeroy, W. B., Martin, C., & Gebhard, P. (1953). *Sexual behavior in the human female*. Philadelphia: W. B. Saunders.

Krane, R. J., Goldstein, I., & Saenz de Tejada, I. (1989). Impotence. *New England Journal of Medicine*, *321*, 1648-1659.

Lazarus, A. A. (1965). The treatment of a sexually inadequate man. In L. P. Ullmann &

L. Krasner (Eds.), *Case studies in behavior modification* (pp. 243–240). New York: Holt, Rinehart & Winston.

Lue, T. F., Hricak, H., Schmidt, R. A., & Tanagho, E. A. (1986). Functional evaluation of penile veins by cavernosography in papaverine-induced erection. *Journal of Urology, 135,* 479–483.

Masters, W. H., & Johnson, V. E. (1970). *Human sexual inadequacy.* Boston: Little, Brown.

Mellinger, B. C., Vaughan, E. D., Thompson, S. L., & Goldstein, M. (1987). Correlation between intracavernous papaverine injection and Doppler analysis in impotent men. *Urology, 30,* 416–419.

Melman, A., Tiefer, L., & Pedersen, R. (1988). Evaluation of first 406 patients in urology based center for male sexual dysfunction. *Urology, 32,* 6–10.

Mohr, D. C., & Beutler, L. E. (1990). Erectile dysfunction: A review of diagnostic and treatment procedures. *Clinical Psychology Review, 10,* 123–150.

Morley, J. E. (1986). Impotence. *American Journal of Medicine, 80,* 897–905.

O'Leary, K. D., & Wilson, G. T. (1987). *Behavior therapy: Application and outcome* (2nd ed.). Englewood Cliffs, NJ: Prentice-Hall.

Paff, B. A. (1985). Sexual dysfunction in gay men requesting treatment. *Journal of Sex and Marital Therapy, 11,* 3–18.

Renshaw, D. C. (1988). Profile of 2376 patients treated at Loyola Sex Clinic between 1972 and 1987. *Sex and Marital Therapy, 3,* 111–117.

Reznichek, R., Price, T., Reznichek, C., & Blackwell, L. (1991, March). *Unreliability of simple doppler for evaluation of penile blood flow.* Paper presented at the annual meeting of the Society for Sex Therapy and Research, Redondo Beach, CA.

Rosen, R. C. (1983). Clinical issues in the assessment and treatment of impotence: A new look at an old problem. *the Behavior Therapist, 6,* 81–85.

Rosen, R. C., & Beck, J. G. (1988). *Patterns of sexual arousal: Psychophysiological processes and clinical applications.* New York: Guilford Press.

Rosen, R. C., & Leiblum, S. R. (1987). Current approaches to the evaluation of sexual desire disorders. *Journal of Sex Research, 23,* 141–162.

Rosen, R. C., Leiblum, S. R., & Hall, K. S. (1987). *Etiological and predictive factors in sex therapy.* Paper presented at the annual meeting of the Society for Sex Therapy and Research, New Orleans.

Schiavi, R. C. (1990). Sexuality and aging in men. *Annual Review of Sex Research, 1,* 227–250.

Schover, L. R., & Jensen, S. B. (1988). *Sexuality problems and chronic disease: A comprehensive approach,* New York: Guilford Press.

Schover, L. R., & von Eschenbach, A. C. (1985). Sex therapy and the penile prosthesis: A synthesis. *Journal of Sex and Marital Therapy, 11,* 57–66.

Slag, M. R., Morley, J. E., Elson, M. K., & Trence, D. L. (1983). Impotence in medical clinic outpatients. *Journal of the American Medical Association, 249,* 1736–1740.

Spector, I. P., & Carey, M. P. (1990). Incidence and prevalence of the sexual dysfunctions: A critical review of the empirical literature. *Archives of Sexual Behavior, 19,* 389–408.

Stekel, W. (1927). *Impotence in the male.* New York: Boni & Liveright.

Tiefer, L. (1986). In pursuit of the perfect penis: The medicalization of male sexuality. *American Behavioral Scientist, 29*, 579–599.

Tiefer, L., & Melman, A. (1989). Comprehensive evaluation of erectile dysfunction and medical treatments. In S. R. Leiblum & R. C. Rosen (Eds.), *Principles and practice of sex therapy* (2nd ed.): *Update for the 1990s* (pp. 207–236). New York: Guilford Press.

Virag, R., Frydman, D., Legman, M., & Virag, H. (1984). Intracavernous injection of papaverine as a diagnostic and therapeutic method in erectile failure. *Angiology, 35*, 79–83.

Wincze, J. P., & Carey, M. P. (1991). *Sexual dysfunction: A guide for assessment and treatment.* New York: Guilford Press.

Wolpe, J. (1958). *Psychotherapy by reciprocal inhibition.* Stanford, CA: Stanford University Press.

Zorgniotti, A. W., & Lefleur, R. S. (1985). Auto-injection of the corpus cavernosum with a vasoactive drug combination for vasculogenic impotence. *Journal of Urology, 133*, 39.

2

The Man behind the Broken Penis: Social and Psychological Determinants of Erectile Failure

BERNIE ZILBERGELD

The man without the erection sees himself as being
less than a man, as an unworthy, as a fraud. It is as if
the flag of his manhood must remain furled for lack of
a mast. Thus the terror, the shame, the withdrawal
spurred by the dysfunction far exceed the reaction to
almost any other medical condition.
—JULTY (1975, p. 15)

Bernie Zilbergeld is among the most insightful and provocative clinicians currently writing about male sexuality. In his classic book on this topic (Male Sexuality, 1978), he articulated the beliefs and assumptions men hold about sexual performance, and illustrated how debilitating and destructive they can be. In the present chapter, Zilbergeld writes with wit and wisdom of the wide variety of psychological reactions experienced by men with erectile difficulties.

Zilbergeld reminds us that male socialization can be detrimental in some instances to adequate sexual performance. For men, in fact, sex is all too often defined as performance, and feelings about one's adequacy as a male are determined in large part by how one functions in bed. Since men are taught to believe that manhood must be won, it is also the case that it can be lost, that it is conditional. Erectile failure can be psychologically devastating—not only because it indicates poor performance, but because it signals loss of masculinity as well.

Men with erectile difficulties experience a variety of negative emotions, ranging from fear and anger (toward their partners as well as themselves) to sexual avoidance and a sense of personal inadequacy. It is not surprising, therefore, that men who present with this complaint often feel fragile, ashamed, and sometimes terrified. Zilbergeld suggests that therapists need to appreciate more fully a man's feelings of shame and embarrassment about initiating therapy, since it can be such a difficult undertaking for some. Zilbergeld concludes his chapter with a number of basic recommendations for achieving more satisfying sex.

Bernie Zilbergeld, Ph.D., is an internationally renowned author and psychologist in private practice in Oakland, California. He is the author of a number of important books in the field, including Mind Power: Getting What You Want through Mental Training *(with Arnold A. Lazarus) and his forthcoming* The New Male Sexuality, *the successor to* Male Sexuality.

The man with an erection problem is a man in serious trouble. His situation is very different from that of a man with almost any other medical or psychological problem, and very different from that of a woman with any sexual problem. His trouble stems not primarily from the fact of a penis that is not working up to expectation, but rather from the heavy symbolic baggage that he, and all of us, attach to the male organ.

To a great extent, of course, the problem that plagues him is a technical one involving blood flow into and out of the penis, hormonal balances, performance anxiety, and so on. It is easy for the health professional to get overinvolved in such issues and almost forget the human being to whom the penis is connected and the psychological burden he is carrying. Too often, I believe, in both medical and therapeutic settings, the man does not receive the understanding he needs and deserves.

In this chapter I hope to explain why men are so concerned about the well-being of their penises, what happens to men when their organs do not perform as desired, and what we as helping professionals can do about it. My thesis, in brief, is that male socialization and cultural expectations place a very heavy burden on a very small portion of the man's anatomy. This burden causes unnecessary anxiety and other bad feelings in both men and women, bad sex, dysfunctional sex, and relationship distress; it also makes it difficult for the man to acknowledge and get help for his problems.

THE MAKING OF ANXIOUS PENIS WATCHERS

Although it is commonly thought by some women and especially some feminists that men have everything going their way in most areas of life, I suggest that this is not the case when it comes to sex. It is certainly true that males of all ages are given more permission and leeway to explore sex than females. Even in these liberated times, it still seems that we are less upset and more forgiving about the sexual explorations, adventures, and infidelities of men than of women. Despite this, however, I hope to show that what men learn about masculinity and sexuality puts them in a precarious and anxious state of mind. Men are in effect taught that in sex they should be able to play well and come out winners against a stacked deck. As any gambler would be happy to point out, there are few victories against stacked decks.

The Male Gender Role

Before learning about sex, boys learn the rudiments of gender identity—what it means to be a man. Regardless of whether they learn the more traditional model of masculinity (exemplified by John Wayne and Rambo) or the newer one (exemplified by Alan Alda and Phil Donahue), sexual performance is an important component. "Performance" is the key word, because performing or achieving is the main theme in male socialization. Whatever else a man may be, he has to be someone who can *do*, who can decide, initiate, strive, and achieve. Given the importance of performing to men, and given that gender identity is learned before the child has much knowledge of sex, it's not surprising that sex, like almost everything else, is turned into a performance.

One important thing the boy learns early on is that while femaleness or womanhood is given by having the right genitals, masculinity or manhood is not; it is conditional. Having the right genitals is necessary but not sufficient. As Norman Mailer (1968, p. 36) put it: "Nobody was born a man; you earned your manhood provided you were good enough, bold enough." Anthropologist David Gilmore notes a recurring notion in a vast variety of societies

> that real manhood is different from simple anatomical maleness, that it is not a natural condition that comes about spontaneously through biological maturation but rather is a precarious or artificial state that boys must win against powerful odds. This recurrent notion that manhood is problematic . . . is found at all levels of sociocultural development regardless of what other alternative roles are recognized. It is found among the simplest hunters and fishermen, among peasants and sophisticated urbanized peoples; it is found in all continents and environments. (1990, p. 11)

The crucial corollary to the rule that manhood must be won is that it can be questioned and lost. A man is always open to the challenge "Are you man enough?" or, as Lady Macbeth says to her husband, "Are you a man?" There is no parallel for women. Femaleness is not open to question or challenge. A woman may be considered unattractive, unladylike, promiscuous, imcompetent, or shrewish, but her essential femaleness is not open to debate. But because a man's masculine identity always remains conditional, he is in a perpetual state of anxiety. Maybe he really isn't good enough or bold enough;

maybe he doesn't have what it takes. Men walk a very thin line. They know it doesn't take much—one act of cowardice, one mistake, one instance of acting too soft or feminine—to be called "girl," "sissy," "lady," or "pussy," terms that carry much more punch than calling a girl "tomboy." For both boys and men, these are fighting words. By using them, one is calling the male's very identity into question. If a male isn't a man, what then is he? From the way most men react, it is clear that their answer is "Nothing at all."

Because the line they walk is so thin and because the consequences of deviance are so grave, males are much more concerned than females with adherence to the rules. Girls and women wear men's clothes, play men's games, and often talk and act like men, but the consequences of a 10-year-old boy's or a 40-year-old man's wearing a dress can be serious. The excess baggage of male identity makes certain things harder for men than for women. A woman who loses her job will be upset because she is not sure how she will pay her bills. A man who loses his job will be upset for the same reason, but in addition he will be upset because one of the pillars of his masculine identity—his ability to be a worker and provider—is now on the line. If worse comes to worst, our unemployed woman will be a poor and maybe homeless woman. The man will be poor and maybe homeless as well, and also not a man. If a woman has a sex problem, she may be upset for a variety of reasons, but neither she nor anyone else considers her less than a woman. However, "An impotent man always feels that his masculinity, and not just his sexuality, is threatened." (Person, 1980, p. 626).

Other themes of male socialization—the emphasis on strength and a corresponding fear of weakness, dependency, and feelings—also affect his view of sex and his ability to deal with sexual problems. I take them up later.

As the boy grows, and especially after he reaches puberty, he is introduced to the model of sex dominant in our culture, aspects of which he has glimpsed even before puberty.

The Fantasy Model of Sex: It's Two Feet Long, Hard as Steel, and Can Go All Night

Some years ago (Zilbergeld, 1978), I used the phrase "the fantasy model of sex" to describe the sexual messages we get in this culture from books, stories, movies, and television shows (whether sexually explicit or not), sexual humor, and other sources. Taken together, these messages constitute our societal model or definition of sex: what sex is, who does what and how, what can be expected, and so on. This model is the blueprint or road map of sexuality. As boys and girls become interested in and attuned to sexual ideas, aspects of the model are what they learn. And these same messages are reinforced continually throughout life.

I have recently updated my analysis; although some small changes are noticeable, by and large the performance demands on men remain the same (Zilbergeld, 1992). Although our culture has certainly opened up sexually, and many more sources of accurate information are available than even two decades ago, boys and girls growing up today are exposed to many of the same sexual messages as were their parents before them.

The fantasy model is centered around male performance, and most of that performance depends on a large, automatically functioning penis. Everything hinges on how well the penis does its job. A hard penis means something, even if it is not necessary to carry out certain acts and even if it is not used at all.

The main message males get is this: "You've got to have good equipment and you've got to use it right. Sex isn't mainly for enjoyment or for expressing love, caring, or even lust; it's mainly to prove that you're a man." This performance orientation explains why men are so obsessed with measurements. If sex were really something to be enjoyed and to enable a man to express personal feelings, then he could just express and enjoy. But if a man has something to prove, then he has to know how he measures up. How big is his erection, how long did it last, how many orgasms were there? The performance orientation also explains why some men brag about sex to their friends. What's the point of a great performance if no one knows about it?

Sexual scenes from two best-selling novels—one 20 years old and one more recent—exemplify the fantasy model. In the first, Harold Robbins's *The Betsy* (1971), the man is a wealthy businessman and the woman works for him. He has just let her know that it's in her interest to have sex with him. With that for introduction and foreplay, we begin:

> Gently her fingers opened his union suit and he sprang out at her like an angry lion from its cage. Carefully she . . . took him in both hands, one behind the other as if she were grasping a baseball bat. She stared at it in wonder. . . .
>
> [After placing his hands under her armpits and lifting her in the air] he began to lower her on him. Her legs came up, circling his waist, as he began to enter her. Her breath caught in her throat. It was as if a giant of white hot steel were penetrating her. She began to moan as it opened her and climbed higher into her body, past her womb, past her stomach, under her heart, up into her throat. She was panting now, like a bitch in heat. . . .
>
> [He then lifts her off him and throws her onto the bed.] Then he was posed over her. . . . His hands reached and grasped each of her heavy breasts as if he wanted to tear them from her body. She moaned in pain and writhed, her pelvis suddenly arching and thrusting toward him. Then he entered her again.
>
> "My God," she cried, "my God!" She began to climax almost before he was fully inside her. Then she couldn't stop them, one coming rapidly after

the other as he slammed into her with the force of the giant body press she had seen working in his factory. She became confused, the man and the machine they were one and the same and the strength was something she had never known before. And finally, when orgasm after orgasm has racked her body into a searing sheet of flame and she could bear no more, she cried out of him: "Take your pleasure . . . Quick, before I die!"

A roar came from deep inside his throat. . . . she felt the hot onrushing gusher of his semen turning her insides into hot, flowing lava. She discovered herself climaxing again. (pp. 101–103)

Here is a different kind of performance, from Erica Jong's *Parachutes and Kisses* (1985):

He heaped the pillows in front of her for her to lean on, and cupping her breasts, he took her from behind, ramming her harder than before. [This is the second time around for these two, the first one having lasted what seemed like 4 hours.] Her cunt throbbed, ached, tingled. She screamed for him to ram her even harder, to smack her, to pound her. . . .

Never had she so surely met her sexual mate—a man who never tired of fucking, who liked to fuck until the point of soreness and exhaustion, a man who had as few hang-ups about sweat and smell and blood as she had. . . .

She had never come before in this position—but when she did, it was as if thirty-nine years of comes were released and she howled and growled like an animal—whereupon he was aroused beyond containment and he began to come with a pelvis and cock gone wild, pounding her fiercely, filling her with come. (pp. 340–341)

Although Jong does not explicitly mention the condition of the man's penis, it's clear from what she does say that it is strong, hard, powerful, and apparently capable of staying that way all night, just like the penis in the Harold Robbins account.

One fascinating characteristic of media accounts of sex is that they almost invariably depict male *performance* and female *pleasure*. He *acts* (rams, pounds, thrusts, bangs) and she *feels* ("unbearable pleasure," "overwhelming joy," "delirious ecstasy")—the usual male–female dichotomy. Although she sometimes performs (she too can thrust and bang), it is rarely clear what he feels and experiences. It's as if his feelings and pleasure are beside the point.

Now let's look at the main performance specifications. *A hard penis is everything.* When males of any age think of sex, they think of what they can do with, or what can be done to, their erections. That's what it's all about. And not any old penis or erection will do. The fantasy model has specifications.

Size

Penises that are shown in X-rated films or described in pornography and other fiction come in only three sizes: large, extra large, and so big guys can't get them through the door. Erections are described as "huge" or "massive," and sometimes lengths such as 10 or 12 inches are given—hardly your average-size penis. Nowhere does one read or hear of average penises.

Hardness

If bigger is better, so is harder. Fantasyland penises are usually described as "hard as steel," "hard as a rock," or "diamond cutters"; something that could cut a diamond, the toughest substance in the world, must really be hard. There is no joy in a penis that's sort of hard, semihard, or only 70% erect.

Functioning

The desired penis functions automatically and predictably, just like a well-oiled machine. It should immediately spring into full readiness whenever its owner decides he will use it. If a man is dancing close with someone, his penis should be fully erect, pressing mightily against his pants and making its presence clearly felt. If a woman unzips his fly, his erection ought to spring out at her. If they kiss, well, here's how one novel put it: "The lingering kiss [the first one that day, it should be said] induced an immediate erection" (Wallace, 1989, p. 226). The way some men talk about it, I have the impression that they think their penises should stand fully erect if a woman even says hello to them. Nowhere does one see or read about a penis that merely moseys out for a look at what's happening.

Automatic functioning means that the penis should function regardless of any other considerations. Neither rain, nor snow, nor sleet shall keep the almighty penis from its appointed rounds. No matter whether a man is sick or well, tired or fresh, anxious or relaxed, preoccupied or fully present; whether he likes his partner or not; whether he is angry or not; or whether he has gotten any stimulation or not—his penis should immediately come to full attention and do its manly thing.

The clear message is that a man showing up at a sexual event without a rock-hard, long-lasting penis is as inappropriate as a carpenter showing up for work without a hammer and tape measure. He simply can't leave home without a stiff dick. Needless to say, these requirements put a bit of pressure on men to have and keep erections. They also create penis envy, but not the kind Freud had in mind. He thought that women envy men's penises and that every woman wishes she had a penis of her own. What is closer to reality is that most men envy the penises in the fantasy model. They assume that some other men (or all other men) have huge, automatically functioning, and long-lasting penises, and wish that they themselves were better endowed. A general state of sexual inadequacy is created in men. Since almost no real penis meets all the specifications, men are always feeling that there's something wrong with them.

This sense of inadequacy helps explain why concerns about penis size are still widespread. Even after exposure to the latest sex research, many men still have a lingering concern that their average-size penises aren't large enough "to do the job," a phrase they often use. After I gave a talk to a college class in human sexuality, one of the students said this to me privately: "I know what Masters and Johnson said. I know what my teacher said. But if I had three wishes, the first would be for a million dollars and the second would be for a larger and harder cock." Many other men have expressed similar sentiments to me.

Results

In the fantasy model, the man's penis produces earth-shaking, bed-breaking, mind-bending effects on his partner: She has endless orgasms; she climaxes "before he was fully inside her"; she howls and growls; she feels "as if her bones were melting"; she experiences "overwhelming pleasure." All this results from the activity of the pounding, magical penis.

Since few women in the real world respond the way the ones in fantasyland do, there is another reason for men to feel inadequate. If only they had better penises, they could melt their partners' bones.

Although most men are unaware of it, the sexual model that they have been indoctrinated into and accepted forces them to play against a stacked deck. Everything—pleasing their partners, success and failure, self-esteem and respect, their very identity as men—hinges on the performance of an organ that they cannot directly control and that is adversely affected by a large number of physical and emotional factors.

What Erection or Lack of It Means

To the man's partner, his erection is seen as a strong indication of his desire for her, her attractiveness, and her ability to turn him on. If the man does not get erect, the partner often takes it to mean that he doesn't find her attractive, that he doesn't love her, or that she doesn't have the skill to turn him on. Whatever the specific interpretation, she is not going to feel good about herself. And this, in turn, will cause her to exert pressure on him—overt or

The reason for this despair is that no other medical condition strikes at the heart of, or is even relevant to, one's sexual identity. The man with, say, diabetes, prostate problems, pneumonia, or even cancer may find his life considerably constrained and even shortened. But having the disease does not make him less of a man in his or anyone else's eyes. The only other condition I can think of that evokes the same horror in men as erection problems is losing one's job. The problem with loss of job and erection difficulties is the same: Both hit at the pillars of masculinity.

Women are often baffled by the agony a man goes through when he fails to get or keep an erection, but they have no parallel experience with which to compare it. A woman's sexual identity is not on the line when she has a sexual dysfunction. And a woman can participate in intercourse or any other sexual act without being aroused or even interested. If she fails to lubricate sufficiently, saliva or artificial lubrication can be brought to the rescue. She may not have an orgasm, of course, but at least she can go through with the act and give her partner pleasure. A man is in a more difficult situation. Because of the belief that sex demands a rigid penis, there is nothing that can rescue him. His "failure" is obvious, dangling in full view. There is no way to fake an erection, and it is difficult (though not impossible) to have intercourse without at least a partial erection.

A man without an erection feels that he has failed as a man. His partner may be sympathetic and supportive, but he may be so consumed with self-loathing that he cannot accept what she offers. Many men distance themselves from their partners after such "failures" and engage in orgies of self-flagellation. The result is usually a miserable time for everyone concerned.

A man with an erection problem is fearful all the time. What he fears most is the moment when she touches his penis and finds it soft. Or, worse yet, when she stimulates it and it doesn't respond. Or when she utters those famous words, "Fuck me," "Take me," or "I want you inside me," and he is unable to comply. What to other men constitutes a success, a moment of great pleasure, or the fulfillment of a favorite fantasy is to him an unbearable demand and the most fearful thing imaginable.

It is easy to think that men are just too performance-oriented, and if they would just relax and not worry so much about their penises, things would be better. Although this idea has a great deal of merit, it is also too simplistic. Men are performance-oriented because that's what they're trained to be. It is true that in recent years we have also added sensitivity to the list of male requirements, but we have not removed the achievement standards. Yes, men should be capable of sensitivity and intimacy, but they also should be strong, be potent, and perform successfully. Men who are merely soft or sensitive are considered wimps, non-men.

Yet another reason why at least some men need to perform is that their partners have certain expectations. I do not mean to suggest that women are responsible for men's erection problems—I do not believe that this is the case—but years of experience have persuaded me that men aren't the only ones exerting pressure for erections. I recently received a call from a woman who had been a client some years ago. She was now dating a man with erection difficulties. They had talked about the situation, and he believed it was getting better and would continue to do so as they spent more time together. And he was, according to her, a caring and sensitive man who was almost always happy to stimulate her to orgasm with hand or mouth. But she was greatly distressed and was thinking of ending the relationship. Her reasons: She liked and missed intercourse; she felt that only intercourse constitutes making love; and, most important of all, even though she knew intellectually she might be wrong, she believed that his problem meant there was "something terribly wrong with me."

This woman is far from the only one. Many women believe, often against their better judgment, that anything more than an occasional lack of erection means that they (the women) are not desired, not loved, not found attractive or sexy. They see themselves as being the cause of the problem, and they find it hard to deal with the implications of that idea. Given all that lack of erection means to these women, it is understandable that they need their partners to have erections and send out pressuring vibrations to that effect, even if they don't say a word about it. And although men can't always identify this extra pressure, they are clearly affected by it.

This situation, of course, has a clear parallel: Many men need their partners to be orgasmic so that the men can feel good about themselves. For a woman who is reliably orgasmic, this is not much of a problem, just as it is not a problem for a man who reliably gets erections that his partner needs him to do this in order for her to feel good about herself. But for men with erection difficulties and women with orgasmic problems, this added pressure does not help and indeed can undermine efforts to resolve the difficulty.

This lesson was obvious in a recent case. The client had been having erection problems for a decade since his divorce. With only one exception, he had never had an erection adequate for intercourse with his woman friend of 6 months. She did not cause the problem—he had had it with several women before he met her—but he felt discouraged about solving it with her because of her desperate need for erections. Intercourse was the only sex act, according to her, and a hard penis was the main way she could feel loved. Because the woman would not participate in therapy, and because the man thought the relationship might not endure, he elected to work with a surrogate partner. After a few months, he was having reliable erections with the surrogate. But no matter what he tried, he couldn't do the same with his friend. When we discussed why things were so different with the two women, he came to this conclusion:

With the surrogate, I don't have to get an erection to make her happy. I can just do what I want and have a good time. If I get hard, terrific. If I don't, no big deal. I still have a good time. Any hassle that may result from not getting hard comes from me, not her. That's real freeing, not having to perform for her. But with my girlfriend, even if she hasn't mentioned it lately, I know getting hard is the only thing that matters. Her whole worth as a woman is riding on how my cock does. I can't get that out of my mind.

This is as good an example as I know of how destructive our sexual model is—how it makes victims of both men and women, and causes people to make each other miserable.

Because so much rides on the functioning of his penis, a man whose penis isn't performing as desired tends to panic. Clear thinking goes out the window. Men in their 50s and even 40s and younger wonder whether they are "over the hill." Men who have never had a homosexual fantasy or experience in their lives wonder whether they are gay. Men who clearly do care for their partners and have reasonably good relationships wonder whether they have "fallen out of love."

In their panic, some men resort to drastic measures. One of these is to have sex with another partner, perhaps an ex-lover. If things go well with her, then at least the man feels that he is not totally washed up. Sometimes an adventure with an ex-lover does go fine and does give the man confidence to come back home and deal more realistically with the problem. With an affair involving a new partner, however, the penis often doesn't operate any better than it does at home. This is not surprising, given all the anxiety the man is carrying into the new relationship, which, like all new relationships, has its own share of anxieties. As a result, his worst fears are confirmed.

Another drastic measure is anger directed at the partner. Yes, there is something wrong and it must be her fault. If she weren't so demanding, critical, passive, fat, or something else, he wouldn't have the problem. Some men verbally abuse their partners with these complaints, most of which in my experience have little or no basis. Even if there is a basis (perhaps she is too critical or passive), the way he expresses himself is not conducive to anything but her retaliating in kind.

Other men simply withdraw in anger and shame. They distance them-selves from their partners and from sex. If there is no sex, they don't have to face the problem. And some women whose partners are having erection problems also withdraw: "I don't want to get myself all worked up and be left hanging." To the suggestion that her man might satisfy her some other way, such a woman may reply, "It's not the same. I'd rather do without." With-drawal, no matter how initiated and by whom, creates more problems. Distance, tension, and hostility build up and often undermine what before was a workable relationship.

Other men do not completely withdraw; they are willing to try sex, but give up as soon as it is clear that they're not going to get hard. Still others will try to satisfy their partners by hand or mouth, but still feel terrible because they don't have an erection.

Many older men simply give up altogether. Having been socialized into sex during a much more repressive time, these are often men whose entire sexual experience is limited to intercourse, who don't know that there are other ways of being sexual, who don't realize that they may need direct penile stimulation to get hard, who can't talk about sex to their partners or anyone else, and who don't realize that a less than 100% erection can be used quite pleasurably in intercourse and other acts.

The wife of an older couple I was seeing for nonsexual issues one day expressed her unhappiness about the absence of sex for the last 8 years. It was very difficult for the man to respond, but he finally said that he was "used up sexually." Further discussion revealed that about 8 years before, he had realized that his penis wasn't as quick to respond as it had previously been, and that his erections weren't as firm. As he worried about these observations, on several occasions he didn't get hard or lost his erection during intercourse. He concluded that he couldn't do himself or his wife "any good any more," and never again initiated sex, despite feeling sad about his wife's disappointment and despite the fact that he had enjoyed the sex they had.

Men in their 60s and older have special problems because the fantasy model has no room for them. It only pertains to young, healthy, beautiful, and acrobatic men and women who have just met. Very little is said or shown in our culture about sex in later years or between a man and a woman who have been together for more than 2 weeks. Nowhere do we hear about the joys of sex for those who have been together for a lifetime and who no longer have the help of fresh flesh to arouse them; for men whose erections are not rock-hard; for women who are not young and immediately lubricating, as well as intensely responsive with cries and screams; and for partners who may both have one or more serious medical conditions.

Fear of Having Problems and Needing Help

Another aspect of male socialization makes it difficult for the man with an erection problem. This is the myth that men should not have any personal problems, and certainly not any problems with sex.

By definition, a man in our culture is someone who is in control of his life. Problems do come up, of course, but a real man quickly resolves them without complaining, whining, or needing outside help. Men understand that women are different. They have lots of problems; they like to talk about them (endlessly, it seems); and they are more than willing to enlist the aid of friends and therapists. But this is not a man's way. Having a personal problem he can't resolve on his own suggests weakness and dependency to a man—two characteristics he has been warned against since early childhood. Once again, his very identity as a male is perceived as under attack.

In the fantasy model of sex, there are few sexual problems or difficulties. It's bad enough for a man to have a problem of any kind, but for his "manhood" not to be in perfect order is an incredible blow. The usual case when a couple comes in for sex therapy is that even if the problem is primarily the man's, he is there only because the woman has dragged him in. He doesn't want to acknowledge the problem; he just wants the whole matter to go away. Needless to say, this just makes the therapy process more difficult and the chances of a successful outcome less likely.

The reality is that men have as many personal problems as women, including problems with sex. But because it is so fraught with meaning if a man has a difficulty, he is in a bind. Not being able to acknowledge it means that he can't try to resolve it on his own or with his partner. She knows there's a problem but can't get him to acknowledge it, which puts her in a bind as well. This kind of situation can drive a woman crazy. If she doesn't do anything, the problem remains. If she keeps bringing it up, she risks feeling like a nag. It doesn't take long before the partners are distant and the relationship deteriorates; in some cases, it is destroyed. This is sad because in the vast majority of these cases the problem could have been easily dealt with, if only it could have been confronted.

My experience with men and women in therapy is that in general it is much harder for men. Just calling and making an appointment is more difficult. And to have to sit and tell someone that they are not up to snuff in the crucial area of sex is incredibly difficult for many of them. I have seen men who sit for a whole session and talk about everything except sex; men who can't talk about much of anything and give only one-word answers to my questions; men who use language so general that it is impossible to tell what they are referring to. I have seen men make their partners into scapegoats, blaming them for everything that is wrong. Other men spend the whole first session, or a large part of it, denouncing therapy and therapists.

In discussing how men present themselves for treatment, it is important to note the contribution of still another feature of male socialization: a difficulty in expressing, or even thinking about, *anything* personal. Delving into personal issues, especially feelings, is something males are warned against from childhood. The result is that the same man who is quite articulate when discussing his job or the fortunes of his favorite athletic team often becomes mute when asked what he is thinking or feeling about something personal.

THE HEALTH PROFESSIONAL AND THE MAN
WITH ERECTION PROBLEMS

Despite the difficulties men have in admitting they have problems, talking about sex, and going for help, increasing numbers are doing all three. And, fortunately, we helping professionals now have a wide variety of tools to offer. Sex therapy and several mechanical and medical interventions (e.g., vacuum devices, penile injections, and penile implants) have been helpful to large numbers of men and their partners.

It is clear that men can change. They can learn to acknowledge problems; to talk about sex with their partners; to go for help; to adopt new ideas, beliefs, and practices. They can learn, in short, to have better sex, to resolve problems, and to feel better about themselves.

But we professionals need to keep in mind that the man with an erection problem needs understanding and support. No one would argue with that statement, of course, because we clinicians like to think that we are always understanding and supportive of our patients, that we take care of them. But I suggest that this is often not the case and that understanding the reasons why may help us to do better.

I think it helps to acknowledge that the man with an erection problem is often not an attractive person. He may be anxious and even panicked. As noted above, he may deny his problem, not want to talk about it, manifest his anxiety as anger at the therapist or his partner, and generally come across as uncooperative or even hostile. Because of his great distress, his thinking may be impaired. He may not be able to collect his thoughts, or may not give a coherent account of his problem or its history. He may not be able to describe what thoughts or feelings he has before or during sex. I have had men referred by a urologist be unable to tell me when they saw the doctor, what tests were done, or even what the doctor's name is. Such a man often finds it difficult to concentrate on what a therapist is saying and may not be receptive to his or her suggestions. Although he says he will do anything to resolve the problem, he often finds it difficult to follow instructions.

From the therapist's point of view, everything the man is doing is wrong. He is putting too much emphasis on his penis; he is working himself up into a lather; he is focusing on the state of his penis rather than on pleasurable sensation; he is not listening to his partner; and he is not expressing himself well. It's easy to get impatient with such a fellow, and, unfortunately, many of us do.

What this amounts to, however, is blaming him for being who he is. What we need to understand is that he really has no choice. He is not getting anxious or holding onto destructive beliefs because he enjoys his problem or because he is trying to thwart his therapist. On the contrary, he is anxious because the situation as he perceives it is anxiety-provoking. He is holding on to destructive beliefs because they are the only beliefs he has. And he can't immediately accept formulations and suggestions because they are new and because he doesn't quite believe them. It is very difficult to overturn the beliefs and ideology that have nurtured a man for 20 or 30 years (or more), and that are supported by the whole culture, just because a therapist says they are wrong. The patient may well be able to learn new ideas and behaviors, but it helps immensely in this task if he feels understood rather than misunderstood or attacked.

One of the main complaints men with erection problems have about doctors and especially urologists is that they do not give them (the patients) enough time and attention. Given who they are, it is very difficult for men to talk about sexual problems. They hate to feel that there are unreasonable time limits and that a doctor is impatient. The bitterness in one man's account of his visit to a urologist is not uncommon:

> It's like he was doing me a favor by giving me a few minutes, as if I wasn't paying for it. He was 25 minutes late, then seemed like he couldn't wait to get me out of the office. He looked annoyed every time I took more than a second to respond to his questions. And it didn't make it any easier for me that he took what seemed like a dozen phone calls while talking with me. Then, before I was done with what I had to say, he stood up and said that the problem seemed psychological rather than physical and I should see a sex therapist. As he was saying that, he was guiding me out of the room. I didn't even have time to ask the questions I had prepared. I never want to go through something like that again.

Another complaint I have heard about many physicians involves their dismissive attitude. A number of men have reported that their doctors responded with something like "Well, what do you expect at your age?" or a perfunctory, conversation-ending "Sounds normal, nothing to worry about" when the men described an erection problem. Such a response, of course, reinforces a man's idea that he is over the hill, that he is not understood, or that his case is hopeless. (Telling the client that what he's going through is normal can be helpful, as I discuss later; before the man can really hear and believe this, however, he needs to feel accepted and understood. Otherwise, the normality message feels dismissive, and the man feels worse instead of better.)

Complaints about therapists usually involve a lack of sensitivity and flexibility. I'm embarrassed to say that I have heard such complaints about myself. I recall one man I found extremely hard to deal with in the first session. He wouldn't answer any question directly, but circumnavigated around every other possible (and irrelevant) topic before even addressing my questions. And before doing that, he said nothing at all for periods of time ranging from several seconds to several minutes. Nothing I did seemed to help, and I was getting impatient. Not wanting to let the impatience get the better of me, I said to him, "It's clear this isn't going well, and I sense I'm not being helpful. What can I do to make it easier?"

That got to him, and with no hesitation he became wonderfully articulate:

> Look, this is the most difficult thing I've ever faced. I've never had a sex problem before, never had to think about sex. I've never been to a shrink before, never considered it. I'm off center and feel like a total zero. I know I'm not answering your questions. I'm not trying to resist you, I just feel lost. And I know I'm making you impatient. If you could just let me go on as I have and not get annoyed, I think it will get better.

I was able to take his advice, and he was right on target. By the next session, he was much more composed, much more accepting of his situation and his need for help, and much better able to express himself.

As I got to know my client better and we talked about our first session, I realized that I had been putting the same kind of performance demands on him in therapy as he felt in sex. I was annoyed by what he was doing, even though it was all that he could do. And, sensing my annoyance, he became angry with me and also with himself for not performing correctly, which just made him feel worse and made talking even more difficult.

Although that case was one of my first and is now many years behind me, and although I like to think that my sensitivity and understanding have grown through the years, I know that there is always a temptation for us as clinicians to expect these men to perform—that is, to do what we want. There is also temptation to be self-righteous about that expectation. After all, if we are to be helpful, they do need to give accurate reports of their experience, to answer our questions in timely fashion, to do the therapy homework or follow the medical regimen. But they may not be able to, at least not right away and perhaps not exactly as we want them to.

Of course, there is another way in which we as therapists put pressure on these men to perform. Like the women discussed earlier, we often need them to get erections so we can feel good about ourselves as therapists, and in one way or another we communicate this to them. I know this from listening to tapes of other therapists and myself, and from the comments of a few men who had failed with other therapists. One of these men put it this way:

> Although his message was just "relax and play," I had the feeling that my having an erection was crucial for his well-being. Whenever I reported on a homework assignment, he'd always ask about how hard I'd gotten. I think he tried to control his reactions, but my impression—and my wife's—was that he was disappointed and even angry when I didn't get hard. The last

session he really lost it. He got furious when I reported three failures and berated me for not doing the homework the way he assigned it. We didn't quit then—we went home and talked about it first—but that's when I realized how I felt pressured by him to have erections. That pressure was defeating the overt message he was giving and I was trying to accept, that pleasure was paramount and erections didn't matter.

It seems important that we not do to men what has already been done to them by the models of masculinity and sex that dominate our culture, and that we not reinforce ways of thinking and being that are already causing them problems. What we need, I believe, is respect, sensitivity, empathy, tolerance, and flexibility. In other words, I think we need to emphasize the *caring* side of our work. We need to treat these men as the fragile and terrified human beings that they frequently are. If "terrified" sounds too strong, I should add that this was the word used by a man who called me recently about his erection problem.

This should not be taken as an argument against technique. Clinicians need to use the most advanced and effective methods of diagnosis and treatment available. But before, during, and afterward, we need to keep in mind and attend to the terrified and fragile human beings we are dealing with. If we forget them, our techniques will be less effective; even when they do work, we will have contributed unnecessarily to the suffering of troubled persons.

Although I have been focusing on the man with an erection problem, everything I've said also applies to his partner. She is also in trouble and needs understanding and sensitivity. If she is "demanding" erections from her partner, a therapist needs to understand that this demand is almost certainly not motivated by a desire to undermine the success of therapy. Rather, it comes from her need to protect her own integrity and well-being. The same is true if she resists certain homework or participation in noninter-course sex. The more the therapist can empathize with her position and not blame or attack her, the greater the likelihood of keeping her cooperation and achieving a positive outcome. In sex therapy, even with effective use of vacuum devices and penile injections, the partner's goodwill and coopera-tion often spell the difference between success and failure. Unfortunately, I know of a number of cases in which the possibility of a successful outcome was lost because the woman felt blamed or not treated fairly.

SOME THINGS MEN (AND THEIR PARTNERS) NEED TO KNOW

If a clinician's sensitivity, understanding, and respect are perceived by the client, the clinician can convey several comforting and otherwise helpful ideas to the man with an erection problem. Since space limitations preclude a comprehensive discussion, and all of the points are treated at greater length elsewhere (Zilbergeld, 1992), I only briefly address them here. An interesting point about these ideas is that they often help despite the man's assertions to the contrary. I have been told numerous times by a man's partner that he was less depressed or upset by his situation after I discussed one or more of these ideas, despite the man's pronouncement during the session that my words didn't make any difference to him.

1. *Talking about sex and one's feelings about it can be helpful in itself.* By this I mean more than just assertiveness, saying what one does and does not want in sex; I also mean one's understandings and feelings. It is not easy for men to listen to and talk about feelings, of course, but they can learn. And they often find out surprising things right away. Many of the men I've worked with, for example, were surprised to learn that their partners were far less upset by the men's erection problems than by their reactions to them (distancing themselves from the partners, being unwilling to try sex that didn't require an erection, being unwilling to touch and kiss, etc.) or their reluctance to talk about the problem and seek help.

Men are also often surprised to find that talking about their own feelings—the burdens and obligations they feel in sex and perhaps elsewhere as well, and the anxiety these produce—often makes them feel better and makes for more closeness in the relationship. Occasionally, just talking about the problem in a real way actually resolves it.

2. *"Good sex" is a much broader category than "intercourse," and erections, though perhaps desirable, are not necessary.* For some men, the idea of sex without intercourse is alien, and it can help them to hear that good sex can consist of one partner's pleasuring the other. Although everyone has at least heard of oral sex or manual stimulation, many people do not understand that these can be the main course and not merely appetizers before intercourse. Since there is a huge concern about being "normal," it can be of great value to have a professional legitimize nonintercourse, nonreciprocal ("my turn, your turn") sexual acts. Some men and their partners also do not realize that stimulation of a soft penis can yield pleasure and even orgasm, provided that neither of them is so intent on producing an erection that they can't enjoy what is going on.

An objection that frequently comes up in discussion of nonintercourse sex is that while "getting off" or "being serviced" is acceptable sometimes, it's not really "making love." My response is that making love, expressing love, and feeling loved are not dependent upon specific acts. Virtually all clients can recall acts of intercourse that felt anything but loving, and virtually all of them can recall other activities, some not even sexual, that felt very loving. I then discuss how one can lovingly buy a gift, write a note, express feelings, give a back rub, and provide sexual stimulation in various ways. If loving feelings are present in the giver and the receiver is open to receiving them, the experience can be very loving. This discussion is usually an eye-opener. It also helps when I say that the more the clients can accept these ideas, the less pressure they will put on the man's penis, and the more likely it becomes that it will behave as they desire.

For clients or partners of clients who still resist the idea of enjoyable sex without erections, the following story often has an effect. Let us say that a man is fortunate enough to have a Mercedes, a car he gets a lot of pleasure from. Then his luck changes and he has to sell the car. What will we think if he rants and raves about not having the Mercedes and refuses to drive any other car or take public transportation—if he says, "If I can't go the right way, I won't go at all"? Aren't we likely to consider him silly or even crazy? Suppose he finally comes to terms with taking buses or driving another car, but his wife refuses to go with him because she considers a bus or Toyota "settling for second best." Doesn't that seem a bit peculiar?

Yet when it comes to sex, people behave in these peculiar ways all the time. Does this make any sense? Should we deprive ourselves of all sexual pleasure because we can't engage in sex in a particular way? There's nothing wrong with wanting a Mercedes and erections and intercourse. But there's also a lot to be said for flexibility. What is first felt to be "second best" often turns out to be not half bad at all.

3. *Sexual anxiety and sex problems are common.* Men are often comforted with the knowledge that they are not alone in their problems and anxieties. I usually begin this discussion by briefly covering the fantasy model of sex, mentioning some of the issues discussed earlier in this chapter. Specifically, men have been led to believe that they should be able to function more or less automatically; that there should be no concerns or difficulties; and that they and their partners should be quite content with their erotic activities, just as it is for people in movies and books. Supposedly this is normal or usual. But in fact it is not.

Many men, being sports fans, respond to my story about Jim Brown, perhaps the greatest running back in the history of American football. Most are aware that Brown's reputation as a lover rivaled his reputation as a ball carrier. And virtually all of them are surprised to hear that he had his own concerns about sexual performance. In his autobiography, Brown (1990, p. 205) complains that even his friends thought he was a superman in bed. But, says Brown, "I was never Superman. I had the same doubts about performing up to expectations that they did." If even Jim Brown, with all his experience, had anxiety about his sexual performances, maybe it's understandable that the rest of us would too. And there's evidence that we do.

After interviewing 125 men of all ages for their book *What Really Happens in Bed* (1989), Steven Carter and Julia Sokol concluded that "all men have sexual anxieties" (p. 310), mostly about the predictability, strength, and staying powers of their erections. In *The Hite Report on Male Sexuality* (1981), Shere Hite reports that a majority of her 7,000 respondents had concerns about getting and keeping erections and ejaculating too quickly. There is good reason to believe, therefore, that *there is nothing abnormal or unusual in men's being anxious about sex.*

Another area in which our ideas of normality are way off base concerns sexual problems. Such problems, most of us think, are rare and hardly the norm. But is that really the case? Seven percent of men—that's several million men—have chronic erection problems, and about 37% suffer from chronic rapid ejaculations (Spector & Carey, 1990). And a large majority of men have sporadic sexual problems. Carter and Sokol (1989) found that "most" of the men they interviewed "have experienced performance failure" (p. 311). In Shere Hite's large sample of men, 65% answered "yes" to the question of whether they had ever had difficulty having an erection when they wanted one, and 70% said that they had ejaculated more quickly than they had wanted to on at least one occasion. *Sex problems are not abnormal or untypical.* They are the norm and are common even among so-called "normal couples" (Frank, Anderson, & Rubinstein, 1978). Most men find this difficult to accept at first, believing that all their buddies are functioning perfectly and never have a problem, but the idea grows on them and is comforting.

I stress that sexual normality is very different from what we imagine it to be. In fact, given the evidence, it seems that our usual definition of "normal" (anxiety-free, problem-free functioning) is itself abnormal. This notion tends to lead many clients to be a bit more tolerant of and generous toward themselves than they have been.

4. *Meeting a man's particular sexual needs or conditions maximizes the probability that his penis will behave the way he wants.* The fantasy model of sex dictates that men be able to function and enjoy without any special requirements. Regardless of who a man is with, how he feels, and what's going on between him and his partner, he should be able to do his job. But the fact is that we all have requirements or conditions in all the important areas of life (Zilbergeld, 1978, 1992). Clients get the point when I ask whether there are any specific circumstances under which they can study or work better, enjoy and digest food better, and even sleep better. I suggest that the same is true in sex, despite the fact that men have been taught they shouldn't have any needs or conditions in that arena.

The point is simple: Certain frames of mind, attitudes toward partner and self, physical and mental stimulation, and a number of other things influence how much we want sex, how aroused we get, how much we enjoy it, and how well we function. Jim Brown put it in his usual blunt way: "Every dick, including mine, has a mind of its own. I never felt like I could fuck any woman, any time. My sexuality hinged on the woman and the situation" (1990, p. 205). This quote has had a significant impact on many clients. The understanding of conditions not only makes men feel better about having them, but also makes them more amenable to having sex only when those conditions are met—an important ingredient in the success of sex therapy.

5. *The less a man and a woman focus on erections and the more they focus on arousal and pleasure, the better things will go.* The man with an erection problem is of course narrowly focused on his penis, monitoring its progress or lack of it in a negative way almost every second during a sexual encounter. Such a focus is inimical to success (Cranston-Cuebas & Barlow, 1990; Masters & Johnson, 1970; Zilbergeld, 1992); however, given how men have been trained, it's understandable why they have become so fixated on their penises. It is also important that we as therapists not come across as if we are blaming them for being this way.

At the same time, however, any change in this situation can be helpful. But just telling men to relax, as so many health professionals do, tends not to work. Many men interpret relaxing as *not* doing; this actually isn't a bad way to look at relaxation, but it isn't enough to hold their attention. And, being men, they tend to want to *do* something. What has worked best for me is to get them to work on increasing arousal and focusing on it. I say that the most important thing in sex is arousal (passion, excitement, "turn-on"): Not only does it feel good, but it is also what mainly controls erections. If other conditions are met and arousal is as high as possible, the penis will be free to do its best. And even if it isn't up to it on occasion, a man and his partner will still have a good time.

I suggest to men that while working at having erections is counterproductive, working at increasing arousal is beneficial. Whatever is going on, I ask men to focus on pleasurable sensations or fantasies and to do whatever seems advisable to increase the arousal. This may mean making changes in the stimulation a man is getting or giving, focusing on a fantasy, or changing the fantasy. The idea of increasing arousal gives men something to work on and to put their nervous energy into; to some extent, it takes their attention off their penises; and it certainly does increase pleasure. All of this can be helpful not only in resolving the erection problem, but also in creating better sex.

6. *There is almost certainly a way of resolving the problem.* Many clients are discouraged about changing their situation and welcome the news that, one way or another, there is almost certainly a satisfactory solution. A number of options—sex therapy, vacuum devices, penile injections, and surgical implants—have proven to be quite effective. Sex therapy clients are often encouraged to hear about the alternatives, even if they don't feel they would go for one. It seems that knowing there is a backup approach if the therapy doesn't work is good news.

Yet another possible solution is to forget about erections and concentrate on putting together a good sex life that does not require them. This option is not attractive to most clients at the beginning, but it is acceptable to some, and I know of several older couples that have adopted it and been satisfied.

The more a man can understand that anxiety about sex is the rule; that erection and other sex problems are widespread and do not necessarily have any disastrous implications; that good sex can be had in many ways, with and without erections; that each man has a set of conditions under which he can function best and enjoy the most; and that there is almost certainly an acceptable solution to his problem, the better the man will feel and the better the clinical outcome. Less anxiety will be generated, clear thinking will be enhanced, and the man and his partner will be better able to work on and resolve their problems.

Given the widespread emphasis in our culture on good sex, it is fortunate that in the last quarter century significant advances have made in both the medical and psychological treatment of sex problems. We have a remarkable technology available, and the vast majority of men with erection problems can be assured of a successful outcome one way or another. But we helping professionals need to remind ourselves continually that the problems we deal with are human problems rather than penis problems, and that the men to whom we apply our methods are frightened and fragile, and very much prisoners of their gender and sexual socialization. To the extent that we keep people—with all their fears, feelings, idiosyncrasies, and limitations—paramount, and adjust our methods to them rather than forcing them to accommodate to the methods, we will be more effective.

We will also do our part to convey an essential lesson that our patients (and indeed our whole culture) need to learn. This message is that in sex people, not organs, relate; the only good sex is that which makes each partner feel good about himself or herself, good about the partner, and good about what they are doing and have done (Ellison, 1988). This is true regardless of how big or hard the penis is, how long the erection lasts, exactly what is done, or how many orgasms there are. All of us, but especially men, need to understand this message. To the extent that we learn it, we can expect men and women to feel better about themselves and each other; we can also expect better sex, perhaps fewer sexual dysfunctions, easier treatment of those that occur, and maybe even better relationships.

REFERENCES

Brown, J. (1990). *Out of bounds*. New York: Zebra.
Carter, S., & Sokol, J. (1989). *What really happens in bed: A demystification of sex*. New York: M. Evans.

Cranston-Cuebas, M. A., & Barlow, D. H. (1990). Cognitive and affective contributions to sexual functioning. *Annual Review of Sex Research, 1,* 119–162.

Ellison, C. R. (1988). Intimacy-based sex therapy. In W. Eicher & G. Kockott (Eds.), *Sexology* (pp. 234–238). Berlin: Springer-Verlag.

Frank, E., Anderson, C., & Rubinstein, D. (1978). Frequency of sexual dysfunction in "normal" couples. *New England Journal of Medicine, 299,* 111–115.

Gilmore, D. D. (1990). *Manhood in the making: Cultural concepts of masculinity.* New Haven, CT: Yale University Press.

Hite, S. (1981). *The Hite report on male sexuality.* New York: Ballantine.

Jong, E. (1985). *Parachutes and kisses.* New York: Signet.

Julty, S. (1975). *Male sexual performance.* New York: Grosset & Dunlap.

Kellerman, J. (1990). *Time bomb.* New York: Bantam.

Mailer, N. (1968). *Armies of the night.* New York: Signet.

Masters, W., & Johnson, V. (1970). *Human sexual inadequacy.* Boston: Little, Brown.

Person, E. S. (1980). Sexuality as the mainstay of identity: Psychoanalytic perspectives. *Signs, 5,* 605–630.

Robbins, H. (1971). *The Betsy.* New York: Pocket Books.

Spector, I. P., & Carey, M. P. (1990). Incidence and prevalence of the sexual dysfunctions: A critical review of the empirical literature. *Archives of Sexual Behavior, 19,* 389–408.

Wallace, I. (1989). *The guest of honor.* New York: Dell.

Zilbergeld, B. (1978). *Male sexuality.* New York: Bantam.

Zilbergeld, B. (1992). *The new male sexuality.* New York: Bantam.

Basic Mechanisms in Male Sexual Response

II

3

Neural and Vascular Control of Erection

ARNOLD MELMAN

In the past decade, major advances have taken place in our understanding of the role of neural and vascular mechanisms in erection. Whereas penile erection was previously believed to be the direct result of parasympathetically mediated vasodilatation effects, recent research has brought to light the role of multiple neurotransmitter substances and complex hemodynamic processes. With the aid of highly sophisticated laboratory techniques, it is now possible to study the microneuroanatomy of the penile bodies, as well as the neuropharamcology of penile innervation. Along with increased understanding of the underlying mechanisms of erection, new medical and surgical treatments have been developed. Among the most prominent investigators in this important area of research is Arnold Melman, author of the present chapter.

The chapter begins with a review of autonomic nervous system mechanisms, and Melman particularly emphasizes the interactive role of sympathetic and parasympathetic control of erection. At the level of the brain, the medial parieto-occipital portion of the limbic system may function as a coordinating center for external sexual stimuli. Spinal mechanisms are also involved, as demonstrated by a series of classic studies in animals and in human patients with spinal cord injury. The neural innervation of the penis itself has recently come under investigation by Melman and others, with several studies confirming the importance of adrenergic innervation of the smooth muscle of the corpora. Additional neurotransmitters, such as vasoactive intestinal polypeptide (VIP) and prostaglandins, are also involved in the mediation of erection, although the identity of the final neurotransmitter has not been confirmed as yet.

The role of arterial and venous mechanisms is considered next. Much controversy existed in the past concerning the role of venous constriction factors in the achievement or maintenance of erection. In reviewing this issue, Melman concludes that the major driving force is decreased vascular resistance in the penile corpora. Venous return is diminished only by means of a passive occlusion of the penile veins *against the tunica albuginea. According to Melman, relaxation of the smooth muscle of the penile corpora is the primary physiological event underlying erection, although increased arterial flow and passive venous occlusion may contribute to erection in a synergistic fashion.*

Given the importance of smooth muscle effects in erection, the final section of this chapter reviews recent studies of the cellular composition of the penile corpora and the effects of various neurotransmitter substances. Clearly, this is an essential area for further research.

Arnold Melman, M.D., is Professor and Chairman of the Department of Urology and Director of the Center for Male Sexuality, Montefiore Medical Center and Albert Einstein College of Medicine, Bronx, New York. He has conducted extensive research on the physiology and pharmacology of male erection, and has published widely in the field.

The advent of successful surgical and medical therapies for treatment of erectile dysfunction has caused an explosion in studies related to an understanding of the physiological mechanisms of human erection. Most recently, researchers in the field have focused their attention on the importance of the interaction of neurotransmitter substances upon the smooth muscle of the penile corpora as the pivotal element in human erection. This chapter integrates past knowledge of male genital anatomy with current basic studies of human erectile mechanisms.

NEURAL MECHANISMS

Neuroanatomic Pathways of the Brain, Spinal Cord, and Peripheral Neurons

The Stimulatory and Inhibitory Centers

Penile erection is initiated by means of a neural stimulus, either at the level of the brain or as a spinal reflex. The event is under the regulation of the autonomic nervous system, and as such is an involuntary response. Since the experiments of Eckhard (1863), the control of erection was thought to be a parasympathetic event, although recent studies have suggested that erection is controlled by both the sympathetic and parasympathetic nerves. Under most conditions, tonic control by the brain results in a flaccid penis. In the awake state, a wide range of visual, auditory, psychic, tactile, and olfactory sexual cues can generate a stimulus that travels down the spinal cord via efferent pathways to the sympathetic and parasympathetic nervous system.

The neural signal causes the penile arteries to dilate, with concomitant relaxation of the corpora, and erection occurs. Inhibitory stimulation reverses the process and penile flaccidity returns. Events that limit inhibitory control by the brain, such as spinal cord transection or anoxia, result in erection. Men who die by hanging are found to have erections.

In an extensive review of the neurological disturbances of sexual functioning, Bors and Comarr (1960) have emphasized the importance of the reticular activating system as the central triage system of the brain. This region facilitates centrifugal and centripetal connections between the spinal cord, cerebellum, hypothalamus, rhinencephalon, and cerebral cortex in the integration of physiological sexual function.

The aforementioned external stimuli (visual, auditory, olfactory) are mediated by the frontal, temporal, parietal, and occipital regions of the cerebral cortex. The medial parieto-occipital portion of the limbic system is a more primitive region of the brain that "coordinates sensory events with visceral needs that regulate automatic functions concerned with feeding, sex, fight, flight, and the emotion provoking situations in the body and its environment" (Papez, 1958). The interaction of neural events in these regions cannot be overemphasized. Thus, in the human sexual response, the centers from which reflex stimuli initiate the autonomic responses necessary for a sexual act, are mediated by more primitive centers that are essentially inhibitory in nature. The man with severe performance anxiety is in a "flight mode," and the resultant penile flaccidity is a consequence of the level of control of excitatory stimulation.

Experiments employing electrical stimulation of the brain in primates have demonstrated that erections can be elicited with stimulation of the lateral, dorsolateral, hypothalamic, medial preoptic, and anterior hypothalamic regions. Lesions placed experimentally in those areas (or observed in patients with Parkinson's disease or stroke) have been associated with erectile failure (Steers, 1990).

The Spinal Cord

The spinal tracts through which the nerve fibers that are concerned with erection pass can best be divided into afferent and efferent pathways. The peripheral stimuli that enhance erection (e.g., light touch and friction of the penile skin), as well as the inhibitory stimuli of pain, cold, and heat, travel up through the dorsal columns. The somatic efferents, on the other hand, travel in the decussating cortico-regulating tracts from the cortex to the anterior horn cells of the cord. The visceral efferents descend through the region of the pyramidal tracts of the lateral columns. There are two primary terminations, in the thoracolumbar cord and in the sacrum where the preganglionic neurons originate. Bors and Comarr (1960) identify an additional efferent pathway, the fasciculus parependymalis, which travels from the hypothalamus, midbrain, and medulla on either side of the central canal. The neurons may connect the sexual centers of the brain directly with the lumbosacral cord.

The extraspinal peripheral pathways travel to the penis from regions classically considered as sympathetic and parasympathetic. The sympathetic nerves arise from the thoracolumbar outflow, and travel in the inferior mesenteric and superior hypogastric plexus through the hypogastric nerve to the pelvic plexus and through the cavernous nerve to the penis (see Figure 3.1).

Eckhard (1863) produced erection in the dog by stimulation of the pelvic parasympathetic nerves, which he termed the "nervi erigentes." For years following this finding, it was assumed that erection was under parasympathetic control only. In 1902, however, Muller demonstrated that there were two different ways to stimulate erection in the dog. He transected the spinal cord of dogs at the lower thoracic level, and then demonstrated that

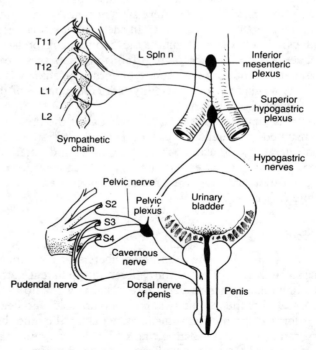

FIGURE 3.1.   Schematic representation of the efferent nerve supply to the penis and bladder. The upper portion of the figure shows sympathetic innervation of the pudendal artery. The lower portion of the figure shows parasympathetic nerve supply to the corpora.

the animals did not achieve normal erections when in the presence of an estrous female. But these same dogs did have full erections in response to direct penile stimulation. When the entire sacral cord and most of the lumbar cord was resected, the dogs no longer produced erections secondary to penile stimulation, but could still have an erection when placed with an estrous female.

This experiment was taken one step further by Root and Bard (1947), who performed surgical studies in cats. They also showed that erections were maintained after ablation of the lower thoracic and sacral spinal cord, but that when the sympathetic supply was also destroyed, erection could not be achieved. In a series of surgical procedures in humans, Whitelaw and Smithwick (1951) performed sympathectomies in patients with severe hypertension. In patients undergoing T_2 through T_{12} sympathectomies, 57% had a disturbance of sexual function, and if the surgery was performed between L_1 and L_3, 63% had erectile dysfunction.

Bors and Comarr (1960) interviewed a large number of patients with spinal cord injuries. None of the patients with an absence of sacral reflex activity had erections secondary to genital stimulation, whereas 24% of these patients experienced erections after psychological stimulation. These authors found that only a small percentage of patients with injuries of the cervical and thoracic spinal cord had erections secondary to psychological stimulation, but more than 80% of these patients had erections after direct genital stimulation. In contrast, the majority of patients with injuries of the lumbar cord had erections after psychological stimulation, and 100% had erections after direct physical stimulation. Taken together, these studies strongly suggest that the motor control of erection is exerted via both sympathetic and parasympathetic fibers.

Autonomic and Peripheral Nerves of the Penis

The gross anatomy of the relationship of the nerves to the corpora of the pelvic organ has been recently described (Lue, Zeineh, Schmidt, & Tanagho, 1984). As a result of those new studies, the risk of impotence as a complication of radical pelvic surgery is reduced if strict anatomic principles are applied during surgery. The lessened risk of erectile dysfunction as a complication of surgery has increased patient acceptance and has fostered the extensive use of radical prostatectomy as a definitive treatment for prostate cancer.

The parasympathetic fibers to the penis emerge from the anterior foramina of S_2 to S_4 and join the fibers from the hypogastric nerve to form the pelvic plexus. The most inferior fibers of the pelvic plexus travel along the posterolateral aspect of the prostate; these are the cavernous nerves, the nerves responsible for efferent control of erection. At the proximal prostatic urethra, the nerves are distant from the prostatic capsule; however, at the apex of the prostate, they lie in close approximation to the prostatic capsule at the 5 o'clock and 7 o'clock positions. In the area of the membranous urethra, the nerves form several bundles at the 3 o'clock and 9 o'clock positions, external to the striated muscles. Distal to the membranous urethra, some fibers of the cavernous nerve penetrate the tunica albuginea of the corpus spongiosum to innervate the corpus cavernosum and glans. The remainder of these nerves ascend gradually at the 1 o'clock and 11 o'clock positions to the area in which the corpora cavernosa join, after which they travel with the corporal vessels.

The microneuroanatomy of the penis has been well outlined by Benson, McConnell, Lipshultz, Corriere, and Wood (1981). Acetylcholinesterase fibers appear in only limited numbers in the human corpora cavernosa and corpus spongiosum. These fibers are often organized in small bundles that sometimes course near arterioles. In fact, most arterioles are approached by acetylcholin- esterase-positive fibers and frequently demonstrate acetylcholinesterase- positive structures thought to be cholinergic terminals in their outer tunic. Histofluorescence for glyoxylic acid fibers indicates the presence of adrenergic nerves. These fibers have been found to be numerous in the corpora caver- nosum. They take a circuitous course through the trabeculae and often appear to approach the walls of the cavernous spaces. Many blood vessels demon- strate adrenergic varicosities in their outer tunic (Benson et al., 1981).

Wagner, Gerstenberg, and Levin (1989) and Stief et al (1990) have re- corded electrical activity from the smooth muscle of the corpora. Electrical spike potentials were observed during penile flaccidity, but these disappeared during erection provoked by visual sexual stimulation. The authors theorized that there is either an inhibition of adrenergic tone or release of a smooth muscle relaxant that inhibits spontaneous electrical responses during erection.

The recent recrudescence of interest in the composition and anatomic pathways of the nerves that control erection has had a major impact in modern vascular and genitourinary surgery. Our increased understanding of these nerves has resulted in the modification of diagnostic procedures and of the surgical approach to pelvic organs. Moreover, the investigation of those nerves and pathways has, in the past decade, been extended to the interac- tion with the effector organ of the penis, the trabecular smooth muscle.

Neuropharmacology

After Eckhard's (1863) early study, it was presumed that the cholinergic parasympathetic system had total control over the physiology of penile erection. However, this has been disproved through the surgical studies outlined above. In addition, it has been shown in both animals and humans that atropine administration does not prevent erections (Dorr & Brody, 1967; Wagner & Brindley, 1980), nor does the infusion of acetylcholine result in erection.

Several studies have further suggested a role for adrenergic neurotransmitters in erectile physiology. For example, a colleague and I (Melman & Henry, 1979) demonstrated a high concentration of norepinephrine in the blood vessels and smooth muscle of corporal tissue, as well as a significant diminution of norepinephrine concentration, in patients with insulin-dependent diabetes who had erectile dysfunction. Benson et al. (1981) treated muscle strips of cavernosal tissue with norepinephrine and acetylcholine. Norepinephrine induced contractions in all the strips tested, which were blocked by phentolamine but unaffected by propranalol. Acetylcholine, on the other hand, produced minimal contractions in 2 of the 24 strips tested, and this effect was blocked by atropine.

One of the peptides currently being considered as possible neurotransmitter is vasoactive intestinal polypeptide (VIP). this compound, a potent vasodilator, has been localized in cavernosal tissue (Polak, Mina, Gu, & Bloom, 1981), and "VIP-ergic" nerves have been found to be depleted in the corpora of impotent men with diabetes (Gu et al., 1984). My colleagues and I (Haberman, Valcic, Christ, & Melman, 1991) also found a significant decrease in corporal VIP content of insulin-dependent diabetic men with impotence. Nevertheless, we did not observe any correlation of VIP content with degree of erectile capacity.

Endothelium-derived relaxing factor is a substance that is released by the endothelium of blood vessels and that relaxes vascular smooth muscle (Furchgott & Zawadski, 1980). This substance may be released by the endothelium in response to stimulation by a neutotransmitter, such as acetylcholine, causing relaxation of the trabeculae. Saenz de Tejada, Goldstein, Azadozi, Krane, and Cohen (1989) have shown a reduction in the release of endothelium-derived relaxing factor in the erectile tissue of impotent men with diabetes.

Prostaglandins have also been shown to be produced by human corporal tissue (Roy, Tan, Kottegoda, & Ratnam, 1984). Prostaglandins are known to modulate autonomic nerve function and the effect of vasoactive hormones that contribute to the myogenic tone of vascular smooth muscle. The release of prostaglandins in the corpora has been shown to be under muscarinic control (Jeremy, Morgan, Mikhailidis, & Dandona, 1986). It is possible that release of prostaglandins is the final step in relaxation of the corporal smooth muscle, which in turn causes erection.

It is evident that neither a cholinergic nor an adrenergic neurotransmitter system is wholly in control of the physiology of erection. At the present time, the identity of the final transmitter is not entirely clear. Taken together, the studies to date strongly suggest that during penile detumescence the smooth muscles of the corpora are under the control of vasoconstrictor transmitters. The passage to the erect state is a result of diminished vasoconstrictor output and active smooth muscle relaxation caused by one or more neurotransmitters.

THE VASCULAR ANATOMY

Gross Anatomy of the Penis

Arterial Tree

Blood flow to the penis is derived from the aorta to the common, and then to the internal iliac arteries with direct continuation as the pudendal arteries. The pudendal arteries exit the bony pelvis through Alcock's canal and enter the perineum medial to the crura of the penis (see Figure 3.2). At that point, the arteries trifurcate and form the arteries to the bulbous urethra, the cavernous arteries, and the dorsal arteries of the penis. The deep artery enters the medial crus and runs through the entire length of the penis. Similarly, the dorsal artery passes over the medial aspect of the crus beneath Buck's fascia and travels along the entire length of the corpora. The blood supply to the glans is supplied by the urethral artieris traveling within the corpora spongiosum and is separate from the cavernosal blood supply. In fact, the glans can be completely separated surgically from the cavernous bodies without affecting its viability.

These small arteries (less than 1 mm in diameter during penile flaccidity) are extremely vulnerable to obstruction as a result of either atherosclerosis or injury. The region most vulnerable to external trauma is the point of exit of the pudendal artery from Alcock's canal, where a pelvic fracture or blunt compression (such as a straddle injury) to the perineum can cause total arterial obstruction.

Intracorporal Penile Circulation

After the deep arteries pass through the tunica albuginea, they are centrally located in the cavernous bodies and travel down the entire pendulous portion of the penis. Two types of arterial branches are given off along the course of their distribution. One branch traverses the framework of the corpora, giving nourishment to the smooth muscle and nerve bundles of the spongy trabecular tissue. The other branch is a series of helicine arteries. These are the serpentine vessels that end directly in the corporal sinusoids— the structures that fill with blood during tumescence. The shape and extra length of the helicine arteries allow the penis both to elongate and to increase

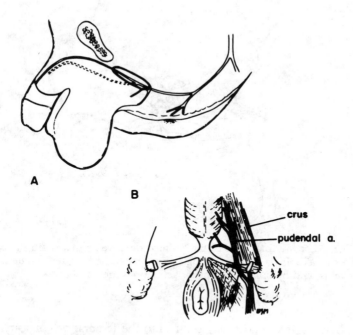

FIGURE 3.2. Schematic representation of the location of the penile arteries. The upper portion of the figure (A) shows the longitudinal relationship of the pudendal artery as it exits the bony pelvis and trifurcates prior to entry into the penis. The lower portion of the figure (B) presents a perineal view of the penile arterial system, showing the relationship of the penile artery to the anus, penile crus, and bulbous urethra.

in diameter without compromising the blood supply to the corpora during erection.

Venous Anatomy

The venous anatomy of the penis plays an important role in the production of an erection. There are three major sets of veins in the human penis: the superficial, the intermediate, and the deep veins (see Figure 3.3).

The subcutaneous veins of the penis drain the skin and the subcutaneous tissues superficial to Buck's fascia, and then coalesce to form the superficial dorsal vein. This is usually a single vessel, but it may be multiple or forked. The superficial dorsal vein usually empties into either the left or the

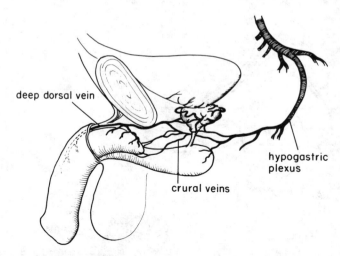

deep dorsal vein

hypogastric
plexus

crural veins

FIGURE 3.3.   Longitudinal view of the primary deep veins that drain the corpora.
The deep dorsal vein is usually a single vein that is fed by the circumflex and
emissary veins, and by numerous smaller veins from the corpora.

right saphenous vein, but it may drain into the femoral or epigastric veins
instead.

The intermediate veins are between Buck's fascia and the tunica albuginea. The main vessel in this group is the deep dorsal vein. This vein is
formed by the convergence of 6 to 15 short, straight vessels in the glans.
These vessels form a retrocoronal plexus, and it is from this plexus that the
deep dorsal vein is formed. The deep dorsal vein runs toward the pubis in
the sulcus between the corpora cavernosa, being fed along its length by the
circumflex and the emissary veins, and by numerous small perforating veins
from the corpora. The deep dorsal vein is usually single, and it empties into
the pudendal plexus in the pelvis. The intermediate system, then, drains the
glans and the corpora cavernosa, and contributes to the drainage of the
corpus spongiosum.

The deep veins of the penis drain the major portion of the corpus
spongiosum. The veins in this set are the bulbar and urethral vessels. In the
proximal part of the penis, numerous veins leave the corpus spongiosum
and merge into several trunks, which enter either the pudendal vein or the
pudendal plexus. Distally, the urethral veins are divided into anterior and
posterior groups. The anterior veins perforate the tunica with four or five
branches joining to form trunks, which in turn join with the posterior emissary
veins to form the circumflex veins. The posterior urethral veins form a plexus
that either joins the bulbar veins or drains directly into the pudendal plexus.

The emissary veins are short veins that pierce the tunica. The anterior emissary veins empty directly into the deep dorsal vein. A similar number of posterior emissary veins open into the sulcus between the corpus spongiosum and corpus cavernosum, where six to eight vessels form a single trunk that joins the anterior urethral veins to form the circumflex veins. The circumflex veins run between the tunica and Buck's fascia, and empty into the deep dorsal vein. Finally, there are anastomotic channels between the superficial dorsal veins and the deep dorsal vein, located proximally to the coronal sulcus and just distal to the pubic bone.

Using scanning electron microscopy, Fournier, Jueneman, Lue, and Tanagho (1987) demonstrated that there is an extensive subalbugineal venular plexus that drains the corpora cavernosa of the dog. These venula run an oblique course between the tunica and the cavernosal tissue, and then coalesce to form several emissary veins, which then pierce the tunica albuginea in the area surrounding the entrance of the cavernosal artery. No muscular deep veins have been identified to date within the corpora cavernosa.

The Hemodynamics of Erection

The penile anatomy outlined above has multiple functions, all of which must occur for the successful production of a rigid erection. These are as follows: (1) increased arterial inflow, (2) decreased corporal resistance, and (3) decreased venous return. Again, none of these reactions alone is responsible for erection; they are components of a complex integrated system of physiological responses that results ultimately in penile erection (see Figures 3.4 and 3.5).

Goldstein and Krane (1983) showed that a reduction in arterial inflow during nerve stimulation prevented erection from occurring in dogs. Newman and Northup (1981) cannulated the dorsal penile artery in a cadaver, and produced an erection in the cadaver with a flow rate of 25 ml/min. Furthermore, they were able to cause erections in other cadavers by directly perfusing the corpora. These studies show that an increased arterial inflow can cause an erection, and that decreased venous return alone is not sufficient to produce an erection.

Many investigators now believe that the driving force for the increase in arterial flow to the penis is the decrease of resistance to flow in the corpora themselves. Dorr and Brody (1967) showed that during an erection created by pelvic nerve stimulation, arterial pressure in the major arteries was unchanged. From this they concluded that the increased flow to the penis must thus be due to decreased vascular resistance. Lue, Zeineh, Schmidt, and Tanagho (1983) have also shown that there is minimal increase in the intra-

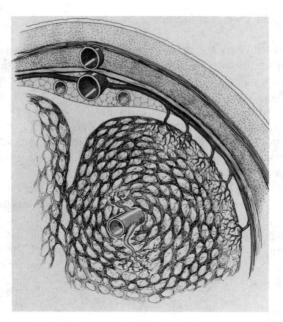

FIGURE 3.4. Cross-sectional schema of the flaccid penis. The smooth muscles of the trabeculae are contracted and the sinusoids empty of blood. The subtunical venous plexus is open and draining into the deep dorsal vein.

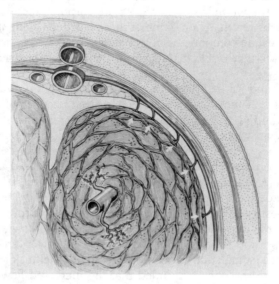

FIGURE 3.5. Cross-sectional schema of the erect penis. The sinusoidal spaces are compressed (arrowheads), with minimal drainage from the corpora.

aorta pressure during erection in the primate, despite increase in blood flow to the penis. The increased flow, then, can only be explained by decreased distal resistance in the corpora cavernosa.

Restriction of venous outflow is necessary for the attainment and maintenance of an erection. The pelvic musculature was thought to play a major part in the obstruction of the venous outflow of the penis, but this theory has long since been disproved. Semans and Langworthy (1939), for example, resected the ischiocavernosus and bulbocavernosus muscles in the cat, and were still able to produce nerve-stimulated erections. In humans, erections often occur in patients with spinal cord injuries, who have paralyzed pelvic floors. Kollberg, Peterson, and Stener (1962) have shown, using electromyography, that erection can occur in the human without the active participation of these muscles.

Other studies have demonstrated the importance of decreased venous return in causing erection. Newman and Northup (1981) found that application of a penile cuff to the base of the penis for as long as 10 minutes, at a pressure greater than diastolic but less than systolic blood pressure, produced cyanosis and edema but no erection. And it is important to remember (as noted above) that no muscular veins have been identified to date in the human corpora. Thus, it can safely be concluded that the penile veins themselves do not actively constrict to prevent blood flow to the corpora.

Passive venous occlusion, though, should not be excluded. Wagner (1981) used xenon washout before and during visual sexual stimulation to prove that there is a marked decline in venous outflow during tumescence. Cavernosography performed after intrapenile injection of papaverine also shows decreased venous outflow with the pharmacologically induced erection. Furthermore, in the dog model, Fournier et al. (1987) have demonstrated that the subalbugineal venous plexus is compressed between the tunica albuginea and the sinusoidal tissue after an intracavernosal injection of papaverine.

Most investigators now agree that erectile hemodynamics rely heavily on the proper interaction of the three systems just described. The most plausible theory at this time is that the cavernous smooth muscles of the corpora, under neurological control in a constant state of contraction, relax. This lowers the vascular resistance of the corpora and results in a significant increase in blood flow to the penis. The dilated corporal spaces then cause passive occlusion of their venous drainage, allowing blood to pool in the corpora at systemic pressures, and thereby producing erection.

The theory that corporal relaxation is the mechanism of erection has prompted the specific investigation of the cellular composition of the corporal smooth muscle and its surrounding supportive structures. We (Luangkhot, Rutchik, Agarwal, Bhargava, & Melman, 1991), for example, have shown that the cavernous bodies contain approximately 50% collagen. Of particular interest is that there is an abundance of type IV collagen in the corpora. Type IV collagen is normally secreted by the vascular endothelium and lines the basement membrane of most blood vessels. The presence of type IV collagen, as well as the presence of an endothelium lining the sinusoids of the cavernous spaces, lends credence to the theory that the penis is a specialized vascular organ. In that same study, we found no significant differences in collagen content with aging, diabetes, or venous corporal incompetence. Patients with Peyronie's disease did show an increased content of collagen (as high as 80%).

In a study of the pharmacology of human erectile tissue (Christ, Maayani, Valcic, & Melman, 1990), we characterized the erectile tissue as having primarily alpha-1 adrenoceptors. Levin and Wein (1980) had previously reported that alpha receptors (contractile) outnumbered beta receptors by a 10:1 ratio. We reported further that erectile smooth muscle demonstrated significant changes with age and disease. Age changes included an increased EC_{50} (the concentration of drug necessary for one-half of the maximal tissue response), an increased maximal contraction for diabetic tissue obtained from older patients, and a decreased rate of contraction for tissue obtained from nondiabetic patients. Furthermore, the erectile tissue was shown to be exquisitely sensitive to concentration of calcium *in vitro*. The removal of calcium from the organ bath caused total tissue relaxation.

The subject of calcium transport effects on smooth muscle is relevant to our understanding of intracorporal pharmacotherapy for the treatment of erectile dysfunction. Calcium is the specific ion that triggers contractile responses in smooth muscle cells. Drugs that stimulate calcium influx will cause the smooth muscle of the penis to contract (the physiological result is detumescence). Certain agonists (e.g., norepinephrine, prostaglandin F_2 alpha) stimulate cell surface membrane receptors to open calcium channels, with resultant increased contraction. *In vitro*, calcium channel blockers (e.g., nifedipine) reduce maximal smooth muscle contraction, as well as the rate of contraction. In contrast, drugs that antagonize the effect of alpha contractile agents (e.g., phentolamine, dibenzyline) cause relaxation of the smooth muscle. In this situation, the cells relax because there is a continuous basal production of cyclic adenosine monophosphate (cAMP). Smooth muscle relaxation is induced by increased levels of intracellular cAMP or cyclic guanosine monophosphate (cGMP). Drugs that enhance the concentration of cAMP (prostaglandin E, VIP) or cGMP (endothelium-derived relaxing factor) cause the smooth muscle of the penis to relax, and the physiological result is tumescence or erection.

My colleagues and I (Moreno et al., 1991) have provided a further elucidation of the potential cellular mechanism of penile detumescence and rigidity. We described the presence of cell gap junctions in the membranes of the smooth muscle of the penile corpora. This was the first demonstration of gap junctions in vascular smooth muscle. Gap junctions are specialized structures composed of protein molecules that lie in apposition on cell surface membranes; they allow transfer of intracellular molecules and electrical currents from one cell into the adjacent cell. Thus, the presence of the gap junctions in the corporal tissue suggests that the tissue may be functioning as a syncytial (i.e., coordinated) network responsive to neurotransmitter stimulation within each corpus.

SUMMARY AND CONCLUSIONS

Over the past several years, research and clinical efforts to influence erectile mechanisms have been directed at increasing our understanding of the relationship of the penile nerves to the erectile structures of the corporal. The recognition of the importance of the penile smooth muscle and its supporting structures to the erectile mechanism has revolutionized medical therapy. Future efforts will be directed to the interaction of neurotransmitters on the smooth muscle of the penis. The virtual explosion of the use of intracavernous pharmacotherapy to treat both organic and psychogenic erectile failure has promoted the search for more efficient agents and methods of delivery of agents, which will readily result in controlled penile erection with a minimum of risk.

REFERENCES

Benson, G. S., McConnell, J. A., Lipshultz, L. I., Corriere, J. N., Jr., & Wood, J. (1981). Neuromorphology and neuropharmacology of the human penis. *Journal of Clinical Investigation, 65*, 506–513.

Bors, E., & Comarr, A. E. (1960). Neurologic disturbances of sexual function with special reference to 529 patients with spinal cord injury. *Urologic Survey, 10*, 191–222.

Christ, G. J., Maayani, S., Valcic, M., & Melman, A. (1990). Pharmacological studies of human erectile tissues: Characteristics of spontaneous contractions and alterations in alpha-adrenoceptor responsiveness with age and disease in isolated tissues. *British Journal of Pharmacology, 101*, 375–381.

Dorr, L. D., & Brody, M. J. (1967). Hemodynamic mechanism of erection in the canine penis. *American Journal of Physiology, 213*, 1526–1531.

Eckhard, C. (1863). Untersuchungen über die erection des penis beim hunde. *Beitrage zur Anatomie und Physiologie, 3*, 123–150.

Fournier, G. R., Jr., Jueneman, K.-P., Lue, T. F., & Tanagho, E. A. (1987). Mechanisms of venous occlusion during canine penile erection: An anatomic demonstration. *Journal of Urology, 137*, 163–167.

Furchgott, R. F., & Zawadski, J. V. (1980). The obligatory role of endothelial cells in the relaxation of arterial smooth muscle cells by acetylcholine. *Nature, 288*, 373–376.

Goldstein, I., & Krane, R. J. (1983). Effects of hypotension on the hemodynamics of erection. *Surgical Forum, 34*, 662–664.

Gu, J., Lazarides, M., Pryor, J. P., Blank, M. A., Polak, J. M., Morgan, R., Marangos, P. J., & Bloom, S. R. (1984). Decrease of vasoactive intestinal polypeptide (VIP) in the penises from impotent men. *Lancet, ii*, 315–317.

Haberman, J., Valcic, M., Christ, G., & Melman, A. (1991). Vasoactive intestinal polypeptide and norepinephrine concentration in the corpora cavernosa of impotent men. *Journal of Impotence Research, 3*, 21–28.

Jeremy, J. Y., Morgan, R. J., Mikhailidis, D. P., & Dandona, P. (1986). Prostacycline synthesis by the corpora cavernosa of the human penis: Evidence for muscarinic control and pathological implications. *Prostaglandins, Leukotrienes and Medicine, 23*, 211–216.

Kollberg, S., Peterson, I., & Stener, I. (1962). Preliminary results of an electromyographic study of ejaculation. *Acta Chirugica Scandinavica, 123*, 478–483.

Levin, R. M., & Wein, A. J. (1980). Adrenergic alpha-receptors outnumber beta-receptors in human penile corpus cavernosum. *Investigative Urology, 18*, 225–226.

Luangkhot, R., Rutchik, S., Agarwal, V., Bhargava, G., & Melman, A. (1991). *Collagen alterations in the corpus cavernosum of impotent men.* Manuscript in preparation.

Lue, T. F., Zeineh, S. J., Schmidt, R. A., & Tanagho, E. A. (1983). Physiology of penile erection. *World Journal of Urology, 1*, 194–196.

Lue, T. F., Zeineh, S. J., Schmidt, R. A., & Tanagho, E. A. (1984). Neuroanatomy of penile erection: Its relevance to iatrogenic impotence. *Journal of Urology, 131*, 273–280.

Melman, A., & Henry, D. (1979). The possible role of catecholamines of the corpora in penile erection. *Journal of Urology, 121*, 419–421.

Moreno, A. P., Christ, G. J., Campos deCarvalho, A. C., Melman, A., Roy, C., Hertzberg, E. L., & Spray, D. C. (1991). *Gap junctions between human corpus cavernosal smooth muscle cells: Identity of the connexin type and unitary conductance events.* Manuscript in preparation.

Muller, L. R. (1902). Klinische und experimentelle studien uber die innervation der blase, des mastdarms, und des genitalapparates. *Deutsche Zeitschrift für Nervenheilkunde, 21*, 86–154.

Newman, H. F., & Northup, J. D. (1981). Mechanism of human penile erection: An overview. *Urology, 17*, 399–407.

Papez, J. W. (1958). Visceral brain, its component parts and their connections. *Journal of Nervous and Mental Disease, 120*, 40–56.

Polak, J. M., Mina, S., Gu, J., & Bloom, S. R. (1981). VIPergic nerves in the penis. *Lancet, ii*, 217–219.

Root, W. S., & Bard, D. (1947). The mediation of feline erection through sympathetic pathways with some remarks on sexual behavior after deafferentation of the genitalia. *American Journal of Physiology, 151*, 80–90.

Roy, A. C., Tan, S. M., Kottegoda, S. R., & Ratnam, S. S. (1984). Ability of the human corpora cavernosa muscle to generate prostaglandin and thromboxanes *in vitro*. *International Research Communications System Medical Science, 12*, 608–609.

Saenz de Tejada, I., Goldstein, I., Azadzoi, K., Krane, R. J., & Cohen, R. A. (1989). Impaired neurogenic and endothelium-mediated relaxation of penile smooth muscle from diabetic men with impotence. *New England Journal of Medicine, 320,* 1025-1030.

Semans, J. H., & Langworthy, O. R. (1939). Observations on the neurophysiology of sexual function in the male cat. *Journal of Urology, 40,* 836-846.

Steers, W. D. (1990). Neural control of penile erection. *Seminars in Urology, 8,* 66-79.

Stief, C. G., Djamilian, M., Schaebsdau, F., Truss, M. C., Schlick, R. W., Abicht, J. H., Allhof, E. P., & Jonas, U. (1990). Single potential analysis of cavernous electric activity: A possible diagnosis of autonomic impotence. *World Journal of Urology, 8,* 75-79.

Wagner, G. (1981). Erection: Physiology, and endocrinology. In G. Wagner & R. Green (Eds.), *Impotence: Physiological, psychological, surgical diagnosis and treatment* (pp. 21-36). New York: Plenum Press.

Wagner, G., & Brindley, G. S. (1980). The effect of atropine, a and b blockers on human penile erection: A controlled pilot study. In A. Zorgniotti & J. Rossi (Eds.), *Vasculogenic impotence: International symposium on corporal revascularization.* Springfield, IL: Charles C Thomas.

Wagner, G., Gerstenberg, T., & Levin, R. J. (1989). Electrical activity of corpus cavernosum during flaccidity and erection of the human penis: A new diagnostic method. *Journal of Urology, 142,* 723-725.

Whitelaw, G. P., & Smithwick, R. H. (1951). Some secondary effects of sympathectomy with particular reference to disturbance of sexual function. *New England Journal of Medicine, 245,* 121-130.

4

Hormonal Determinants
of Erectile Function

JULIAN M. DAVIDSON AND RAYMOND C. ROSEN

Hormonal influences on male sexual behavior are complex and pervasive. The word "hormone" comes from the Greek hormon, which means "to arouse or set in motion." Hormones are involved in multiple ways in the initiation and maintenance of sexual behavior. In recent years, clinical research has focused increasingly on hormonal correlates of desire disorders, as well as on antiandrogenic treatments for individuals with hyperactive sexual desire. In contrast, research on the hormonal correlates of erectile disorders has yielded a complex and largely inconclusive pattern of results.

Our understanding of hormone physiology has evolved greatly in recent years. Steroid receptor mechanisms, in particular, have come under intense investigation, as have the roles of various neurotransmitter mechanisms. The relevance of these advances to our understanding of hormonal aspects of sexual behavior, however, remains uncertain.

Research with hypogonadal men has highlighted the effects of subnormal levels of testosterone on male arousal and libido. Interestingly, these men may be capable of having erections with visual erotic stimulation, but not during spontaneous fantasy or rapid eye movement (REM) sleep. This has led Bancroft (1989) and others to speculate about the existence of a two-pathway mechanism for control of erectile function. These key issues are addressed in some detail in the introductory sections of this chapter.

Another area in which hormonal effects have been studied is the treatment of sex offenders with antiandrogenic therapy. Again, a suppression of circulating testosterone levels is associated with a loss of nocturnal penile tumescence and fantasy-induced erections. Some of these men, however, report satisfactory erections with partner stimulation.

Effects of hormone levels in aging men are discussed primarily by Segraves and Segraves in Chapter 5 of this volume.

In contrast to the research on hypogonadal men, laboratory studies with eugonadal males have produced largely unreliable and inconsistent findings. Earlier studies on testosterone levels in normal male volunteers failed to show a predictable association between hormone levels and various measures of sexual arousal and orgasm. More recently, plasma oxytocin levels have been found to correlate with levels of sexual arousal in the laboratory. Again, the clinical significance of these findings is yet to be demonstrated.

Turning to clinical issues, this chapter presents a detailed discussion of hormonal assessment in the evaluation of erectile disorders. Although there is ongoing controversy concerning the specific tests to be employed, current standards necessitate attention to endocrine evaluation in most, if not all, cases of erectile dysfunction.

Hormone replacement therapy is highly effective in the treatment of men with clear-cut hypogonadal syndrome (Davidson & Meyers, 1988). In eugonadal male patients, however, the results of testosterone administration have been inconsistent to date. Clearly, more research is needed in this important area.

Julian M. Davidson, Ph.D., is Professor of Molecular and Cellular Physiology at Stanford University. He is a distinguished contributor to the field of sexual endocrinology, and has conducted critical research on topics such as aging effects on sexuality, hypogonadal syndrome, and hormonal correlates of arousal.

Raymond C. Rosen, Ph.D., is Professor of Psychiatry and Medicine, and Co-Director of the Sexual Counseling Service at Robert Wood Johnson Medical School. He is the Past President of the International Academy of Sex Research, and is widely known for research on sexual psychophysiology and drug effects on sexuality.

Although hormonal factors in erectile dysfunction have frequently been a subject of speculation, there has been a dramatic upsurge of interest in the topic since the publication of a report by Spark, White, and Connolly (1980). This study, in which 37 of 105 men with erectile dysfunction were found to have demonstrable abnormalities of the hypothalamic–pituitary–gonadal axis, has been liberally interpreted by the popular press as showing that the majority of impotence cases are physical in origin. In the decade since, hormonal screening has become a routine procedure in the clinical evaluation of erectile disorders (Krane, Goldstein, & Saenz de Tejada, 1989), and interest is rapidly growing in the use of exogenous hormones for treatment of erectile failure (Carani et al., 1990; Nankin, Lin, & Osterman, 1986; O'Carroll & Bancroft, 1984).

Despite these advances in the clinical area, our understanding of the basic mechanisms by which hormones control sexual behavior in the human male has, unfortunately, advanced little in the past two decades. If anything, research in several areas indicates that hormonal effects on sexual behavior are far more complex than was previously recognized. This is the case at both the physiological and the behavioral levels.

A major goal of this chapter is to review the current state of knowledge concerning the impact of hormones on male erectile function. Beginning with a brief discussion of physiological properties and mechanisms of action, we consider the effects of hormonal variation on male sexual function in the eugonadal male, as well as conditions of reduced testicular function (e.g., castration, aging, hypogonadism). We also consider a variety of clinical issues, including the role of hormonal screening in assessment, and the use of hormone replacement therapy in the treatment of male erectile disorders.

Several limitations of the present chapter need to be stated at the outset:

1. Although this chapter is intended to consider the effects of hormones in general on erectile function, most of the presentation is focused on the effects of androgens, especially testosterone, in this regard. Other hormones, such as prolactin, estrogen, and oxytocin, are more briefly considered, since testosterone continues to be the focus of most research on male sexual response (Davidson & Myers, 1988; Bancroft, 1989).

2. We also restrict our discussion primarily to hormone effects in humans. Despite the considerable body of literature on hormones and sexual behavior in subhuman species, the relevance of these findings to sexual behavior in the human male is uncertain, and largely beyond the scope of the present chapter.

3. Another limitation of the present chapter is that little attention is given to the role of hormones in the control of hypersexuality or paraphilic sexual behavior in males. Rather, our overall goal in this chapter is to consider the effects of hormones on hyposexual conditions in general, and erectile disorders in particular.

CURRENT CONCEPTS IN HORMONE PHYSIOLOGY

Recent research has identified a bewildering array of chemical modulators of behavior, of which hormones are only one particular class. Readers should bear in mind the classic definition of a hormone: a chemical agent produced by specialized organs (endocrine glands) and released into the bloodstream to act on target tissues at a distance from the site of secretion. Hormones travel widely, and their actions do not depend on the sites of production, such as the pituitary, thyroid, parathyroid, gonads, adrenals, and pancreas.

Chemically, the sex hormones are classified as steroids or peptides. The steroids originate from three steroid-producing endocrine glands: the testis and ovary (gonads) and the adrenal cortex. The principal steroid hormones consist of the androgens, estrogens, and progestins, of which the most important are testosterones, estradiol, and progesterone, respectively. The peptide (or protein) hormones relevant to sexual function are gonadotropin-releasing hormone (GnRH) from the hypothalamus, and follicle-stimulating hormone (FSH), luteinizing hormone (LH), and prolactin (PRL) from the anterior pituitary. An additional posterior-pituitary peptide hormone, oxytocin, has been implicated in several laboratory studies of sexual arousal (Carmichael et al., 1987; Murphy, Seckl, Burton, Checkley, & Lightman, 1987).

Among the steroid hormones, primary attention has been given to testosterone in the control and regulation of male sexual behavior. Testosterone secreted by the testes can be considered a prohormone, as two of its active metabolites are of importance. First, there is its conversion by the enzyme aromatase to the estrogen estradiol; second, testosterone is converted by the enzyme 5-alpha reductase to dihydrotestosterone (DHT), a more potent androgen than testosterone itself. In various species, sexual differentiation of the brain by testosterone is achieved via its conversion to estrogen (Kemper, 1990). However, it has not been established that conversion is necessary for the activating effects of testosterone on adult sexual behavior. Whereas conversion of testosterone to DHT is required for adequate differentiation and growth of certain tissues (particularly the prostate, the external genitalia, and the skin hair follicles), aromatization may not be required for the major effects of testosterone on the central nervous system (Bancroft, 1989).

Developmentally, the secretion of testosterone *in utero* causes early differentiation of the primordial structures into male internal and external genitalia, as well as enlargement of the phallus during the third trimester. At puberty, an increase in testosterone has obvious and profound effects on both morphology and physiology of the male (Snyder, 1984). After puberty, most males exhibit relatively stable testosterone levels until the fifth or sixth decade of life. Recent studies, however, have indicated a notable decline in testosterone levels after age 65–70 (Schiavi, 1990), as discussed by Segraves and Segraves in Chapter 5 of this volume.

In understanding testosterone's effects on male sexual response ("activational effects"), three specific factors need to be taken into consideration: (1) cyclical and pulsatile effects; (2) bioavailability of free and bound testosterone; and (3) negative feedback mechanisms. Testosterone levels show marked circadian variation, with the highest levels being reached during rapid eye movement (REM) sleep and the early morning hours (Schiavi, Fisher, White, Beers, & Szechter, 1982). Pulsatile effects have also been observed, with short spikes in testosterone occurring at least six or seven times per day (Schwartz, Kolodny, & Masters, 1980). For this reason, a single sample of testosterone may not be a reliable indicator of the overall level. Similarly, measures of total testosterone may not reflect the amount of bio-available or unbound testosterone in the plasma. Approximately 30–60% of total testosterone is bound by sex-hormone-binding globulin (SHBG) and is physiologically inactive, while an additional 40–70% is loosely bound to albumin (Manni, Pardridge, & Cefalu, 1985). Only 5% or less of the total testosterone is completely unbound, and recent evidence suggests that albumin-bound testosterone is freely available to tissues. Many laboratories nowadays are able to measure "bioavailable" testosterone, which is the sum of the free plus albumin-bound fractions in plasma.

Finally, testosterone levels in the blood are closely regulated by the effects of homeostatic or negative feedback mechanisms (see Figure 4.1). At a central level, the hypothalamus regulates hormone production by secretion of a modulating hormone, GnRH. In turn, GnRH stimulates the basophilic cells of the anterior pituitary to produce LH, which acts on the interstitial cells of the testes to produce testosterone. Homeostatic regulation of the system occurs when increased testosterone levels in the bloodstream cause the hypothalamus to decrease the rate of secretion of GnRH, which results in a lower level of LH secretion from the pituitary.

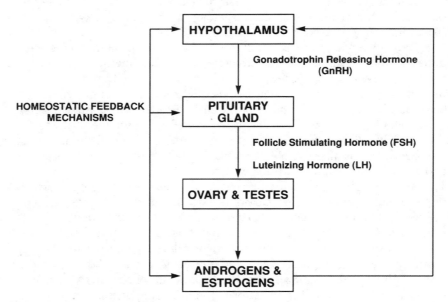

FIGURE 4.1.   Schematic representation of homeostatic mechanisms involved in the regulation of steroid hormones in men and women. Adapted from Segraves (1988).

TESTOSTERONE EFFECTS ON SEXUAL RESPONSE

The role of testosterone in initiating and maintaining sexual behavior in the male has been established through research in many species. In particular, the loss of sexual function when testosterone is removed by surgical ablation, or through seasonal regression, seems to be universal among mammals. With castration, sexual behavior in the male typically declines: A loss of ejaculation occurs first, followed by loss of intromission and finally of mounting behavior (Beach, 1948; Hart, 1974). Androgen replacement is generally effective in restoring these actions in reverse order (Bancroft, 1989). Among humans, however, the role of testosterone in sexual arousal is far more complex and controversial. In particular, the effects of testosterone on the cognitive-affective or libidinal aspects of sexual response have been a major focus of inquiry in recent years (Davidson & Myers, 1988; Segraves, 1988).

Evidence concerning testosterone's effects on sexual arousal in males is derived from several sources, including studies of hormone replacement therapy in hypogonadal males, antiandrogenic treatment of sex offenders, and laboratory studies of sexual arousal in eugonadal (healthy) males. Although certain trends are apparent in this research, it is equally clear that many questions remain unanswered at the present time.

The first major finding from studies of hypogonadal males is that sexual desire levels and the capacity for seminal emission are closely tied to androgen withdrawal and replacement (Davidson, Camargo, & Smith, 1979; Luisi & Franchi, 1980). Within 3–4 weeks of androgen withdrawal, sexual interest and desire are markedly reduced in hypogonadal patients. Similarly, sleep erections (nocturnal penile tumescence, or NPT) and spontaneous or fantasy-based erections are clearly androgen-dependent in these individuals, and are rapidly abolished when testosterone therapy is withdrawn (Davidson, Kwan, & Greenleaf, 1982).

Though hypogonadal men are deficient in orgasm and ejaculation, there is no solid evidence that either of these functions requires testosterone in adulthood. Of course, semen production (or, more precisely, the functioning of the accessory sexual glands) is dependent on testosterone, in that both semen and spermatogenesis require the active presence of the hormone. The seminal emission and ejaculation proper utilize the smooth muscle of the genital tract and the striated muscle of the penis, respectively. But perhaps the major role of testosterone in orgasm may simply be to make possible a more robust level of sexual arousal, enough to trigger orgasm. Such a trigger-like effect could involve testosterone, albeit in a more indirect fashion.

In contrast to the effects on desire or orgasm, it has been repeatedly shown that testosterone has little or no effect on erections elicited by external stimuli, such as erotic videotapes. Normal responses to such stimuli occur in hypogonadal men and are not changed with androgen replacement (Bancroft & Wu, 1983; Kwan, Greenleaf, Mann, Crapo, & Davidson, 1983). Thus, erectile failure occurring in an androgen-deficient man may be interpreted as a reaction to the hormonally related loss of sexual desire, and not as a direct consequence of androgen deficiency per se.

Similar results were obtained in an earlier study of antiandrogenic therapy in sex offenders (Bancroft, Tennent, Lucas, & Cass, 1974). After administration of cyproterone acetate, a potent antiandrogenic drug, subjects continued to show normal erections in response to an erotic film, although there was little or no response to fantasy. Taken together, these findings suggest that two differentially regulated types of erections occur: (1) non-androgen-dependent erections that are elicited by tactile stimuli or in response to erotic films (i.e., externally mediated stimuli); and (2) erections occurring "spontaneously" during sleep or waking, which are internally generated and are strongly androgen-dependent.

We must presume that the neural pathways subserving spontaneous daytime erections and NPT diverge from those involved in erections induced by erotic stimulation. It appears increasingly likely that the former, but not the latter, are directly dependent on testosterone. These androgen-dependent neural pathways seem to be bypassed when the stimulus is explicitly sexual, as in laboratory presentation of erotic film stimuli, and probably direct stimulation by a sexual partner (Davidson & Myers, 1988). Erotic tactile sensitivity also does not appear to be androgen-dependent; in fact, the evidence, such as it is, shows that the sensitivity of both the penis and the index finger is lower in hypogonadal men (Burris, Graceley, Carter, Sherins, & Davidson, in press; see below).

Bancroft (1989) has summarized recent clinical and experimental findings on the relationship between androgens and erectile function as follows:

> Erection is seen as a response at a late stage of a sequence of events in the system. Interference with erection can occur at various points in this sequence. Within the brain (and possibly spinal cord) . . . an androgen-dependent neurophysiological substrate [is postulated] for both sexual interest, or desire, and spontaneous erections, such as occur during sleep. . . . In addition, external stimuli mediated by specific sensory systems in the brain may lead to erections by means of pathways which are not androgen-dependent and hence are independent of the central arousability system. (p. 126)

Overall, the most consistent androgen-related effect on sexual behavior is that of increasing libido (Segraves, 1988). These libidonic (cognitive-experiential) and motivational responses are little understood, but are highly significant determinants of sexual arousal in both men and women (Levine, 1988; Leiblum & Rosen, 1988). Sexual desire, it should be emphasized, is influenced itself by other components of sexual response, including the anatomic, physiological, and behavioral events of erection and climax, as well as other psychological and interpersonal factors (Levine, 1988). Whereas the effects of testosterone on libido are certain, at least in the case of hypogonadal male patients, the relationship between androgen and erectile function appears to be more complicated and may involve a variety of mediating factors, such as cognitive focus or perceptual influences (Davidson et al., 1982; Kemper, 1990).

Given the essential role of touch in sexual activity, it is surprising how little is known about the influence of testosterone on erotic sensitivity. In one recent study (Burris et al., in press), vibrotactile sensitivity of the penis was related to androgen levels in several patient groups. Penis and index finger sensitivity were studied. Standard psychophysical methodology was used for determining the threshold of sensitivity (Green & Swets, 1966) and intensity (Graceley, Dubner, & McGrathe, 1982). Four different groups were evaluated: an untreated hypogonadal group, a treated hypogonadal group, a group of normal volunteers, and an additional control group of infertile patients.

Untreated hypogonadal men (i.e., those never treated or those not treated for many years) had the lowest threshold of vibrotactile perception when compared with normal volunteers, treated hypogonadal patients, and infertile men. Moreover, when tested for intensity of touch, the untreated hypogonadal group perceived the stimuli as more intense than all other groups did. Treatment with testosterone in hypogonadal men was associated with a decline in perceived intensity of vibrotactile stimulation. However, at the highest levels of vibrotactile stimulation, these testosterone effects disappeared.

These data suggest that testosterone does *not* enhance the touch sense in penis or finger skin. On the contrary, it appears that the effect of testosterone is inhibitory, at least as far as vibrotactile stimulation is concerned. Obviously, the androgenic eroticization of skin in sexual situations is not related to quantitative skin perception, but presumably to other qualitative factors involved in sexual arousal. It remains to be determined how testosterone levels or changes in testosterone relate to these effects.

HORMONE LEVELS IN NONDYSFUNCTIONAL MEN

Does testosterone level affect sexual desire or performance in healthy (eugonadal) males? One early study (Brown, Monti, & Corriveau, 1978) correlated questionnaire ratings of sexual interest and activity with testosterone levels in 101 healthy young men. There was no correlation between the variables in this population. Surprisingly, Kraemer, Becker, Brodie, Doering, and Hamburg (1976) reported a negative relationship between self-reported frequency of orgasm and testosterone levels in 20 healthy male volunteers. On the other hand, Knussman, Christiansen, and Couwenbergs (1986) subsequently reported positive inter- and intraindividual correlations (generally in the range of .20 to .30) between serum testosterone levels and orgasm frequency.

Several studies by other investigators have examined hormone–behavior relationships in sexual interaction situations. For instance, Rowland et al. (1987) investigated psychophysiological and hormonal changes during sexual arousal to a series of erotic videotapes shown in the laboratory. Subjects were 16 healthy males aged 18–40. Results showed clearly that LH levels were increased by about 45 minutes after onset of sexual arousal. Testosterone concentration was also positively correlated with higher levels of erectile response, although it did not appear to rise over repeated presentations, as predicted. Cortisol levels were correlated with self-reported worry, and testosterone with relaxation.

Elevated PRL levels have been associated with decreased sexual arousal, as occurs with administration of phenothiazine drugs (Rubin, Poland, & Tower, 1976; Ghadirian, Chouinard, & Annable, 1982). PRL levels are highly responsive, in turn, to dopaminergic activity in the pituitary (Bancroft, 1989). Hyperprolactinemia in men occurs with or without decreased testosterone function, and is an additional important cause for erectile failure (Spark et al., 1980; Krane et al., 1989).

Finally, the relationship between oxytocin, a neuropeptide hormone, and sexual response has been investigated in a number of recent studies (Carmichael et al., 1987; Murphy et al., 1987; Murphy, Checkley, Seckl, & Lightman, 1990). In its peripheral rather than cerebral role, oxytocin's effects are involved in reproductive functions. In women, oxytocin facilitates smooth muscle contractions of the uterus during parturition, and contractions of the myoepithelial cells for milk ejection during lactation.

Two studies demonstrate that oxytocin levels are markedly increased during stimulation of sexual arousal in both men and women (Carmichael et al., 1987; Murphy et al., 1987). In the first study, plasma oxytocin levels were measured prior to, during, and after masturbation to orgasm in 9 male and 13 female volunteers. Results showed a marked increase in plasma oxytocin during sexual arousal and orgasm in both male and female subjects, although mean plasma levels prior to and during orgasm were higher in women than in men (Carmichael et al., 1987). In women, the mean plasma oxytocin level increased from 2.0 to 3.6 pg/ml during orgasm.

Murphy et al. (1987) reported results from a similar study of oxytocin release during sexual arousal in 13 healthy young males. Although subjects showed little oxytocin response to the presentation of an erotic film stimulus, a highly significant increase in oxytocin was observed during masturbation-induced orgasm. Considering the differences in subjects, and methods used for achieving sexual arousal, these findings are generally consistent in demonstrating oxytocin's role in sexual arousal.

The most recent study involved oxytocin and naloxone, an opioid receptor antagonist (Murphy et al., 1990). Healthy male subjects again masturbated to orgasm, preceded by either infusion of naloxone or placebo in counterbalanced order. Results showed a definite inhibition of plasma oxytocin levels during orgasm in association with naloxone treatment. Although naloxone had no effect on heart rate or blood pressure at orgasm, a decrease in the level of subjective arousal and pleasure at orgasm was noted. The authors concluded that opioid receptor blockade with naloxone has an inhibitory effect on the neural pathways mediating the oxytocin response at orgasm. This was associated with noticeable changes in subjective arousal in this study.

EFFECTS OF AGING

As discussed in Chapter 5 of this volume by Segraves and Segraves, decreasing androgen levels in aging have been correlated with declining sexual frequency, although the causal relationship between these factors is not at all clear (Schiavi, 1990). Along with the hormonal decrements comes a loss of reproductive activity, including diminished activity of Sertoli cells and inhibin. Moreover, Leydig cells decrease in number; SHBG increases with age, which reduces bioavailable testosterone. DHT, interestingly, shows relatively little change with aging. In rats, it has been demonstrated that the failure of sexual behavior in aging is associated with decreases in GnRH and the endogenous opiate beta-endorphin (Dorsa, Smith, & Davidson, 1984).

ENDOCRINE EVALUATION FOR ERECTILE DISORDERS

Over the past decade, there has been increasing emphasis in the clinical literature on the role of hormonal studies in the clinical evaluation of erectile dysfunction. The importance of hormonal screening was dramatically underscored by Spark et al. (1980), who, as noted at the beginning of this chapter, reported that 37 (35%) of the 105 patients referred to their center with complaints of erectile failure had previously unsuspected disorders of the hypothalamic–pituitary–gonadal axis. A large number of these individuals (27 of 105) were found to have either hypo- or hypergonadotropic hypogondadism, and a smaller number had hyperprolactinemia (8 of 105) or occult hyperthyroidism (2 of 105). Many of these patients had previously been diagnosed as psychogenic, and in some instances had been referred for several years of psychological counseling. Once the endocrinopathy had been detected, and appropriate medical treatment provided, however, 33 of the 37 patients recovered erectile function.

Although this study has been criticized on the grounds of selection biases in the sample (patients were all referred by physicians to a specialized endocrine laboratory) and the lack of placebo controls in the evaluation of treatment effects (Kavich-Sharon, 1980), its impact on the field has been considerable. Similar findings were reported by other authors in the early 1980s (e.g., Slag et al., 1983; Davis, Viosca, & Guralnik, 1985), and the role of hormonal screening in assessment of erectile failure has taken on increasing significance in the clinical literature. Despite this emphasis, widespread disagreement exists over a number of basic issues, such as the overall incidence of endocrinopathy in this population, the value of routine endocrinological screening in all cases of erectile failure, the etiological and prognostic significance of hormone abnormalities, and the pros and cons of specific hormonal assays. We briefly review current theory and practice in each of these areas.

What is the likely incidence of endocrine disorders in men with erectile failure? Despite a number of large-scale clinical studies in the past 10 years, incidence estimates continue to vary widely. Perhaps the most important determining factor is the role of subject selection factors (Kavich-Sharon, 1980), and it is therefore important to consider findings from studies of different age groups and clinical populations.

The first study to evaluate the incidence of hormone abnormalities in a general outpatient setting was reported by Slag et al., (1983). These authors evaluated 100 men with erectile dysfunction (mean age = 59.4 years), who were drawn from a broad sample of male patients in a general medical outpatient clinic. Each of the patients identified was subjected to a comprehensive psychiatric and medical assessment, including screening for total testosterone, PRL, FSH, and LH, as well as thyroid function tests (T3, T4, and T3U). Primary hypogonadism, defined as elevated LH or FSH with associated low or low-normal testosterone values (<400 ng/dl), was found in 10% of the sample. Secondary hypogonadism (low FSH or LH levels with subnormal testosterone values) was found in a further 9% of the patients. Four percent had elevated PRL levels, and an additional 5% of the sample had previously undiagnosed hypothyroidism. Taken together, these findings suggest that approximately 25% of male patients with erectile failure in this age group show evidence of abnormal endocrine function.

The major advantage of this study is that subjects were selected from patients in a general outpatient clinic, thus avoiding the selection biases of Spark et al. (1980) and most other studies in the area. On the other hand, the investigators used a rather liberal definition of hypogonadism (testosterone < 400 ng/dl) and failed to show a positive effect of treatment of hormonal abnormalities, as in the Spark et al. study. Among the patients with hyperprolactinemia (4%), three were diabetic and one was taking phenothiazine medications; in other words, no pituitary tumors were identified in this sample. Based upon these findings, the authors recommend routine screening for total testosterone, FSH, LH, and thyroid function in all cases of erectile dysfunction. Inclusion of PRL assessment is viewed as optional, given the uncertain relevance of the PRL findings in this study.

In a similar study, Nickel, Morales, Condra, Fenemore, and Surridge (1984) conducted a comprehensive evaluation of 256 patients (mean age = 51.5 years) referred to a Canadian urology clinic. A total of 45 patients (17.5%) were found to have significant abnormalities of the hypothalamic-pituitary–gonadal axis, inlcuding 18 patients (7%) with hypergonadotropic hypogonadism, 16 patients (6.2%) with hypogonadotropic hypogonadism, 16 patients (6.2%) with hyperprolactinemia. Among the patients with hyperprolactinemia, 5 patients were also found to have depressed testosterone levels (<300 ng/dl) and were included in the hypogonadotropic hypogonadal category. Two of the hyperprolactinemic patients were found to have previously unsuspected pituitary tumors (prolactinomas), which required surgery. Only one patient with occult hypothyroidism was identified on routine hormonal screening.

An important finding from this study was that 8 of the 45 patients with abnormal endocrine values qualified for a diagnosis of psychogenic erectile failure, based upon concurrent assessment of NPT, adequate early morning erections, and a positive response to psychotherapy. An additional 6 patients had known vascular or neurological disorders that were viewed as primary causes for erectile failure. After other causes had been eliminated, only 31 patients (12.1%) were found to have endocrine abnormalities that could be considered as the major determinants of erectile failure in this sample. Furthermore, Nickel et al. (1984) suggest that more than 90% of patients with endocrine-related organic impotence can be detected from a combination of careful history taking, physical examination with emphasis on testicular volume, and a single determination of serum testosterone values. According to these authors, complete hormonal assessment (including determination of gonadotropin and PRL levels) should be reserved only for patients with clinical evidence of hypogonadism or decreased total testosterone levels.

A follow-up study by the same group (Leonard, Nickel, & Morales, 1989) investigated in greater depth the role of hyperprolactinemia as a determining factor in erectile failure. After reviewing evaluations of 1,236 consecutive patients at the Queens University Urology Clinic, the authors found 5.3% of these patients to have elevated PRL levels. Among the various causes of hyperprolactinemia in this sample were medication use, pituitary adenomas, chronic renal failure, and a large number of cases diagnosed as "idiopathic hyperprolactinemia." PRL levels were markedly higher (mean = 20.9 ng/dl) in the 15% of patients with pituitary adenomas, all of whom responded positively to a trial of bromocriptine therapy. Given that all patients with significant hyperprolactinemia in this study were also found to have other signs of hypogonadism, the authors continue to argue that comprehensive endocrine evaluation should be reserved for only those patients with abnormal serum testosterone levels.

In a comprehensive study of 49 male patients in a British sexual dysfunction clinic, Friedman, Clare, Rees, and Grossman (1986) reported a relatively low rate of abnormal endocrine findings. Although 10 of the 49 patients had at least one endocrine value outside the normal range, only 1 patient had subnormal testosterone levels. Five patients had elevated SHBG levels, and 4 patients had elevated levels of gonadotropins. A positive response to testosterone therapy was noted in 4 of the 5 patients with elevated SHBG levels, and in the single patient with subnormal testosterone. None of the patients with elevated gonadotropin levels responded to hormone therapy.

From the low rate of hypogonadism and apparent absence of hyperprolactinemia in the sample, the authors conclude that endocrine screening is only of limited value in the diagnostic evaluation of erectile failure. However, these findings should be cautiously interpreted, in view of the relatively small sample size ($n = 49$) and the fact that the median age (46 years) of patients in this study was significantly lower than in most other studies to date. On the other hand, the relatively high rate of elevated SHBG levels in this study, and the positive response in most of these patients to testosterone therapy, are noteworthy findings that warrant further investigation.

More recently, Baskin (1989) conducted an intensive evaluation of 600 consecutive patients (mean age $= 58$ years), who had been referred to a specialized endocrine clinic for evaluation of erectile failure. As in the original Spark et al. (1980) study, which was conducted on a similar sample, a high overall number of patients (32%) in this study were found to have significant endocrinopathy, including 14% with primary testicular failure, 13% with secondary hypogonadism, 6% with unsuspected hypothyroidism, and 3% with hyperprolactinemia. Seven of the 20 patients with elevated PRL levels were found to have pituitary microadenomas, and were successfully treated with bromocriptine therapy. All of the patients with occult hypothyroidism responded positively to levothyroxine replacement therapy.

In an effort to predict which of the hypogonadal patients in his study were most likely to respond to testosterone therapy, Baskin (1989) developed a novel index of androgen function, termed the "androgen quotient" (AQ). This value was calculated independently for each subject by multiplying FSH by LH values, and dividing the product by serum testosterone level, as follows:

$$AQ = \frac{FSH \ (mIU/ml) \times LH \ (mIU/ml)}{Testosterone \ (ng/dl)} \times k$$

According to this formula, the normal AQ is less than 0.19, and the constant (k) is 1. Patients with primary testicular failure, as expected, had low testosterone levels with normal or elevated gonadotropins, resulting in AQs below 0.19. In assessing the subsequent effects of hormone replacement therapy, Baskin found that a high AQ was more accurate than testosterone level alone in predicting a positive response to treatment. Patients with normal or low AQs generally showed little benefit from testosterone therapy. Based upon these findings, the author recommends that use of the AQ in screening can reduce the risk of unnecessarily giving testosterone to male patients who may be at risk for prostatic cancer.

In reviewing the results of the studies described above, we can advance a number of tentative conclusions:

1. The incidence of hormone abnormalities in men with erectile failure is closely linked to the age of the sample and source of recruitment (i.e., general outpatient clinic vs. specialized endocrine evaluation unit). In all of the studies to date, however, it appears that at least 10–20% of men referred for evaluation are likely to show abnormalities of the hypothalamus–pituitary–gonadal axis. A much higher percentage of men referred for specialized endocrine assessment will show such abnormalities.

2. In addition to hypo- and hypergonadotropic hypogonadism, several studies have shown a significant (albeit much lesser) incidence of hyperprolactinemia and hyper- or hypothyroidism in these patients. Moreover, patients with these disorders appear to show a good sexual response to appropriate medical treatment.

3. Although most authors acknowledge the need for endocrine screening in such cases, there is widespread disagreement on the specific tests to be employed or the interpretation thereof. For example, Leonard et al. (1989) recommends initial assessment with serum testosterone alone, to be followed by a more comprehensive evaluation only when an abnormal testosterone level is reported. In contrast, Baskin (1989) and others have argued for routine assessment of FSH, LH, and PRL, as well as thyroid function tests, in all cases of erectile failure. Still others (e.g., Lakin, 1988) advise assessment of only testosterone and PRL in all cases.

What recommendations can be made at this time for clinicians and sex therapists? To begin with, the potential role of endocrine abnormalities should be considered in *every* case of erectile failure. Depending upon the type of clinical facility and the nature of the patient population, however, clinicians may opt for routine administration of more or less complete screening batteries. Cost may be a difficulty in some cases, as complete endocrine batteries can run as high as $300–400 in some centers. Of course, this should be balanced against the potentially much greater costs (both medical and financial) of misdiagnosis and resulting inadequate or inappropriate treatment.

Overall, we concur with Segraves (1988), who recommends routine evaluation of serum testosterone and PRL levels in all male patients with erectile failure or low libido. According to Segraves, "attempts to minimize patient costs by utilizing serum testosterone alone are ill advised" (p. 285), given the risk of misdiagnosis of occasional patients with hyperprolactinemia. Furthermore, patients who are found to have low testosterone levels on initial screening should *always* be referred for a more comprehensive evaluation, including FSH, LH, and SHBG testing, before any treatment recommendations are made. Clinicians should also be extremely sensitive to the possibility of hypo- or hyperthyroidism in these cases; where possible, thyroid function tests should be included in the early stages of assessment.

ENDOCRINE THERAPY FOR PATIENTS WITH ERECTILE DISORDERS

Hormonal treatments for erectile dysfunction have been recommended in various forms for several decades now. In the 1950s, for example, a popular medical remedy for erectile failure was a compound known as Afrodex, which consisted of a combination of testosterone, yohimbine, and strychnine (Margolis, Prieto, Stein, & Chin, 1971). More recently, it is generally accepted that although hormone therapy is of major value in the treatment of clear-cut endocrinopathies (e.g., hypogonadism), it has little value in the treatment of erectile failure in eugonadal males. The effects of treatment on three specific patient groups needs to be considered. These groups are (1) hypogonadal men; (2) patients with hyperprolactinemia; and (3) sexually dysfunctional eugonadal men.

Patients with Hyper- and Hypogonadotropic Hypogonadism

Testicular failure may be a cause of primary or hypergonadotropic hypogonadism. Alternatively, hypogonadism can be determined by specific abnormalities of the hypothalamus–pituitary–gonadal axis (McClure, 1988). Secondary hypogonadism is defined as a defect at the hypothalamic and/or pituitary level, in which serum LH and FSH levels are inappropriately low and serum testosterone is also low (hypergonadotropic hypogonadism). Elevated gonadotropin levels are the characteristic response of an intact hypothalamus–pituitary system to testicular failure. Several studies have examined hormone replacement therapy effects on sexual function in both of these diagnostic subgroups.

Davidson et al. (1979) administered testosterone enanthate to six male hypogonadal patients aged 32–65. Four of the six had secondary hypogonadism, and two had primary testicular failure. Using a double-blind, crossover evaluation, the authors demonstrated significant improvements in sexual desire and performance in five of the six patients (see Figure 4.2). As shown in the figure, different effects on the various measures of arousal and orgasm in the study were observed for 100-mg and 400-mg doses of testosterone enanthate. From these results, it appears that there are different androgen

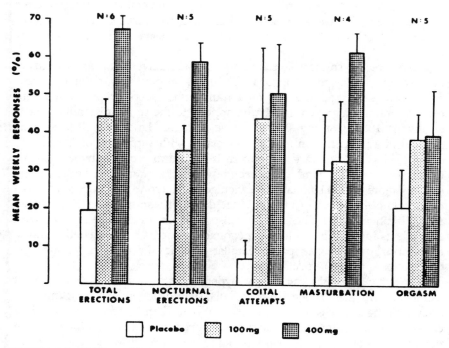

FIGURE 4.2.   Effects of hormone replacement therapy (100 mg, i.m.; 400 mg, i.m.; placebo) on core parameters of sexual arousal, coitus (including unsuccessful attempts), masturbation, and orgasm. Data are from six adult hypogonadal males aged 32–65. From "Effects of Androgen on Sexual Behavior in Hypogonadal Men" by J. M. Davidson, C. Camargo, and E. R. Smith, 1979, *Journal of Clinical Endocrinology and Metabolism*, 48, 955–958. Copyright 1979 by the Endocrine Society. Reprinted by permission.

threshold effects for the individual components of sexual response (Rosen & Beck, 1988).

Several additional studies have demonstrated the value of androgen replacement therapy for hypogonadal men. For example, Skakkebaek, Bancroft, Davidson, and Warner (1981) evaluated the effects of double-blind treatment with testosterone undecanoate or placebo in six hypogonadotropic and six hypergonadotropic men with hypogonadism. The researchers reported that increases in sexual desire were observed first, followed by improvements in ejaculation and erectile function. Changes in sexual function were similar between the two groups. It should be noted that the undecanoate form of testosterone used in this study is available in Europe, but not in the United States for this purpose.

Snyder (1984) recommends the use of long-acting intramuscular injections of testosterone ester (either testosterone enanthate or testosterone cypionate) for androgen replacement therapy. Daily oral ingestion of methyl testosterone is also available. Both of these methods, however, carry a significant risk of adverse side effects such as gynecomastia, liver function abnormalities, and edema.

More recent studies have investigated alternative methods of testosterone administration for hypogonadal patients. In particular, several publications have described the use of a transdermal preparation with a thin testosterone-impregnated membrane applied to the scrotum (Findlay, Place, & Snyder, 1987; Conway, Boylan, Howe, Ross, & Handelsman, 1988). This method of administration may be associated with supraphysiological levels of DHT, however, which is of concern in regard to prostatic hyperplasia or cancer. On the other hand, it has been reported that transdermal testosterone delivery more closely simulates the average testosterone production rate than do periodic injections of much higher doses of testosterone (Carey, Howards, & Vance, 1988). These authors also reported an absence of significant side effects in a sample of four hypogonadal patients being treated with the transdermal testosterone patch. Similar findings have been reported by Conway et al. (1988) in Australia.

In some instances, secondary hypogonadism may be associated with external factors, such as the use of anabolic steroids for athletic competition or body building (Jarow & Lipshultz, 1990). When taken in large doses or for an extended period of time, anabolic steroids can cause feedback inhibition of the hypothalamus and pituitary gland, resulting in decreased secretion of both LH and FSH. Some users of anabolic steroids develop hypogonadotrophic hypogonadism and resulting erectile dysfunction, as illustrated by one recent case.

Case Vignette

Joe P. was a 27-year-old Hispanic construction worker and competitive body builder. Two years prior to entering treatment Joe had committed himself to an intensive body-building program, which included the use of high doses of an illegally obtained anabolic steroid, methandrostenolone (Danabol). With increasing use of the drug in subsequent months, Joe experienced a gradual loss of libido and intermittent episodes of erectile failure. His wife, Maria, attributed their sexual difficulties to a loss of interest in the marital relationship, and possible sexual attraction to other women. At this time, she was unaware of his increasing use of anabolic steroids.

Endocrine evaluation indicated abnormally low levels of LH (1.6 ng/ml) and FSH (2.8 ng/ml), in addition to diminished serum testosterone (226 ng/ml). PRL was within normal limits (8.7 ng/ml). Physical examination was unremarkable, although the patient's testes appeared mildly atrophied. On the basis of these findings, Joe was strongly advised to discontinue his use of Danabol, as well as to adopt a less rigorous training schedule. Over the following months, his sexual desire gradually returned, and the couple were able to resume intercourse in time.

Several sessions of couples counseling were provided in order to reestablish trust in the relationship, and to overcome Joe's performance anxiety in regard to intercourse. Six months later, Maria had become pregnant, and therapy was discontinued.

Patients with Hyperprolactinemia

Elevated PRL levels may be a cause of both low desire and erectile failure, just as normalization of PRL is associated with a return of potency in a high percentage of cases (Schwartz, Bauman, & Masters, 1982; Johnston, Prescott, Kendal-Taylor, Hall, & Cook, 1983). Although high PRL levels are most often associated with low testosterone, in some cases hyperprolactinemia will lead to arousal or desire deficits *despite* the presence of a normal serum testosterone level (Sheeler & Lakin, 1988). This observation leads us to recommend independent assessment of PRL in most cases.

Common causes of hyperprolactinemia include microadenomas or PRL-secreting tumors of the pituitary, use of dopamine-blocking drugs (e.g., phenothiazines), and other factors. PRL levels are closely related to dopaminergic activity in the pituitary: Specifically, PRL levels rise when dopaminergic activity is inadequate (Bancroft, 1989). Drugs used in the treatment of hyperprolactinemia are dopamine agonists, such as bromocriptine (Parlodel). Bromocriptine is usually given at dosages ranging from 2.5 mg to 5 mg per day, but may be increased to 40 mg/day in order to normalize PRL levels. Sexual function typically improves within a few days of initiating treatment. Alternative treatments include pituitary surgery or irradiation. Overall, it is not clear whether sexual function improves in these patients because of the direct effects of lowering PRL levels, or because of a change in dopaminergic transmission in the nervous system. Psychological factors may coexist with neuroendocrine causes for sexual dysfunction (Bancroft, O'Carroll, McNeilly, & Shaw, 1984).

Normalization of PRL is typically associated with rapid changes in all facets of sexual response. The close relationship between hormone levels and sexual function is nicely illustrated in the following case:

> A 71-year-old man had a 3-year history of decreased potency, decreased libido, and anorgasmia. Initial testing revealed a testosterone level of 185 ng/dl and a prolactin level of 81.3 ng/ml. Treatment with bromocriptine (Parlodel), 2.5 mg twice a day restored his libido, potency, and orgasms within 3 weeks of starting therapy. Tests done 6 weeks after he began bromocriptine treatment showed a prolactin level of 9.8 ng/ml and a testosterone level of 334 ng/dl. (Sheeler & Lakin, 1988, p. 125)

Sexually Dysfunctional Patients without Hormone Abnormalities

Although androgen therapy has frequently been recommended in the past for sexually dysfunctional men with normal testosterone levels, there are surprisingly few controlled studies of this form of therapy in the literature. Cooper (1980) evaluated the effects of parenterally administered androgen treatment (mesterolone) in a group of 25 males with psychogenic impotence and normal plasma testosterone levels. Although the author reported a "slight trend" toward clinical improvement in these patients, no significant effects were observed on either plasma testosterone levels or measures of sexual function.

Given the association between hormone levels and sexual desire, however, it is possible that androgen therapy will be of value to male patients with erectile difficulties secondary to hypoactive sexual desire. This hypothesis was directly investigated in a well-controlled British study of testosterone treatment in men with either low sexual interest ($n = 10$) or erectile dysfunction ($n = 10$) (O'Carroll & Bancroft, 1984). Surprisingly, men with low libido in this study were found to have *higher* baseline levels of testosterone than men with erectile dysfunction. The testosterone therapy had little or no effect on erectile function, although the men with low desire experienced a significant degree of improvement with intramuscular testosterone therapy (Sustanon) given every 2 weeks, compared to double-blind placebo. Only 3 of 10 patients in the low-desire group experienced *clinically significant* improvements following testosterone therapy. The authors concluded: "Androgens are relevant to sexual interest, but not erectile function, as those men whose principal problem was erectile dysfunction failed to respond to testosterone therapy even though their testosterone levels were significantly lower than those in the low sex interest group" (O'Carroll & Bancroft, 1984, p. 149).

In a subsequent study of patients with medical illness and secondary impotence complaints, Nankin et al. (1986) evaluated the effects of testosterone cypionate therapy on sexual function and circulating testosterone levels, in a group of 10 impotent men with complex medical histories and low baseline testosterone levels. All subjects had mean morning testosterone concentrations below 420 ng/dl. Patients were given either 200 mg testosterone cypionate or placebo intramuscularly every 14 days, for a total of six injections in each condition (12 weeks). The average testosterone level on placebo was 320 ± 81 ng/dl, and was increased to 377 ± 103 ng/dl with testosterone administration. Significant improvements in sexual interest and potency (i.e., erectile function) were observed in the testosterone treatment condition. Of the 10 patients, 7 reported definite improvements in libido, and 5 noted that potency returned and vaginal intercourse was resumed while they were on testosterone therapy. Clearly, androgen therapy is of value to some men in the lower range of normal circulating testosterone levels.

Most recently, Carani et al. (1990) evaluated the effects of oral testosterone undecoanate in two groups of sexually dysfunctional men ($n = 14$), with and without signs of mild hypogonadism. Significant improvements were found in subjects with low baseline serum testosterone levels, as in the studies reported above. Little or no change, however, was observed in patients with relatively normal baseline levels.

Taken together, these studies strongly suggest that androgen therapy is of little value for eugonadal males with erectile dysfunction. To judge from the findings of at least one study (O'Carroll & Bancroft, 1984), hormonal treatment may be mildly beneficial for male patients with low desire, but little or no effect has been observed to date for patients with erectile dysfunction alone.

CONCLUSION

In recent years our understanding of the physiology of hormonal function has been greatly enriched by developments in molecular biology. In particular, researchers such as Jean Wilson at Dallas have reported that genes of the three major proteins in androgen physiology have been cloned. These include isolation of the cDNAs for the androgen receptor, the 5-alpha reductase enzyme, and the aromatase enzyme. The 5-alpha reductase enzyme eluded purification for many years because of its extensive hydrophobicity. Recently, however, the androgen receptor gene has been successfully cloned and is being fully characterized. The impact of these advances on our understanding of hormonal effects on behavior awaits further investigation.

At the behavioral level, an equally complex picture of the effects of androgens on sexual desire, arousal, and orgasm has emerged (Davidson & Myers, 1988; Bancroft, 1989). Although certain aspects of sexual response, such as libido and spontaneous arousal, are strongly dependent on hormonal influences, these factors may have little or no effect on erectile capacity. Our understanding of these processes will undoubtedly increase in the years to come.

REFERENCES

Bancroft, J. (1989). *Human sexuality and its problems*. New York: Churchill Livingstone.

Bancroft, J., O'Carroll, R., McNeilly, A., & Shaw, R. W. (1984). The effects of bromo-criptine on the sexual behavior of hyperprolactinemic men: A case study. *Clinical Endocrinology, 21*, 131–137.

Bancroft, J., Tennent, T. G., Lucas, K., & Cass, J. (1974). Control of deviant sexual behavior by drugs: Behavioral effects of estrogens and anti-androgens. *British Journal of Psychiatry, 125*, 310–315.

Bancroft, J., & Wu, F. C. (1983). Changes in erectile responsiveness during replace-ment therapy. *Archives of Sexual Behavior, 12*, 59–66.

Baskin, H. J. (1989). Endocrinologic evaluation of impotence. *Southern Medical Jour-nal, 82*, 446–449.

Beach, F. A. (1948). *Hormones and behavior*. New York: Hoeber.

Brown, W. A., Monti, P. M., & Corriveau, D. P. (1978). Serum testosterone and sexual activity and interest in men. *Archives of Sexual Behavior, 7*, 97–103.

Burris, A. S., Graceley, R. H., Carter, S. C., Sherins, R. J., & Davidson, J. M. (in press). Testosterone therapy is associated with reduced tactile sensitivity in human males. *Hormones and Behavior*.

Carani, C., Zini, D., Baldini, A., Della Casa, L., Ghizzani, A., & Marrama, P. (1990). Effect of androgen treatment in impotent men with normal and low levels of free testosterone. *Archives of Sexual Behavior, 19*, 223–234.

Carey, P. O., Howards, S. S., & Vance, M. L. (1988). Transdermal testosterone treatment of hypogonadal men. *Journal of Urology, 140*, 76–79.

Carmichael, M. S., Humbert, R., Dixen, J., Palmisano, G., Greenleaf, W., & Davidson, J. M. (1987). Plasma oxytocin increases in the human sexual response. *Journal of Clinical Endocrinology and Metabolism, 64*, 27–31.

Conway, A. J., Boylan, L. M., Howe, C., Ross, G., & Handelsman, D. J. (1988). Randomized clinical trial of testosterone replacement therapy in hypogonadal men. *International Journal of Andrology, 11*, 247–264.

Cooper, A. J. (1980). A clinical and endocrine study of mesterolone in secondary impotence. *Journal of Psychosomatic Research, 24*, 275–279.

Davidson, J. M., Camargo, C., & Smith, E. R. (1979). Effects of androgen on sexual behavior in hypogonadal men. *Journal of Clinical Endocrinology and Metabolism, 48*, 955–958.

Davidson, J. M., Kwan, M., & Greenleaf, W. (1982). Hormonal replacement and sexuality in men. *Clinics in Endocrinology and Metabolism*, *11*, 599–624.

Davidson, J. M., & Myers, L. S. (1988). Endocrine factors in sexual psychophysiology. In R. C. Rosen & J. G. Beck, *Patterns of sexual arousal: Psychophysiological processes and clinical applications* (pp. 158–186). New York: Guilford Press.

Davis, S. S., Viosca, S. P., & Guralnik, M. (1985). Evaluation of impotence in older men. *Western Journal of Medicine*, *142*, 499–505.

Dorsa, D. M., Smith, E. R., & Davidson, J. M. (1984). Immunoreactive-beta-endorphin and LHRH levels in the brains of aged male rats with impaired sex behavior. *Neurobiology of Aging*, *5*, 115–120.

Findlay, J. C., Place, V. A., & Snyder, P. J. (1987). Transdermal delivery of testosterone. *Journal of Clinical Endocrinology and Metabolism*, *64*, 266–271.

Friedman, D. E., Clare, A. W., Rees, L. H., & Grossman, A. (1986). Should impotent males who have no clinical evidence of hypogonadism have routine endocrine screening? *Lancet*, *i*, 1041.

Ghadirian, A. M., Chouinard, G., & Annable, L. (1982). Sexual dysfunction and plasma prolactin levels in neuroleptic-treated schizophrenic outpatients. *Journal of Nervous and Mental Disease*, *170*, 463–467.

Graceley, R. H., Dubner, R., & McGrathe, P. A. (1982). Fentanyl reduces the intensity of painful tooth pulp sensations: Controlling for detection of active drugs. *Anesthesia and Analgesia*, *61*, 751–755.

Green, D. M., & Swets, J. A. (1966). *Signal detection theory and psychophysics*. New York: Wiley.

Hart, B. L. (1974). Gonadal androgen and sociosexual behavior of male mammals: A comparative analysis. *Psychological Bulletin*, *81*, 383–400.

Jarow, J. P., & Lipshultz, L. I. (1990). Anabolic steroid-induced hypogonadotropic hypogonadism. *American Journal of Sports Medicine*, *18*, 429–431.

Johnston, D. G., Prescott, R. W., Kendall-Taylor, P., Hall, K., & Cook, D. B. (1983). Hyperprolactinemia: Long-term effects of bromocriptine. *American Journal of Medicine*, *75*, 868–874.

Kavich-Sharon, R. (1980). Impotence is not always psychogenic [In reply]. *Journal of the American Medical Association*, *244*, 1558–1559.

Kemper, T. D. (1990). *Social structure and testosterone*. New Brunswick, NJ: Rutgers University Press.

Knussman, R., Christiansen, K., & Couwenbergs, C. (1986). Relations between sex hormone levels and sexual behavior in men. *Archives of Sexual Behavior*, *15*, 429–445.

Kraemer, H. C., Becker, H. B., Brodie, H. K., Doering, C. H., & Hamburg, D. A. (1976). Orgasmic frequency and plasma testosterone levels in normal human males. *Archives of Sexual Behavior*, *5*, 125–132.

Krane, R. J., Goldstein, I., & Saenz de Tejada, I. (1989). Impotence. *New England Journal of Medicine*, *321*, 1648–1659.

Kwan, M., Greenleaf, W. J., Mann, J., Crapo, L., & Davidson, J. M. (1983). The nature of androgen action on male sexuality: A combined laboratory/self-report study on hypogonadal men. *Journal of Clinical Endocrinology and Metabolism*, *57*, 557–562.

Lakin, M. M. (1988). Diagnostic assessment of disorders of male sexual function. In D. K. Montague (Ed.), *Disorders of male sexual function* (pp. 26–43). Chicago: Year Book Medical.

Leiblum, S. R., & Rosen, R. C. (1988). Changing perspectives on sexual desire. In S. R. Leiblum & R. C. Rosen (Eds.), *Sexual desire disorders* (pp. 1–20). New York: Guilford Press.

Leonard, M. P., Nickel, C. J., & Morales, A. (1989). Hyperprolactinemia and impotence: Why, when and how to investigate. *Journal of Urology, 142*, 992–994.

Levine, S. B. (1988). Intrapsychic and individual aspects of sexual desire. In S. R. Leiblum & R. C. Rosen (Eds.), *Sexual desire disorders* (pp. 21–44). New York: Guilford Press.

Luisi, M., & Franchi, F. (1980). Double-blind group comparative study of testosterone undecanoate and mesterolone in hypogonadal male patients. *Journal of Endocrinological Investigation, 3*, 305–308.

Manni, A., Pardridge, W. M., & Cefalu, W. (1985). Bioavailability of albumin bound testosterone. *Journal of Clinical Endocrinology and Metabolism, 61*, 705–710.

Margolis, R., Prieto, P., Stein, L., & Chin, S. (1971). Statistical summary of 10,000 male cases using Afrodex in the treatment of impotence. *Current Therapeutics and Research, 13*, 616–621.

McClure, R. D. (1988). Endocrine evaluation and therapy. In E. A. Tanagho, T. F. Lue, & R. D. McClure (Eds.), *Contemporary management of impotence and infertility* (pp. 84–94). Baltimore: Williams & Wilkins.

Murphy, R. M., Checkley, S. A., Seckl, J. R., & Lightman, S. L. (1990). Naloxene inhibits oxytocin release at orgasm in men. *Journal of Clinical Endocrinology and Metabolism, 71*, 1056–1058.

Murphy, R. M., Seckl, J. R., Burton, S., Checkley, S. A., & Lightman, S. L. (1987). Changes in oxytocin and vasopressin secretion during sexual activity in men. *Journal of Clinical Endocrinology and Metabolism, 75*, 738–741.

Nankin, H. R., Lin, T., & Osterman, J. (1986). Chronic testosterone cypionate therapy in men with secondary impotence. *Fertility and Sterility, 46*, 300–307.

Nickel, J. C., Morales, A., Condra, M., Fenemore, J., & Surridge, D. H. (1984). Endocrine dysfunction in impotence: Incidence, significance and cost-effective screening. *Journal of Urology, 132*, 40–46.

O'Carroll, R., & Bancroft, J. (1984). Testosterone therapy for low sexual interest and erectile dysfunction in men: A controlled study. *British Journal of Psychiatry, 145*, 146–151.

Rosen, R. C., & Beck, J. G. (1988). *Patterns of sexual arousal: Psychophysiological processes and clinical applications*. New York: Guilford Press.

Rowland, D. L., Heiman, J. R., Gladue, B. A., Hatch, J. P., Doering, C. H., & Weiler, S. J. (1987). Endocrine, psychological, and genital response to sexual arousal in men. *Psychoneuroendocrinology, 12*, 149–158.

Rubin, R. T., Poland, R. E., & Tower, B. B. (1976). Prolactin-related testosterone secretion in normal adult men. *Journal of Clinical Endocrinology and Metabolism, 42*, 112–116.

Schiavi, R. C. (1990). Sexuality and aging in men. *Annual Review of Sex Research, 1*, 227–250.

Schiavi, R. C., Fisher, C., White, D., Beers, P., & Szechter, R. (1982). Hormonal variations during sleep in men with erectile dysfunction and normal controls. *Archives of Sexual Behavior, 11*, 189–200.

Schwartz, M. F., Bauman, J. E., & Masters, W. H. (1982). Hyperprolactinemia and sexual disorders in men. *Biological Psychiatry, 17*, 861–876.

Schwartz, M. F., Kolodny, R. C., & Masters, W. H. (1980). Plasma testosterone levels of sexually functional and dysfunctional men. *Archives of Sexual Behavior, 5*, 355–366.

Segraves, R. T. (1988). Hormones and libido. In S. R. Leiblum & R. C. Rosen (Eds.), *Sexual desire disorders* (pp. 271–312). New York: Guilford Press.

Sheeler, L. R., & Lakin, M. M. (1988). Hypogonadism and hyperprolactinemia. In D. K. Montague (Ed.), *Disorders of male sexual function* (pp. 120–127). Chicago: Year Book Medical.

Skakkebaek, N. E., Bancroft, J., Davidson, D. W., & Warner, P. (1981). Androgen replacement with oral testosterone undecanoate in hypogonadal men: A double blind controlled study. *Clinical Endocrinology, 14*, 49–61.

Slag, M. F., Morley, J. E., Elson, M. K., Trence, D. L., Nelson, C. J., Nelson, A. E., Kinlaw, W. B., Beyer, H. S., Nuttall, F. Q., & Shafer, R. B. (1983). Impotence in medical clinic outpatients. *Journal of the American Medical Association, 249*, 1736–1740.

Snyder, P. J. (1984). Clinical use of androgens. *Annual Review of Medicine, 35*, 207–217.

Spark, R. F., White, R. A., & Connolly, P. B. (1980). Impotence is not always psychogenic: Newer insights into hypothalamic–pituitary–gonadal dysfunction. *Journal of the American Medical Association, 243*, 750–755.

5

Aging and Drug Effects on Male Sexuality

R. Taylor Segraves and Kathleen B. Segraves

As life expectancy increases, and large numbers of individuals are maintained on chronic drug therapy, the impact of these factors on sexual function has become a critical concern for researchers and clinicians alike. In this chapter, R. Taylor Segraves and Kathleen B. Segraves provide a highly informative critique of clinical research in each of these areas, as well as clinical guidelines for evaluating erectile difficulties associated with drugs or aging.

Although several studies have documented an overall decline in sexual desire and performance in elderly men, the specific mechanisms involved are not well understood at present. Certainly, it is clear that older men have decreased penile sensitivity, lower serum testosterone levels, and diminished nocturnal penile tumescence (NPT), although a causal connection with erectile dysfunction per se has not been established. Psychological factors are equally important, as unrealistic expectations and self-defeating attitudes may undermine sexual adjustment in many elderly males. In addressing these issues, the authors advise considerable caution in interpreting test results, as well as in conducting clinical interviews with elderly male patients.

Evaluating drug effects on sexual function is similarly complex and challenging. For instance, the sexual side effects of a specific drug may vary greatly, depending upon the dosage level and duration of use, as well as the patient's age, health status, and previous level of sexual functioning. Certain categories of drugs (e.g., antihypertensives, neuroleptics) are frequently associated with erectile dysfunction, although some individuals appear more susceptible to these effects than others. In other instances, erectile difficulties may be mistakenly attributed to past or present medication use. In light of these difficulties, the authors present both empirical data and clinical guidelines for evaluating adverse drug effects in a given individual. Overall, this chapter provides an unusually detailed and comprehensive review of both prescription and nonprescription drug effects on male sexual response.

While the search for the perfect aphrodisiac continues, several oral medications (e.g., yohimbine, apomorphine) have recently been shown to have positive effects on erectile capacity. Although the mechanisms involved have not been sufficiently studied, these agents offer a potential alternative to more invasive treatments, such as intracorporal injections or a surgical implant. These drugs may also play an increasing role in the treatment of psychogenic erectile difficulties, as illustrated by the final case vignette in the chapter.

R. Taylor Segraves, M.D., Ph.D., is Associate Director of the Department of Psychiatry, Cleveland Metropolitan General Hospital, and Professor of Psychiatry at Case Western Reserve University School of Medicine. He is the past president of the Society for Sex Therapy and Research, and has published widely in the area of medical and psychological evaluation of erectile disorders.

Kathleen B. Segraves, Ph.D., is Director of Behavioral Medicine in the Department of Psychiatry, MetroHealth Medical Center, and Assistant Professor of Psychiatry at Case Western Reserve University School of Medicine. She is on the Advisory Committee for the World Association for Sexology, and has published widely in the areas of behavioral medicine and sexual disorders.

Two ubiquitous influences exerting possible deleterious effects on the erectile response are aging and drugs. According to the 1980 census, 11% of the U.S. population was over 65 years of age. By the year 2000, slightly less than 20% of our population will be over 65. Americans aged 85 or over constitute the fastest-growing segment of our population (Leiblum & Segraves, 1989; Labby, 1985). With increasing life expectancy and decreased societal taboos regarding sexuality, many of these older individuals are turning to physicians and sex therapists for advice and assistance. Clearly, the professional needs to be aware of the "natural" effects of aging in order to counsel such individuals and to know when a complaint appears to go beyond the natural consequences of aging and merits a full medical evaluation.

The advances of modern medicine have contributed to the longevity of our population. Many commonly prescribed pharmacological agents were unimaginable several decades ago. The histamine H_2 blockers have drastically reduced the need for major abdominal surgery for duodenal ulcers. Antihypertensive drugs have increased longevity by reducing the incidence of stroke and other forms of cardiovascular disease. The pharmacological capacity to induce penile erections in men with organic erectile impairment has restored sexual function to many men. Drugs are now available to combat baldness, and in 1990 the Food and Drug Administration approved a drug for the treatment of obsessive–compulsive disorder. The list of new agents is seemingly endless. However, most of our pharmacological agents have influences on multiple organ systems as well as the target organ, and we are becoming increasingly aware that many drugs adversely influence the sexual system. Nonprescription drugs are also used by a large segment of society, and many of these agents may also adversely affect sexual function.

The purpose of this chapter is to summarize the evidence concerning both aging and drug effects on the erectile response.

AGING AND MALE SEXUALITY

It is well known that the prevalence of erectile failure increases with age, and that disease processes and the treatments of the disease account for a large percentage of this increased prevalence. However, a number of studies have indicated a progressive decline in sexual function in "healthy" aging men. Because other chapters in this text address the effect of disease on sexual function, this section focuses on the decline in function that is due presumably to age and not to disease.

A number of studies have documented a gradual decline in sexual activity after age 50, with a more precipitous decline in the frequency of coital activity after age 70 (Hegeler & Mortensen, 1977; Pfeiffer, 1974; Kinsey, Pomeroy, & Martin, 1948; Verwoerdt, Pfeiffer, & Wang, 1969; Davidson, Kwan, & Greenleaf, 1982). For example, Pfeiffer (1974) found that about 70% of the men surveyed were sexually active at age 68. By age 78, the number who were sexually active dropped to 25%. Similar findings were reported by Hegeler and Mortensen (1977) in their questionnaire study of 1,163 Danish men between the ages of 51 and 95. In the 51- to 55-year-old group, 94% were sexually active. Corresponding percentages at ages 66–70, 78–80, and 91–95 were 75%, 36%, and 3%, respectively. Pearlman and Kobashi (1972) questioned 2,801 men seen in the private practice of urology about their sexual activity. Although 86% of patients under 20 years old and 80% of patients in their 40s reported weekly sexual activity, only 50% in the sixth decade and 10% in the eighth decade of life indicated this level of activity. Masters and Johnson (1966, 1977) compared the sexual response of 20 men aged 50–70 years with that of men aged between 20 and 40 years, and noted a number of changes in the older group; these included greater latency to erection, less turgid erections, less forceful ejaculation, decreased ejaculatory demand, and a longer refractory period.

A number of studies of nocturnal penile tumescence (NPT) have demonstrated an age-related decline in nocturnal erections (Kahn & Fisher, 1969; Reynolds et al., 1989; Karacan, Hursch, & Williams, 1972; Karacan, Williams, Thornby, & Salis, 1975), with the major decrement occurring after age 60 (Schiavi & Schreiner-Engel, 1988; Schiavi, Schreiner-Engel, Mandeli, Schanzer, & Cohen, 1990). Schiavi and Schreiner-Engel (1988) noted a discrepancy between self-reports of continued sexual activity in older men and NPT records demonstrating erectile impairment. They suggested that NPT monitoring may yield false impressions of organicity in some elderly patients. They also noted that NPT may be a reflection of central sexual arousal processes. The influence of aging on NPT is covered more fully by Schiavi in Chapter 6 of this text. Because erection in the human is mediated by both a thoracolumbar outflow mediating psychogenic erections and a sacral outflow mediating reflexogenic erections, NPT may not measure erections mediated by tactile sensation. Other research has also indicated a decrease in penile tactile sensitivity with age, the change being precipitous after age 65 (Newman, 1970). Recent investigation has documented the association of decreased penile sensation with decreased erectile function (Gerstenberg, Nordling, Hald, & Wagner, in press). Although the relative contribution of sensory sensitivity to erectile function has been minimally investigated to date, sexual arousal is probably partially maintained by penile tactile sensation. Age-related decrements in penile sensitivity may be another factor contributing to decreased sexual activity in aging males.

Thus, research has demonstrated an age-related decline in sexual activity, in NPT, and in penile sensitivity. An age-related decline in sexual desire has also been documented (Schiavi, 1990b). Numerous investigators have searched for the explanation for this decline in male sexual behavior. Because androgens are related to sexual behavior, sexual libido, and penile sensitivity (in lower animals at least), and because androgens also demonstrate an age-related decline, numerous researchers have questioned whether declining androgen levels may explain decreased sexual activity in elderly men.

Research has clearly indicated that total serum testosterone and serum free testosterone levels decrease progressively with age. The mean testosterone level in the ninth decade is usually approximately only two-thirds of that in the third decade (Neaves, Johnson, Porter, Parker, & Petty, 1984; Bancroft, 1983). After the sixth decade, mean plasma levels tend to decline rather rapidly (Vermeulen, Rubens, & Verdonck, 1971). Nankin and Calkins (1986) pointed out that bioavailable testosterone includes both free testosterone and albumin-bound testosterone. An estimate of bioavailable testosterone can be obtained by precipitating sex-hormone-binding globulin (SHBG). The supernatant non-SHBG-bound testosterone is thus a good estimate of bioavailable testosterone. This measure of testosterone also declines with age. Tissue concentration of free testosterone has also been shown to decrease with age, signifying a decreased availability of androgens to peripheral tissue in elderly patients (Deslypere & Vermuelen, 1981). This decrease in serum androgens with aging is thought to result primarily from decreased testicular production of androgen (Neaves et al., 1984), although other investigators have proposed that the decreased testosterone production is secondary to changes with aging in the hypothalamic–pituitary complex, which regulates sex hormone production (Vermeulen, 1986).

Clearly, there is evidence of a decline in serum testosterone with aging, as well as clear evidence of a decline in sexual function with aging. A logical question is whether the decline in serum testosterone causes the decline in sexual activity with age. The available data are not clear. In the Baltimore Longitudinal Study on Aging (Tsitouras, Martin, & Hartman, 1982), 183 men aged 60–79 were extensively studied. Sexual histories, serum testosterone, and various other parameters were studied. Although serum testosterone did not decrease with age, sexual activity declined in a predictable fashion. The authors suggested that the findings of a relationship between testosterone and sexual activity in older men might indicate that higher testosterone levels are necessary to overcome target tissue insensitivity produced by aging. Somewhat similar findings were reported by Davidson et al. (1982). Hormonal and behavioral measures were studied in 220 men aged 41–93. Although small correlations were found between hormonal and sexual behavior variables, a multiple-regression analysis indicated that hormone level accounted for only a minor portion of the behavioral variance. A much larger part of the variability in sexual behavior was accounted for by age. These authors suggested that the sexual decline with age may reflect a change in androgen sensitivity in the target tissue, rather than a change in androgen production. Schiavi (1990b) also reported a relationship between aging and declining bioavailable testosterone. Bioavailable testosterone and various aspects of sexual behavior were also significantly interrelated.

Although research has consistently shown that androgen levels decrease with aging and that this decrease corresponds with a decrease in sexual function, the available evidence does not permit a definitive statement as to the relative role played by declining androgens in the decline of male sexual behavior with aging. The available evidence also does not permit a statement as to the relative importance of decreased circulating androgen versus decreased target sensitivity.

CLINICAL SIGNIFICANCE OF AGING EFFECTS

It is important to emphasize that the age of onset and rate of decline of sexual function are widely variable. A small number of men in their 70s might have an intercourse frequency equivalent to that of men in their 30s or 40s. Unfortunately, most men in their 70s will not. The decline in the responsivity of the genitals to sexual stimuli need not represent a total cessation of activity or failure of function unless physical disease intervenes. Clinically, one may encounter men of advanced years who are trying to force themselves to perform at a level more characteristic of younger men. These men may not have successfully dealt with their feelings about growing older and may require brief supportive psychotherapy before they are able to accept information about the impact of aging on male sexual function.

It is imperative that the neurophysiology laboratory evaluating the patient be experienced in the evaluation of older men, and thus interpret a record demonstrating impaired NPT with some degree of skepticism. The assessment of erectile problems in aging males is complicated. It is often quite difficult to distinguish between pathology and normal physiological variation associated with aging, as discussed more fully in Chapter 6 by Schiavi. On numerous occasions, we have been made aware of the difficulties associated with the use of NPT studies in the assessment of erectile capacity in older males. For example, one of us (R.T.S.) referred a 73-year-old carnival worker with a complaint of erectile dysfunction to our neurophysiological laboratory for evaluation. The NPT record was read as consistent with biogenic erectile dysfunction. On two nights of testing, the patient demonstrated minimal erectile capacity. His maximum erection of 1.8 cm was judged as 60% of full and of insufficient turgidity for vaginal penetration. The patient listened carefully as R.T.S related the report to him and explained the various treatment options available. R.T.S. then inquired whether the patient would like an appointment to pursue one of these options with a urologist. He replied that this would not be necessary. When R.T.S. inquired why the patient did not wish to pursue this further, he replied that the sleep test had "cured" him! He had resumed successful intercourse with his partner.

In evaluating the elderly patient, it is critical that the clinician take a very careful history. As in younger patients, the clinician should search in the history for specific indications of disease processes. For example, a patient with diabetes mellitus should receive a careful neurological evaluation. In addition, the clinician should inquire carefully regarding sexual drive, and should distinguish between subjective libido and societally generated expectations. For example, a 66-year-old plumber married to a 48-year-old beautician sought treatment in our pharmacological erection program because of erectile failure. He claimed strong libido and a desire for daily coitus. His wife rolled her eyes at this statement, inviting the therapist to query her about her apparent disbelief. She revealed that his desired frequency for coitus had increased significantly after his retirement, and that he had also become increasingly competitive with their sons. The therapist then inquired as to what she thought this meant. She replied, "He wants to be sure he's still a man." This gradually led to a discussion of normal aging and the gradual diminution of libido with age. The plumber kept watching his watch, and was clearly relieved when the hour was over. The therapist thought that the hour was wasted. However, 2 weeks later, he received a call from the beautician. She stated that they had had a big argument on the way home and she had told him that "acting like a baby over getting older didn't make him a bigger man in her eyes." The next evening, he had attempted coitus. She had assisted him manually in maintaining his erection. Approximately 1 week later, they had again engaged in coitus.

DRUG EFFECTS ON ERECTILE FUNCTION

Within the last decade, sex therapists and physicians in general have come increasingly to realize that many commonly prescribed pharmacological agents may adversely affect sexual functioning (Papadopoulos, 1989; Segraves, 1989; Jarowenko & Bennett, 1982). It is critical for clinicians to be aware of these drug side effects on sexual function, because they represent easily reversible causes of sexual disturbance. Failure to recognize these effects may also lead to treatment noncompliance in many patients. More importantly, the clinical presentation of drug side effects may resemble symptoms of organic impotence, and misdiagnosis may lead to unnecessary surgical intervention.

For most of the drugs whose use appears to be associated with sexual problems, the quality of the evidence for this association is less than optimal. Controlled double-blind studies are the exception rather than the rule in this area of inquiry. Most generalizations are based upon case reports and clinical series of different agents in heterogeneous populations. The methodology employed has varied widely, from sexual questionnaires and standardized interviews, to simple records of the frequency of unsolicited patient complaints. For many drugs that have been available for some time, our knowledge base is relatively secure: The sheer number of case reports and/or repeated independent studies of large numbers of men experiencing these problems makes the association highly probable.

Although specific drugs have been demonstrated to have an adverse effect on most aspects of sexual function, this section focuses on drug effects on erectile function.

Hypotensive Agents

More than 60 million people in the United States have elevated blood pressure (Joint National Committee on Detection, Evaluation and Treatment of High Blood Pressure, 1984). Because hypertensive arterial disease is associated with a higher risk for cerebral vascular accident, myocardial infarction, congestive heart failure, and renal failure, most physicians treat hypertensive disease vigorously. Our knowledge of the frequent association of hypotensive medication with sexual dysfunction may represent the prevalence of this disorder and the frequency with which hypotensive agents are prescribed, rather than an unusual propensity for these agents to cause erectile dysfunction. It is also noteworthy that 8–10% of untreated hypertensive patients have erectile problems (Oaks & Moyer, 1972). The information concerning the effects of antihypertensive drugs on erectile function is summarized in Table 5.1.

Diuretics

Diuretics are generally the first agents utilized in the treatment of essential hypertensive, with other drugs added to the treatment regimen if diuretics alone provide insufficient control of blood pressure (McMahon, 1978). In the past, it was thought that diuretics rarely caused impotence (Segraves, Mad-

TABLE 5.1.   Antihypertensive Drugs and Erectile Failure

Drug	Class[a]	Effect[b]
Hydrochlorothiazide	Diuretic	3
Chlorthalidone	Diuretic	3
Spironolactone	Diuretic	3
Methyldopa	Central antiadrenergic	4
Clonidine	Central antiadrenergic	4
Reserpine	Central antiadrenergic	4
Guanethidine	Peripheral antiadrenergic	4
Prazosin	Peripheral antiadrenergic	1
Hydralazine	Vasodilator	2
Propranolol	Beta blocker	4
Atenolol	Beta blocker	2
Pindolol	Beta blocker	2
Metoprolol	Beta blocker	2
Nadolol	Beta blocker	1
Acebutolol	Beta blocker	1
Timolol	Beta blocker	2
Labetalol	Mixed blocker	2
Captopril	ACE inhibitor	1
Enalapril	ACE Inhibitor	1
Lisinopril	ACE inhibitor	1
Nifedipine	Ca channel blocker	2
Verapamil	Ca channel blocker	3

[a]ACE, angiotensin-converting-enzyme; Ca, calcium.
[b]1, unlikely to cause erectile problems; 2, uncertain; 3, probable; 4, highly probable.

sen, Carter, & Davis, 1985). However, some investigators suspect a relationship between diuretic use and erectile dysfunction. There have been several case reports of impotence associated with hydrochlorothiazide (Keidan, 1976; Boyden, Nugent, & Ogihara, 1980). Bulpitt and Dollery (1973) administered a questionnaire to 477 hypertensive patients and found that 31% of men on diuretics alone complained of impotence. Hogan, Wallin, and Baer (1980), in a questionnaire study of 861 male hypertensives, reported that 9% of men taking hydrochlorothiazide alone complained of erectile failure. Williams, Croog, Levine, Testa, and Sudilovsky (1987) reported that the addition of hydrochlorothiazide to patients on methyldopa, captopril, or propranolol significantly increased the incidence of sexual dysfunction. The propranolol–diuretic combination had the greatest impact on sexual function. The Veterans Administration Cooperative Study Group on Antihypertensive Agents (1982) also reported as increased incidence of impotence in patients taking hydrochlorothiazide, as compared to pretreatment. However, Bauer, Baker, and Hunyor (1978) found no difference in the incidence of erectile dysfunction in chlorothiazide-treated men, as compared to placebo-treated patients.

The Medical Research Council of Great Britain (Medical Research Council Working Party on Mild to Moderate Hypertension, 1981) examined the effect of bendrofluozide on sexual function and reported that 23% of men on this drug complained of impotence, as compared to 10% for placebo. Chlorthalidone, a thiazide-like diuretic, has also been reported to cause erectile problems (Stressman & Ben-Ishay, 1980; Pillay, 1976). In a study of 31 normotensive men and 19 patients on chlorthalidone, Geissler, Turnlund, and Cohen (1986) found that men on chlorthalidone reported erectile dysfunction and impaired libido more often than controls.

From the available evidence, it is impossible to state definitively that any of the diuretics causes erectile dysfunction, although there does seem increasing evidence of an association. The evidence regarding hydrochlorothiazide is conflicting, and there is relatively little evidence concerning bendrofluozide and chlorthalidone. The mechanism whereby diuretics might impair erectile function is unclear. Zinc depletion has been proposed (Papadopoulos, 1989); however, chlorthalidone usage has been shown to be associated with elevated serum and hair zinc levels.

Spironolactone is an aldosterone antagonist and acts as a potassium-sparing diuretic (Moss & Procci, 1982). This drug has been reported to cause gynecomastia (Spark & Melby, 1968), diminished libido (Spark & Melby, 1968), and impotence (Spark & Melby, 1968; Brown et al., 1972; Greenblatt & Koch-Weser, 1973; Zarren & Black, 1975). Several investigators have reported that impotence associated with spironolactone remits when the drug is discontinued. In one clinical series of 42 patients with hyperaldosteronism, 30% reported "relative impotence" while engaged in high-dose spironolactone therapy (Spark & Melby, 1968). In another series, only 1 out of 26 men on spironolactone therapy developed impotence (Brown et al., 1972).

From the available information, it is impossible to ascertain the frequency with which spironolactone causes erectile problems. Sexual side effects of the drug appear to be mediated by its anti-androgenic effects (Loriaux, Menard, Taylor, Pita, & Santen, 1976).

Methyldopa

Methyldopa is one of the most commonly used antihypertensive medications and is frequently employed as a "second-step" drug if diuretics alone do not control blood pressure. Its mechanism of action is activation of inhibitory alpha-adrenergic receptors in the brain, decreasing sympathetic outflow. Whereas some investigators have found minimal or no effects of methyldopa on erectile capacity (Bulpitt & Dollery, 1973; Curd et al., 1985; Prichard, Johnston, Hill, & Rossenheim, 1968; Bauer, Hull, & Stokes, 1973; Johnson, Kitchin, & Lowther, 1966), others have reported that methyldopa frequently causes erectile impairment (Pillay, 1976; Newman & Salerno, 1974; Kolodny, 1987; Alexander & Evans, 1974).

An interesting report by Alexander and Evans (1974) may explain discrepancies in the literature. They found that 53% of hypertensives, when directly questioned, complained of impotence while taking methyldopa. However, only 7% volunteered this information on a questionnaire. In general, studies employing direct questioning have reported higher frequencies of sexual disorders on methyldopa than those employing questionnaires or relying on patients' volunteering of information (Stevenson & Umsted, 1984; Moss & Procci, 1982). Recent studies by Lipson and colleagues (Lipson, Moore, Pope, Todd, & Avila, 1981; Lipson, 1985) provide more evidence that methyldopa interferes with erectile function. In the first study, utilizing detailed sexual questioning, 75% of diabetes on methyldopa and hydrochlorothiazide had erectile problems. When prazosin was substituted for methyldopa, 79% showed improvement. In the second study, a single-blind, placebo-controlled, crossover study examined the effect of methyldopa and prazosin on erectile function. Placebo and prazosin caused significantly less impairment than methyldopa. This finding was confirmed by subsequent NPT studies. A recent multicenter, randomized, double-blind clinical trial (Croog, Levine, Sudilovsky, Baume, & Clive, 1988) has reported that methyldopa plus a diuretic is associated with an increased incidence of both erectile and ejaculatory problems.

Although methyldopa has clearly been shown to be associated with erectile failure, the mechanism by which this occurs remains obscure. Animal research has suggested that the effects of methyldopa on erectile function in rats is mediated by inhibitory effects on the central nervous system (Melman, Fersel, & Weinstein, 1984).

Clonidine

Clonidine is believed to reduce blood pressure by its stimulation of hypothalamic and medullary alpha receptors, a mechanism similar to that of methyldopa. Sexual dysfunction has been reported less frequently with clonidine than with methyldopa, and various investigators have suggested that clonidine has minimal or no sexual side effects (Raftos, Bauer, & Lewis, 1973; Saunders & Kong, 1980; Amery, Verstraete, & Bossaert, 1970; Ferder, Inserra, & Medina, 1987). However, numerous authors have reported that small numbers of patients become impotent while taking clonidine (Segraves et al., 1985). Mroczek, Davidou, and Finnerty (1972) reported that 17% of patients on this drug experienced impotence. Using a patient interview, Onesti, Bock, and Heimsoth (1971) found that 24 out of 59 patients (41%) complained of erectile dysfunction while taking clonidine. This represented a significant increase from the pretreatment frequency of such complaints. Clonidine has recently been found to decrease the duration of NPT in a prospective placebo-controlled study in hypertensive patients (Kostis et al., 1990). Finally, a recent study has shown that injection of clonidine into the internal pudendal artery of dogs suppressed penile intracorporeal pressure (Lin et al., 1988).

Reserpine

Reserpine is used for the treatment of mild hypertension or as an adjunctive treatment with other drugs to treat moderate to severe hypertension. The use of reserpine in the treatment of hypertension has declined dramatically. Its mechanism of action is presumed to be similar to that of methyldopa and clonidine. Case reports have linked reserpine administration with complaints of impotence (Boyden et al., 1980; Bulpitt & Dollery, 1973; Laver, 1974; Veterans Administration Cooperative Study Group on Antihypertensive Agents, 1977; Tuchman & Crumpton, 1955) and difficulty with ejaculation (Bulpitt & Dollery, 1973; Laver, 1974; Girgis, Etriby, & El-Hefnawy, 1968). However, it is unclear how frequently these side effects are encountered. Bulpitt and Dollery (1973) reported that 33% of patients on reserpine complained of erectile failure. However, a similar number of patients on diuretics alone expressed similar complaints. Laver (1974) reported that 46% of patients on reserpine had significant sexual impairment. In a study of veterans (Participating Veterans Administration Medical Centers, 1982), the incidence of impotence in patients taking reserpine was dose-related, with a higher incidence at the 0.25-mg dose.

Guanethidine

Guanethidine is used to treat moderate to severe hypertensive disease. It is believed to exert its hypotensive action through interference with norepinephrine release by peripheral nerve terminals. Although its major side effect appears to be failure of ejaculation or delayed ejaculation (Girgis et al., 1968; Moser, Prandoni, & Orison, 1974; Schinger & Gifford, 1962; Bulpitt & Dollery, 1973; Brahma, Chowdhury, & Sarkar, 1966), erectile failure also appears to be associated with guanethidine use. In a previous publication (Segraves et al., 1985), nine separate studies of the effect of guanethidine on impotence were reviewed. In these studies, 222 patients were investigated, and 54 patients (24%) complained of erectile failure. In a large-scale multiple-site study of experience treating hypertensive disease, 5,485 patients were studied (Curd et al., 1985). Of the six drugs studied, guanethidine had the largest number of patients withdrawing because of erectile failure or retrograde ejaculation. The mechanism by which guanethidine causes erectile failure is unclear. However, the corpora cavernosa contain adrenergic as well as cholinergic terminals.

Prazosin

Prazosin is believed to exert its hypotensive action by blockade of postsynaptic alpha-adrenergic receptors, resulting in relaxation of peripheral arterioles (Brogden, Heel, Speight, & Avery, 1977). Most investigators report that this drug is minimally associated with erectile insufficiency (New Zealand Hypertension Study Group, 1977; Stokes & Oates, 1978; Pitts, 1974), and some investigators have even reported priapism with this agent (Bhalla, Hoffbrand, & Phatak, 1979; Burke & Hirst, 1980; Adams & Soucheray, 1984; Banos, Bosch, & Farre, 1989). In the Veterans Administration Cooperative Study Group on Antihypertensive Agents (1981), prazosin had a significantly elevated incidence of sexual dysfunction as compared to hydralazine. Unfortunately, this study did not specify the type of sexual dysfunction indexed. Thus, the results of this otherwise well-conducted study are uninterpretable for the purposes of this review. Quite different results were reported by Lipson (1985). In a single-blind crossover study, prazosin and placebo were equal in the frequency of erectile impairment, and both had lower frequencies than methyldopa. This absence of an effect of prazosin on erectile function was confirmed by NPT recording (portable home recording devices). Because prazosin is an alpha-1 blocker (Luther, 1989), and as the flaccid state of the penis is presumably mediated by alpha-1 receptors (Segraves, 1989), one would expect prazosin to be associated with priapism rather than erectile failure.

Hydralazine

Hydralazine lowers blood pressure by directly relaxing arteriolar smooth muscle. There have been relatively few reports of sexual dysfunction associated with this drug, and a few investigators have suggested that this drug may facilitate erectile function. Ahmad (1980b) reported a case of a patient who developed impotence when hydralazine was added to a treatment regimen of propranolol and furosemide. When the hydralazine was discontinued, erectile function returned to baseline. When the patient was rechallenged with hydralazine, the impotence recurred. Keidan (1976) reported a case of a patient on hydrochlorothiazide who became impotent when hydralazine was added to the regimen; the impotence remitted when both drugs were discontinued. In the Veterans Administration Cooperative Study (1981), 8.5% of patients on hydralazine reported impotence for at least two visits. However, the absence of a comparison group makes this data difficult to interpret. It is also of note that there has been a report of priapism possibly related to hydralazine therapy (Rubin, 1968). Davies (1979) reported the return of libido and erectile function in a man taking oxprenolol when hydralazine was substituted for hydrochlorothiazide.

Beta Blockers

Beta-blocking agents can be subclassified by their affinity for beta-1 receptors (located in the heart) or for beta-2 receptors (located on arteries, arterioles, and other tissues); by their tendency to cross the blood–brain barrier (lipophilic vs. hydrophilic); and by the presence or absence of intrinsic sympathomimetic activity. For the reader's convenience, the major beta blockers and their characteristics are listed in Table 5.2. The obvious significance of this information is that if an agent that is lipophilic causes erectile dysfunction and another agent that is hydrophilic does not, one has suggestive evidence that the ability of the drug to cross the blood–brain barrier may be related to its propensity to cause sexual dysfunction. This has both theoreti-

TABLE 5.2. Characteristics of Beta Blockers

Name	Cardioselective?	Lipophilic?	Intrinsic sympathetic activity?
Propranolol	No	Yes	No
Nadolol	No	No	No
Timolol	No	—	No
Pindolol	No	Yes	Yes
Metoprolol	Yes	Yes	No
Atenolol	Yes	No	No
Acebutolol	Yes	—	Yes

cal (i.e., central vs. peripheral mechanism of action) and practical (switching to the hydrophilic drug) significance.

Propranolol, a nonselective lipophilic drug, has been the major beta blocker used in hypertension control, and the majority of reports associating erectile failure with beta blockers concern propranolol (Bansal, 1988). A number of investigators relying on patient self-reports or questionnaires have reported that erectile dysfunction is associated with propranolol therapy for hypertensive disease (Williams et al., 1987; Medical Research Council Working Party on Mild to Moderate Hypertension, 1981; Bauer et al., 1978; Warren, Brewer, & Orgain, 1976; Warren & Warren, 1977; Burnett & Chanine, 1979; Knarr, 1976; Miller, 1976; Hogan et al., 1980).

Burnett and Chanine (1979) used a semistructured interview to assess sexual function in 46 patients treated with propranolol. Patients reporting prior sexual dysfunction were excluded from the study. Fifteen percent complained of complete erectile failure, and another 28% complained of diminished erectile quality. Those complaining of more severe sexual difficulties were on higher dosage schedules. A threshold effect for producing erectile impairment appeared to occur at about 160-180 mg per day. Sexual side effects occured within 1-4 weeks after therapy was initiated. Hollifield, Sherman, and Vanderzwagg (1976) also reported a higher frequency of sexual difficulties at higher dose levels. In a comparison of propranolol and labetalol in the treatment of hypertension, Due, Giguere, and Plachetka (1986) reported impotence to occur significantly more often with propranolol.

In the most elegantly designed study to date, Rosen, Kostis, and Jekelis (1988) studied the effect of atenolol (100 mg q.d.), metoprolol (200 mg q.d.), pindolol (20 mg q.d.), and propranolol (160 mg q.d.) in 30 normotensive males in a double-blind placebo-controlled study. Erectile function was assessed by NPT testing and by questionnaires. Minimal effects were noted on sexual function. The absence of observed effects on erectile function is probably attributable to the brevity of the exposure to propranolol. However, two recent studies have provided evidence that propranolol causes erectile impairment. In a double-blind multicenter study (Croog et al., 1988), erectile problems were more common with propranolol. In another study (Kostis et al., 1990), propranolol was found to decrease the amplitude of NPT.

The current evidence is highly suggestive that higher doses of propranolol taken for 1-4 weeks produce erectile failure (Moss & Procci, 1982). The mechanism by which this occurs is uncertain. It has been suggested that propranolol-induced impotence may be due to central nervous system beta-adrenergic blockade (Moss & Procci, 1982) and to reduction of central sympathetic outflow (Stevenson & Umsted, 1984). Propranolol has also been shown to decrease serum testosterone (Rosen et al., 1988).

It has been suggested that beta blockers with less lipophilicity, and thus less central nervous system penetration, should have a lessened propensity to cause erectile dysfunction (Sharifi, 1982). Atenolol is a hydrophilic beta blocker. Although there have been case reports of impotence associated with atenolol (Simpson, 1977; Douglas-Jones & Cruickshank, 1976; Ambrosini, Costa, & Montebugnoli, 1983), Bathen (1978) reported a case of erectile impairment on propranolol, which was relieved by the substitution of atenolol.

In one series, Zacharias, Cowan, and Cuthbertson (1977) reported that one out of 543 patients taking atenolol developed impotence. In another series, Zacharias (1980) reported that the incidence of impotence on this drug did not differ from the incidence on placebo. However, Suzuki, Tominaga, Kumagai, and Saruta (1988), measuring sexual side effects by a self-administered questionnaire, reported that 26% of 39 patients on 50–100 mg atenolol developed erectile impairment. During placebo treatment, only 5% reported such impairment.

Pindolol is a nonselective lipophilic beta blocker. There is relatively little information concerning sexual side effects with this drug. This reflects perhaps relatively little clinical experience with this drug, rather than an absence of such side effects. In a multicenter European study, however, the incidence of impotence with pindolol was only 0.03% (Rosenthal, 1979).

Metoprolol is another lipophilic beta blocker. Materson et al., (1989), in a double-blind comparison of dilevalol and metoprolol, reported that 4 of 137 patients on metoprolol developed impotence during the drug trial. The method by which sexual side effect information was obtained was not specified.

Nadolol is a hydrophilic beta blocker that has rarely been reported to be associated with erectile failure. Three independent large series have all reported the incidence of impotence to be less than 1% on this agent (Jackson, 1980; Schimert & Buschbeck, 1981; Alexander, Christie, Vernam, Fand, & Shafer, 1984). The Veterans Administration Study Group on Antihypertensive Drugs (1983) reported that 5 out of 132 patients on 80–240 mg of nadolol developed impotence during the multicenter trial.

There is minimal information concerning sexual side effects with acebutolol. One investigation reported erectile impairment to occur in 2% or fewer of patients on this drug (Wahl, Turlapaty, & Singh, 1985). Similarly, little evidence is available concerning sexual side effects with timolol. Impotence has been reported after the use of timolol eye drops to decrease intraocular pressure (McMahon, Shaffer, & Hoskins, 1979; Fraunfelder & Meyer, 1985). In one large series of patients treated with timolol for hypertension, fewer than 1% developed impotence (Attalla, Saheb, & Randall, 1981).

Labetalol is a lipid-soluble drug with mixed nonspecific beta blockade and alpha-1 antagonism. The ratio of its beta to alpha blockade is approximately 3:1 (MacCarthy & Bloomfield, 1983). Although Stokes, Mennie, Gellatly, and Hill (1983) reported erectile and ejaculatory problems to be more common with labetalol than with metoprolol or prazosin, other investigators have reported that erectile problems with this drug are very infrequent (Tcherdakoff, 1983) and that this drug causes a lower incidence of erectile difficulties than propranolol (Due et al., 1986; Burris et al., 1986).

Angiotensin-Converting-Enzyme Inhibitors

The synthesis of angiotensin-converting-enzyme inhibitors introduced a new class of drugs in the treatment of arterial hypertension. Drugs such as captopril, enalapril, and lisinopril are believed to exert their antihypertensive effect through inhibition of the renin–angiotensin–aldosterone system. Very little is known about the sexual side effect profile of these drugs. In a double-blind study of enalapril (an angiotensin-converting-enzyme inhibitor) and atenolol in 16 men, Ohman and Karlberg (1984) reported the absence of sexual side effects until hydrochlorothiazide was added to the treatment regimen. In the large multicenter study reported by Croog et al. (1988), captopril did not adversely influence any aspect of male sexual function.

Calcium Channel Blockers

Calcium channel blockers include drugs such as verapamil, nifedipine, and diltiazem. These drugs selectively antagonize calcium movements and are used in the treatment of hypertension, angina, and certain cardiac arrhythmias. There is relatively little information concerning the sexual effects of these drugs. There have been case reports of impotence associated with verapamil (Fogelman, 1987, 1988; King et al., 1983), and impotence has been reported to be infrequent with nifedipine (Marley & Curram, 1989; Marley, 1989). Suzuki et al. (1988) reported impaired ejaculation to be common with slow-release nifedipine.

Clinical Significance of the Effects of Hypotensive Agents

As is obvious from this rather extensive review, a large number of commonly prescribed hypotensive agents may cause erectile problems. Although this review indicates that certain agents (e.g., propranolol, methyldopa, clonidine, and guanethidine) are highly likely to have sexual side effects, and that other agents (e.g., prazosin, hydralazine, atenolol, labetalol, and especially captopril) are unlikely to be associated with erectile dysfunction, it is important to stress that any agent may cause erectile difficulties in certain patients. For example, if the patient has moderate occlusive disease of the hypogastric–cavernous arterial bed, the decrease in systemic blood pressure produced by any effective hypotensive agent may result in decreased perfusion pressure in the lacunar spaces, thus reducing penile rigidity (Krane, Goldstein, & Saenz de Tejada, 1989). It is also important to stress that there is considerable individual variation in vulnerability of erectile function to different drugs. In other words, the existing literature can only serve as a general guide to patient management.

Determining whether a given hypotensive agent is responsible for erectile impairment in a given patient may prove exceedingly difficult. Arterial hypertensive disease is a chronic disease. This means that the patient who complains of erectile failure may have been treated for hypertensive disease for 10 years prior to seeking a consultation for this problem. During this time period, he may have had numerous drug and dosage adjustments and may have switched physicians numerous times. He probably will not be able to remember reliably when the dose adjustments occurred, or even when his erectile difficulties began.

Other Nonpsychiatric Drugs

Other nonpsychiatric drugs possibly affecting erectile capacity are listed in Table 5.3.

Disopyramide

Disopyramide is an older antiarrhythmia drug. Several case reports have documented impotence on this drug, which remitted with drug discontinuation (Ahmad, 1980a) or lowering of the dose (McHaffie, Guz, & Johnson, 1977). We ourselves have encountered two patients who developed erectile failure on this drug and whose sexual function normalized upon drug discontinuation. These cases have not been previously reported.

Amiodarone

Amiodarone is another antiarrhythmia drug. There have been several case reports of impotence on this drug (Heger, Solow, Prystowsky, & Zipes, 1984; Anastasiou-Nana et al., 1986). However, the evidence at present is insufficient to permit us to evaluate the significance of these reports.

Perhexiline

Perhexiline is an antiangina drug. In one series, 12 out of 16 men on this drug complained (upon direct questioning) of erectile dysfunction. However, drug discontinuation did not result in return of function (Howard & Rees, 1976). In another series, 8 out of 43 men developed impotence on 400 mg

TABLE 5.3. Other Medical Drugs and Erectile Failure

Drug	Class	Effect[a]
Disopyramide	Antiarrhythmic	3
Amiodarone	Antiarrhythmic	2
Perhexiline	Antiangina	2
Clofibrate	Hypolipidemic	3
Digitalis	Cardiac drug	3
Cimetidine	Antiulcer	4
Ranitidine	Antiulcer	1
Acetazolamide	Glaucoma drug	3
Ethoxzolamide	Glaucoma drug	3
Dichlorphenamide	Glaucoma drug	3
Methazolamide	Glaucoma drug	3
Indomethacin	Prostaglandin inhibitor	2
Primidone	Seizure drug	2
Thiabendazole	Trichinosis drug	2
Methantheline	Anticholinergic	2
Baclofen	Antispasmodic	2
Ketoconazole	Antifungal	2
Disulfiram	Alcohol treatment	3

[a]1, unlikely to cause erectile problems; 2, uncertain; 3, probable; 4, highly probable.

per day of perhexiline. Three of these men discontinued use of the drug, and sexual function normalized in two of the three (Pilcher et al., 1973).

Clofibrate

Clofibrate is one of the widely used hypolipidemic drugs. There have been case reports of erectile dysfunction with this drug (Schneider & Kaffarnik, 1975; Blane, 1987). In the report by Schneider and Kaffarnik, drug discontinuation yielded return of erectile function. In a large series of 1,065 patients on clofibrate and 2,695 on placebo (Coronary Drug Project Research Group, 1975), 14.1% of the clofibrate patients and 10% of the placebo patients complained of impotence. This difference was statistically significant.

Digitalis

Long-term use of digitalis has been reported to be associated with gynecomastia (LeWinn, 1953) and decreased sexual function (Neri, Aygen, Zuckerman, & Baharh, 1980; Neri, Zuckerman, Aygen, Lidor, & Kaufman, 1987). In one study, patients on digoxin were compared with a drug-free control group. The patients on digoxin had significantly lower testosterone and luteinizing hormone levels, as well as elevated estradiol levels. The group on digoxin also had significantly elevated frequencies of desire and erectile problems (Neri et al., 1980). Similar findings were reported in a later study (Neri et al., 1987).

Histamine H₂ Antagonists

Histamine H_2 Antagonists

In the United States, the drugs most commonly used to treat peptic ulcer disease are the antacids and the H_2 receptor antagonists cimetidine and ranitidine (Zimmerman, 1984). Cimetidine administration has been reported to be associated with decreased libido (Biron, 1979; Gifford, Aeugle, Myerson, & Tannenbaum, 1980), gynecomastia (Jensen et al., 1984; Hall, 1976; Delle Fave et al., 1977), and impotence (Strum, 1983; Peden, Cargill, Browning, Saunders, & Wormsley, 1979; Collen et al., 1984; Jensen et al., 1983; Wolfe, 1979). Sexual side effects have usually been reported at higher dose levels, such as 2–5 g per day (e.g., Jensen et al., 1983), although they have been reported at doses as low as 600 mg per day (Biron, 1979). With drug discontinuation or lowering of the dose, sexual side effects have usually abated (Biron, 1979; Wolfe, 1979; Peden et al., 1979). In one study (Jensen et al., 1983), cimetidine-induced impotence was confirmed by NPT studies while patients were on the drug. The NPT indices normalized upon drug discontinuation. The frequency with which cimetidine is associated with erectile dysfunction appears dose-related. At doses of 5.3 g per day, Jensen et al., (1983) reported impotence in 9 of 22 patients. In a series of patients on 1 g per day, Long et al., (1985) reported no disturbances of sexual function. In postmarketing surveillance of cimetidine (Gifford et al., 1980; Colin Jones, Langman, Lawson, & Vessey, 1985), reports of erectile difficulties have been low.

Although gynecomastia has been reported with ranitidine (Tosi & Cagnoli, 1982; Jack, Richards, & Granata, 1982), this appears to be an infrequent occurence (Zimmerman, 1984). There has been a case report of impotence with ranitidine (Viana, 1983); however, the causal relationship has been questioned (Smith & Elsdon-Dew, 1983). Other investigators have reported that patients suffering impotence on cimetidine recover erectile function when ranitidine is substituted as the antiulcer drug (Jensen et al., 1983, 1984; Collen et al., 1984).

The mechanism by which cimetidine induces erectile failure is unknown. It has been suggested that cimetidine causes sexual problems more frequently than ranitidine because cimetidine has considerable antiandrogenic action, which is absent or negligible in ranitidine (Jensen et al., 1983). However, both drugs have a number of other pharmacological properties besides their antagonism of histamine H_2 receptors (Gwee & Cheah, 1986). At high doses, cimetidine has ganglion-blocking activity (Gwee, Cheah, & Lee, 1985). Cimetidine has also been found to stimulate prolactin secretion in men (Carlson & Ippoliti, 1977), although this effect is minor at lower therapeutic dosages (Long et al., 1985). Depression has been associated with cimetidine (Billings, Tang, & Rakoff, 1981) and could mediate the effects of this drug on libido. At a peripheral level, Adaikan and Karim (1979) have pointed out that H_2 antagonists can block relaxation of the smooth muscle in the corpora cavernosa.

Other Drugs

A number of other drugs have been reported to be associated with erectile failure. Carbonic anhydrase inhibitors (e.g., acetazolamide, ethoxzolamide, dichlorphenamide, and methazolamide) are used in the long-term management of glaucoma and have been reported to have sexual side effects, such as decreased libido and impotence (Epstein, Allen, & Lunde, 1987; Wallace, Fraunfelder, & Petursson, 1979; Epstein & Grant, 1977). As previously mentioned, another ophthalmological preparation, timolol eye drops, has been also reported to cause erectile difficulties (McMahon et al., 1979).

There have been case reports of impotence with indomethacin, a potent prostaglandin inhibitor (Miller, Rogers, & Swee, 1989); primidone, an anti-seizure medication (Mattson et al., 1985); thiabendazole, a treatment for trichinosis (Hennereuser, Pabst, Poeplau, & Gerok, 1969); methantheline bromide, an anticholinergic agent (Schwartz & Robinson, 1952); baclofen, an antispasticity drug (Hedley, Maroun, & Espir, 1975); and ketoconazole, an oral antifungal drug that is also used in the treatment of prostatic cancer because of its antiandrogenic effect (Pont et al., 1984; Nashan, Knuth, Weidinger, & Nieschlag, 1989). Disulfiram (commonly known as Antabuse), a drug for the treatment of alcohol addiction, has been shown to decrease the number and frequency of nocturnal erections (Snyder, Karacan, & Salis, 1981).

Lastly, a number of pharmacological agents, such as ketamine (Pietras, Cromie, & Duckett, 1979; Gale, 1972), amyl nitrate (Welti & Brodsky, 1980), and terbutaline (Shantha, Finnerty, & Rodriquez, 1989), have been reported to be effective in treatment of intraoperative penile tumescence.

Case Vignette

A 50-year-old diabetic from a rural community sought a consultation for treatment of his erectile dysfunction. He had adult-onset diabetes mellitus, managed by oral hypoglycemic agents; had been prescribed disopyramide by his primary physician because of a cardiac arrhythmia several years ago; and had developed erectile difficulties insidiously over the past 2 years. At about the time he developed erectile problems, his wife had become sexually involved with a neighbor. The primary physician attributed the patient's erectile problem to marital discord and referred the couple to a local psychotherapist. Psychological intervention at first was ineffective. The patient said, "Sure, I'm angry as hell at my wife, but that shouldn't interfere with my ability to masturbate as well. What the hell is going on here?" The primary physician was consulted and asked whether the patient had complained of erectile problems prior to disopyramide and whether the drug could be safely discontinued. The physician said that he was sure that the drug was not responsible but that the patient could discontinue it. Approximately 2 weeks later, the patient reported return of erectile function. He and his wife returned to the psychotherapist for continued marital therapy.

Occupational Pollutants

There is some information concerning the role of occupational pollutants in the genesis of erectile problems; although such pollutants are not "drugs" per se, we discuss them briefly here. Espir, Hall, Shirreffs, and Stevens (1970) reported that four out of five members of a team of farm workers became impotent after using various pesticides. Recovery after cessation of exposure was quite delayed. In one case, it took a year for erectile functioning to return. Because chlorinated hydrocarbon compounds are slowly eliminated from the body, such compounds may have been the etiological factor. Carbon disulfide, a chemical used in the rayon-making process, has been reported to cause impotence. In one study, 10 out of 16 men exposed to high levels of carbon disulfide complained of erectile problems. None of the subjects in a reference group working in a paper mill complained of such difficulties (Wagar, Tolonen, Stenman, & Helpio, 1981). Suskind and Hertzberg (1984) examined 203 men exposed to toxic levels of the herbicide (2,4,5-trichlorophenoxy)acetic acid in a runaway factory reaction, and 163 employees not exposed. The exposed employees had higher levels of impotence and decreased libido. Myeloneuropathy, including impotence, has been reported after prolonged exposure to nitrous oxide (Blanco & Peters, 1983; Layzer, 1978). This may be a particular hazard to dentists working in poorly ventilated offices.

Cancer Chemotherapy

Decreased libido (Armitage, Fyfe, & Lewis, 1984; Shalet, 1980; Chapman, 1982), gynecomastia (Shalet, 1980), and impotence (Armitage et al., 1984; Scheithauer, Ludwig, & Maida, 1985; Chapman, Rees, Sutcliffe, Edwards, &

Malpos, 1979) have been reported during cancer chemotherapy. However, in most of these reports it is difficult to be certain which agent is responsible for the sexual difficulty, as cancer chemotherapy usually involves a combination of agents. In certain cases it is difficult to be certain whether pharmacotherapy is the causative agent, as the patient may also have had surgical intervention or radiation, which independently may have impaired erectile function (Bennett, 1982). Of course, in most of the cases, it is exceedingly difficult to disentangle the sexual impairment resulting from psychological factors from that of the treatment factors (Schover & Jensen, 1988).

Recreational Drugs

The effect of alcohol on sexual function has been reviewed elsewhere (Schiavi, 1990a; Abel, 1985; Buffum, 1982; Leiblum & Rosen, 1984; Wilson, 1981). Thus this section only briefly summarizes the major findings. Acute alcohol ingestion at low dose levels may be associated with a verbal report of increased sexual desire. At higher dose levels, sexual arousal is clearly diminished by alcohol. Problems of sexual desire and arousal are highly prevalent among chronic alcoholic patients and may reflect peripheral neuropathy of the autonomic plexus, as well as reabsorption of estrogens into the blood secondary to advanced alcoholic liver disease.

Both cocaine and amphetamine have been reported to augment erectile capacity acutely (Segraves et al., 1985; Abel, 1985). However, chronic use of both agents has been reported to be associated with decreased libido and erectile problems.

The effect of opiates on sexual functioning has also been reviewed elsewhere (Jarowenko & Bennett, 1982; Segraves et al., 1985; Segraves, 1988a). Narcotic drugs such as methadone and heroin have a marked influence on libido and erectile problems. These problems appear to remit with drug discontinuation.

Neuroleptics and Other Psychiatric Drugs

Ejaculatory impairment, female anorgasmia, and erectile failure have been reported with antipsychotic drugs (Segraves, 1988c). Current evidence suggests that the interference with orgasm is secondary to the alpha-adrenergic blocking activity of these agents, and that the interference with erectile capacity is probably secondary to dopamine blockade (Segraves, 1989). Table 5.4 lists the psychiatric drugs that have been associated with erectile failure.

Case reports and clinical series have documented erectile failure with a variety of neuroleptics, including chlorpromazine (Greenberg, 1971), pimo-

TABLE 5.4. Psychiatric Drugs and Erectile Failure

Drug	Class	Effect[a]
Chlorpromazine	Antipsychotic	3
Pimozide	Antipsychotic	3
Thiothixine	Antipsychotic	2
Thioridazine	Antipsychotic	4
Sulpiride	Antipsychotic	3
Haloperidol	Antipsychotic	2
Fluphenazine	Antipsychotic	3
Diazepam	Tranquilizer	1
Chlordiazepoxide	Tranquilizer	1
Lorazepam	Tranquilizer	1
Alprazolam	Tranquilizer	1
Chlorazepate	Tranquilizer	1
Buspirone	Tranquilizer	1
Lithium	Mood stabilizer	3
Phenelzine	Antidepressant	1
Amitriptyline	Antidepressant	1
Fluoxetine	Antidepressant	1
Imipramine	Antidepressant	2
Clomipramine	Antidepressant	3
Amoxapine	Antidepressant	2
Protriptyline	Antidepressant	2
Desirpramine	Antidepressant	1

[a]1, unlikely to cause erectile problems; 2, uncertain; 3, probable; 4, highly probable.

zide (Ananth, 1982), thiothixine (Charalampous, Freemesser, Maleu, & Flord, 1974), thioridazine (Sandison, Whitelaw, & Currie, 1960; Kotin, Wilbert, & Verburg, 1976; Haider, 1966; Witton, 1962), sulpiride (Weizman, Maoz, Treves, Asher, & Ben-David, 1985), haloperidol (Meco et al., 1985), and fluphenazine (Batholomew, 1968). This effect may be dose-related, as dose reductions have been reported to be associated with the return of erectile function in the case of sulpiride, chlorpromazine, and pimozide. There has been only one double-blind study to date of the effects of neuroleptics on erectile function. Tennett, Bancrott, and Cass (1974), using a low dose of chlorpromazine (125 mg orally) or benperidol (1.25 mg), found no effect on erectile function for either drug.

Although there is evidence that diazepam (Riley & Riley, 1986), chlordiazepoxide (Hughes, 1964), lorazepam (Segraves, 1987), and alprazolam (Uhde, Tancer, & Shea, 1988; Sangal, 1985; Munjack & Crocker, 1986) may

ance. The patient stated that he had stopped his thioridazine because it "took away my manhood." The referring agency suspected that the patient's erectile failure and medication noncompliance were related to his underlying paranoid schizophrenia. The patient's sexual history was remarkable in that all of his sexual experience had been with prostitutes. In the past, when he had attempted masturbation, he had heard voices questioning his manhood and had noted neighborhood men laughing at him the next day. R. T. S. was uncertain as to the cause of this patient's erectile problem. On a trial basis, the thioridazine was discontinued and 5 mg haloperiodol per day was begun. Within 3 weeks, this patient reported that he was again able to have erections during coital activities.

Case Vignette

In another case, a 45-year-old attorney with recurrent major depressive disorder complained of impotence while being treated with amitriptyline (300 mg at hours of sleep). It was difficult to link the erectile problem clearly with amitriptyline, as the patient had been too depressed to be interested in sex prior to pharmacotherapy. Thus, baseline data were unavailable. It was also difficult to ascertain whether the erectile failure and decreased libido were secondary to a partially treated depressive episode, or were side effects of amitriptyline. Because the patient appeared to be more or less free of depressive symptoms at this time, a provisional diagnosis of drug-induced erectile disorder was made. The patient was instructed to decrease his amitriptyline from 300 to 250 mg per day and to return in 3 weeks. At the 3-week follow-up visit, he reported minimal change in his erections. His depressive disorder appeared stable. Therefore, the patient was instructed to decrease his amitriptyline to 200 mg per day and to return again in 3 weeks. At this follow-up visit, the patient reported return of both erectile capacity and his depressive symptomatology. The patient stated, "Being impotent and depression-free is better than being potent and depressed." The consultant replied, "Maybe we can do better than either of these two alternatives." At this point, desipramine was gradually begun as amitriptyline was discontinued. At 250 mg per day of desipramine, this patient became euthymic and potent.

PHARMACOLOGICAL TREATMENT
OF ERECTILE DYSFUNCTION

The use of intracavernosal injections to induce erections artificially, and the effects of exogenous androgens on male sexuality, are discussed elsewhere in this text. Thus this section focuses on orally administered agents that facilitate male erectile behavior.

Since the beginning of recorded history, men have searched for potions that might increase sexual desire, pleasure, or (more importantly) performance. In view of the large number of drugs that have been reported to induce sexual dysfunction, it is possible that other pharmacological agents that influence the same neurobiological substrate may enhance sexual behavior. A number of miscellaneous case reports have suggested possible efficacy for drugs such as trazodone (Lal, Rios, & Thavundayil, 1990), thioridazine and mesoridazine in low doses (Gold & Justino, 1988), levodopa (Segraves, 1989), and fenfluramine (Stevenson & Solyom, 1990).

Controlled studies have focused on drugs with dopaminergic, opioid, and adrenergic action. Two controlled studies (Pierini & Nusimovich, 1981; Benkert, Crombach, & Kockott, 1972) have investigated the efficacy of levodopa in the treatment of idiopathic erectile failure. Whereas one study found this approach to be effective, the other did not. A number of studies have found that apomorphine hydrochloride given either sublingually or subcutaneously in the arm can elicit penile erections about 15 minutes after the drug is administered (Schlatter & Lal, 1972; Lal, Ackman, Thavundayil, Kiely, & Etienne, 1984; Danjou, Alexandre, Warot, LaComblez, & Pvech, 1988; Segraves, Bari, Segraves, & Spirnak, 1991). Unfortunately, side effects such as nausea, dizziness, and hypotension limit the usefulness of apomorphine for treatment of erectile problems.

It is well known that opioid drug use is associated with decreased sexual desire and erectile function. A number of authors have suspected that opioid antagonists may facilitate sexual behavior (Mendelson, Ellingboe, Keuhnle, & Mello, 1979; Goldstein, 1986; Charney & Heninger, 1986). Only one double-blind controlled study has investigated the use of opioid antagonists in the treatment of erectile problems. Fabbri et al. (1989) reported that 50 mg of oral naltrexone for 2 weeks restored erectile function in 11 out of 15 men. The effect of naltrexone was statistically different from that of the placebo condition. Until an independent laboratory confirms this finding, it has to be regarded as tentative support at best for the assumption that opioid antagonists have a role in the treatment of erectile failure.

Of all of the alleged prosexual drugs, yohimbine has received the most study. Yohimbine is a preferential presynaptic alpha-2 antagonist. The presynaptic receptor is believed to regulate norepinephrine release, and yohimbine increases adrenergic activity. Yohimbine was one of the ingredients of a drug known as Afrodex, which was marketed for the treatment of impotence. However, Afrodex was withdrawn from the market in 1973. There have been five double-blind studies of the efficacy of yohimbine in the treatment of erectile failure. Overall, these studies suggest that yohimbine may be effective in idiopathic impotence and perhaps also in milder cases of biogenic impotence. Morales et al. (1987) found no statistically significant difference between yohimbine and placebo in the treatment of biogenic impotence. This study had a high placebo response rate, suggesting that the screening criteria were somehow flawed. Reid et al. (1967) reported that 10 weeks of yohimbine therapy was clearly effective in the treatment of psychogenic erectile disorder. Three other studies (Sondra, Mazo, & Chancellor, 1990; Susset et al., 1989; Riley, Goodman, Kellet, & Orr, 1989) have also reported efficacy of yohimbine in the treatment of patients with erectile disorder.

In these studies, it is difficult to be certain as to the etiology of the erectile problems in many of the patients. The evidence clearly suggests that yohimbine may have a place in the treatment of some men with erectile disorder. Current evidence provides little information as to the indications for its use; there is also minimal evidence concerning the proper dosage. Fortunately, this drug has a relatively benign side effect profile. The mechanism of action of yohimbine is also unclear. It probably has an active metabolite, as yohimbine itself has a very short half-life. Yohimbine probably works by action on the central nervous system rather than by action on peripheral tissue (Sondra et al., 1990).

Case Vignette

A lawyer in his mid-50s consulted one of us (R. T. S.) because of intermittent erectile failure associated with a mild decrease in libido. There was no evidence of affective disorder, and routine evaluation revealed normal testosterone and prolactin levels. Early morning erections and masturbatory erections were reported as normal. His erectile problem began after the last child left the household to begin college. At this point, his wife increased sexual demands, and the patient had difficulty responding. The patient refused to involve his wife in treatment because it was "my problem and I don't want to upset her." His desire to protect his wife was investigated further. It was learned that his wife had been a college beauty queen and was having difficulty adjusting to middle age and the loss of her status as a ravishing beauty. According to the husband, she regarded his erectile failure as a personal rejection of her and a confirmation of her fear that she was no longer attractive.

As the patient's wife was unavailable for treatment, R. T. S. considered a trial of yohimbine. The patient's medical history was benign, and the patient was normotensive. Thus the patient was prescribed yohimbine three times a day for 4 weeks and was given a return appointment at that time. Upon his return, and to R. T. S.'s surprise, the patient reported a return of erectile function accompanied by an increase in libido approximately 20 days after starting the drug. Interpersonal strife at home decreased with the resumption of coitus. Yohimbine was continued for another 2 months prior to being discontinued.

CONCLUSION

Modern medicine has enabled human beings to extend their lifetimes and to live more active and fulfilling lives. However, aging and the drugs that are often needed during the later phase of life can have a profound effect on sexual functioning. Aging and the use of drugs both involve complicated processes, which can result in sexual problems by interacting with multiple systems. Ironically, both of these factors (aging and drugs) have not been systematically studied to determine how they independently and collaboratively affect men's ability to function sexually.

Clinicians who treat aging males must rely on clinical judgment as well as science. The field of sexual medicine is in its infancy, and normative values for various diagnostic procedures and tests are unavailable for the aging male. The aging process involves changes in hormone levels, vascular systems, tactile sensitivity, sleep patterns, and at times decrements in general health that may require medications or surgery. The complexities of evaluating sexual problems in this phase of life are apparent.

Clinicians who are involved in treatment of older men need to form collaborative working relationships with physicians and ancillary personnel with expertise in evaluating this population. Knowledge in treating sexual dysfunctions in the young is not reliably transferable when working with the elderly. Adjustments to our diagnostic and treatment approaches need to be made, given the changes in physiology and the possible effects of concurrent medical treatments. The generalist is ill advised to attempt to forge ahead alone in treating an aging male; he or she would be doing a great disservice to the patient by treating a reversible drug-related sexual dysfunction as if it were a resistant psychogenic sexual dysfunction. Sexual functioning under the best of circumstances is the end product of a complicated dynamic interplay of interrelated systems. The process of aging complicates matters further.

Although there are obvious gaps in our knowledge concerning the effects of age and drugs on erectile function, a suitable data base exists to assist the skilled clinician in his or her assessment of patients. In spite of large areas of missing information, the explosion of information on these topics is gratifying. As more health professionals become concerned with the continuation and quality of life, as well as its complexity, we can expect our knowledge base to continue to expand in the years to come.

REFERENCES

Abel, E. L. (1985). *Psychoactive drugs and sex*. New York: Plenum.

Adaikan, P. G., & Karim, S. M. M. (1979). Male sexual dysfunction during treatment with cimetidine. *British Medical Journal, i*, 1282–1283.

Adams, J. W., & Soucheray, J. A. (1984). Prazosin-induced priapism in a diabetic. *Journal of Urology, 132*, 1208.

Ahmad, S. (1980a). Disopyramide and impotence. *Southern Medical Journal*, 73, 958.

Ahmad, S. (1980b). Hydralazine and male impotence. *Chest*, 78, 358.

Alexander, C. J., Christie, M. H., Vernam, K. A., Fand, R. S., & Shafer, W. B. (1984). Long-term experience with nadolol in treatment of hypertension and angina pectoris. *American Heart Journal*, 108, 1136–1140.

Alexander, W. D., & Evans, J. I. (1974). Side-effects of methyldopa. *British Medical Journal*, ii, 501.

Ambrosini, E., Costa, F. U., & Montebugnoli, L. (1983). Comparison of antihypertensive efficacy of atenolol, oxprenolol and pindolol at rest and during exercise. *Drugs*, 25(Suppl. 21), 30–36.

Amery, A., Verstraete, M., & Bossaert, H. (1979). Hypotensive action and side-effects of clonidine-chlorthalidone and methyldopa-chlorthalidone in treatment of hypertension. *British Medical Journal*, iv, 392–395.

Ananth, J. (1982). Impotence associated with pimozide. *American Journal of Psychiatry*, 139, 1374.

Anastasiou-Nana, M. I., Anderson, J. L., Nanas, J. N., Luz, J. R., Smith, R. A., & Anderson, K. P. (1986). High incidence of clinical and subclinical toxicity associated with amiodarone treatment of refractory tachyarrhythmias. *Canadian Journal of Cardiology*, 2, 138–145.

Armitage, J. O., Fyfe, M. A., & Lewis, J. (1984). Long-term remission durability and functional status of patients treated for diffuse histiocytic lymphoma with the CHOP regime. *Journal of Clinical Oncology*, 2, 898–903.

Attalla, F. M., Saheb, I. V. H., & Randall, R. F. (1981). Timolol-blocadren post marketing surveillance program in hypertension. *Current Therapeutics and Research*, 29, 423.

Bancroft, J. (1983). *Human sexuality and its problems*. Edinburgh: Churchill Livingstone.

Banos, J. E., Bosch, F., & Farre, M. (1989). Drug-induced priapism: Its aetiology, incidence and treatment. *Medical Toxicology and Adverse Drug Experiences*, 4, 46–58.

Bansal, S. (1988). Sexual dysfunction in hypertensive men: A critical review of the literature. *Hypertension*, 12, 1–10.

Bartholomew, A. A. (1968). A long-acting phenothiazine as a possible agent to control deviate sexual behavior. *American Journal of Psychiatry*, 124, 917–922.

Bathen, J. (1978). Propranolol erectile dysfunction relieved. *Annals of Internal Medicine*, 88, 716–717.

Bauer, G. E., Baker, J., & Hunyor, S. N. (1978). Side-effects of antihypertensive treatment: A placebo-controlled study. *Clinical Science and Molecular Medicine*, 55, 3415–3445.

Bauer, G. E., Hull, R. D., & Stokes, G. S. (1973). The reversibility of side-effects of guanethidine therapy. *Medical Journal of Australia*, i, 930–933.

Benkert, O., Crombach, G., & Kockott, G. (1972). Effect of L-dopa on sexually impotent patients. *Psychopharmacology*, 23, 91–95.

Bennett, A. H. (1982). Organic causes of impotence: Surgical. In A. H. Bennett (Ed.), *Management of male impotence* (pp. 135–142). Baltimore: Williams & Wilkins.

Bhalla, A. K., Hoffbrand, B. I., & Phatak, P. S. (1979). Prazosin and priapism. *British Medical Journal*, ii, 1039.

Biron, P. (1979). Diminished libido wih cimetidine therapy. *Canadian Medical Association Journal, 18,* 404–405.

Billings, R. F., Tang, S. W., & Rakoff, V. M. (1981). Depression associated with cimetidine. *Canadian Journal of Psychiatry, 26,* 260–261.

Blanco, G., & Peters, H. A. (1983). Myeloneuropathy and macrocytosis associated with nitrous oxide abuse. *Archives of Neurology, 40,* 416–418.

Blane, G. F. (1987). Comparative toxicity and safety profile of fenofibrate and other fibric acid derivatives. *American Journal of Medicine, 83,* 26–36.

Blay, S. L., Ferraz, M. P. T., & Calil, H. M. (1982). Lithium-induced male sexual impairment: Two case reports. *Journal of Clinical Psychiatry, 43,* 497–498.

Boyden, T. W., Nugent, C. A., & Ogihara, T. (1980). Reserpine, hydrochlorothiazide and pituitary-gonadal hormones in hypertensive patients. *European Journal of Clinical Pharamcology, 17,* 329–332.

Brogden, R. N., Heel, R. C., Speight, T. M., & Avery, G. S. (1977). Prazosin: A review of its pharmacological properties and therapeutic efficacy in hypertension. *Drugs, 14,* 163–197.

Brahma, S. K., Chowdhury, B., & Sarkar, B. K. (1966). Guanethidine in hypertension. *Journal of the Indian Medical Association, 46,* 541–543.

Brown, J., Davies, D. L., Ferris, J. B., Fraser, R., Haywood, E., Lever, A. F., & Robertson, J. I. S. (1972). Comparison of surgery and prolonged spironolactone therapy in patients with hypertension, aldosterone excess and low plasma renin. *British Medical Journal, ii,* 729–734.

Buffum, J. (1982). Pharmacology: The effect of drugs on sexual function. A review. *Journal of Psychoactive Drugs, 14,* 5–44.

Bulpitt, C. J., & Dollery, C. T. (1973). Side-effects of hypotensive agents evaluated by a self-administered questionnaire. *British Medical Journal, iii,* 485–490.

Burke, J. R., & Hirst, G. (1980). Priapism and prazosin. *Medical Journal of Australia, i,* 382.

Burnett, W. G., & Chanine, R. A. (1979). Sexual dysfunction as a complication of propranolol therapy in men. *Cardiovascular Medicine, 4,* 811–815.

Burris, J. F., Goldstein, J., Zager, P. G., Sutton, J. M., Sirgo, M. A., & Plachetka, J. R. (1986). Comparative tolerability of labetalol versus propranolol, atenolol, pindolol, metoprolol, and nadolol. *Journal of Clinical Hypertension, 2,* 285–293.

Carlson, H. E., & Ippoliti, A. F. (1977). Cimetidine, an H_2-antihistamine, stimulates prolactin secretion in man. *Journal of Clinical Endocrinology and Metabolism, 45,* 367–370.

Chapman, R. M. (1982). Effect of cytotoxic therapy on sexuality and gonadal function. *Seminars in Oncology, 9,* 84–94.

Chapman, R. M., Rees, L. H., Sutcliffe, S. B., Edwards, C. R. W., & Malpos, J. S. (1979). Cyclical combination chemotherapy and gonadal function. *Lancet, i,* 285–289.

Charalampous, K. D., Freemesser, G. F., Maleu, J., & Flord, K. (1974). Loxapine succinate: A controlled double-blind study in schizophrenia. *Current Therapeutics and Research, 16,* 829–837.

Charney, D. S., & Heninger, G. R. (1986). α_2-adrenergic and opiate receptor blockade. *Archives of General Psychiatry, 43,* 1037–1041.

Colin Jones, G., Langman, M. J. S., Lawson, D. H., & Vessey, P. (1985). Post-marketing surveillance of the safety of cimetidine in twelve-month morbidity report. *Quarterly Journal of Medicine, 54,* 253–268.

Collen, M. J., Howard, J. M., McArthur, K. E., Raufman, J. P., Cornelius, M. J., Ciarleglio, C. A., Gardner, J. D., & Jensen, R. T. (1984). Comparison of ranitidine and cimetidine in the treatment of gastric hypersecretion. *Annals of Internal Medicine, 100,* 52–58.

Coronary Drug Project Research Group. (1975). Clofibrate and niacin in coronary heart disease. *Journal of the American Medical Association, 231,* 360–381.

Couper-Smartt, T. D., & Rodham, R. (1973). A technique for surveying side-effects of tricyclic drugs with reference to reported sexual effects. *Jouranl of International Medical Research, 1,* 473–476.

Croog, S. H., Levine, S. Sudilovsky, A., Baume, R. M., & Clive, J. (1988). Sexual symptoms in hypertensive patients: A clinical trial of antihypertensive medications. *Archives of Internal Medicine, 148,* 788–794.

Curd, J. D., Borhani, N. O., Blaszkowski, T. P., Zimbaldi, N., Fotiv, S., & Williams, W. (1985). Long-term surveillance for adverse effects of antihypertensive drugs. *Journal of the American Medical Association, 253,* 3263–3268.

Danjou, P., Alexandre, L., Warot, D., LaComblez, L., & Pvech, A. J. (1988). Assessment of erectogenic properties of apomorphine and yohimbine in man. *British Journal of Clinical Pharmacology, 26,* 733–739.

Davidson, J. M., Kwan, M., & Greenleaf, W. J. (1982). Hormonal replacement and sexuality in men. *Clinics in Endocrinology and Metabolism, 11,* 559–623.

Davies, I. B. (1979). Hydralazine as an aphrodisiac. *British Medical Journal, ii,* 1367.

Delle Fave, G. F., Tamburrano, G., DeMagistris, L., Natoli, C., Santoro, M. I., Carratu, R., & Torsoli, A. (1977). Gynaecomastia with cimetidine. *Lancet, i,* 1319.

Deslypere, J. P., & Vermeulen, A. (1981). Aging and tissue androgens. *Journal of Clinical Endocrinology and Metabolism, 53,* 430–434.

Douglas-Jones, A. P., & Cruickshank, J. M. (1976). Once-daily dosing with atenolol in patients with mild to moderate hypertension. *British Medical Journal, i,* 990–991.

Due, D. L., Giguere, G. C., & Plachetka, J. R. (1986). Postmarketing comparison of labetalol and propranolol in hypertensive patients. *Clinical Therapeutics, 8,* 624–631.

Epstein, D. L., & Grant, W. M. (1977). Carbonic anhydrase inhibitor side-effects. *Archives of Ophthalmology, 95,* 1378–1382.

Epstein, R. J., Allen, R. C., & Lunde, M. W. (1987). Organic impotence associated with carbonic anhydrase inhibitor therapy. *Annals of Ophthalmology, 19,* 48–50.

Espir, M. L. E., Hall, J. W., Shirreffs, J. G., & Stevens, D. L. (1970). Impotence in farm workers using toxic chemicals. *British Medical Journal, i,* 423–425.

Everett, H. C. (1975). The use of bethanechol chloride with tricyclic antidepressants. *American Journal of Psychiatry, 132,* 1202–1204.

Fabbri, A., Jannini, E. A., Gnessi , L., Moretti , C., Ulisse, S., Franzese, A., Lazzari, R., Fraioli, F., Frajese, G., & Isidori, A. (1989). Endorphins in male impotence: Evidence for naltrexone stimulation of erectile activity in patient therapy. *Psychoneuroendocrinology, 14,* 103–111.

Ferder, L., Inserra, F., & Medina, F. (1987). Safety aspects of long-term antihypertensive therapy (10 years) with clonidine. *Journal of Cardiovascular Pharmacology*, *10*(Suppl. 12), 5104–5108.

Fogelman, J. (1987). Verapamil may cause depression, confusion and impotence. *Texas Medicine*, *83*, 8.

Fogelman, J. (1988). Verapamil caused depression, confusion, and impotence *American Journal of Psychiatry*, *145*, 380.

Fraunfelder, F. T., & Meyer, S. M. (1985). Sexual dysfunction secondary to topical ophthalmic timolol. *Journal of the American Medical Association*, *253*, 3092–3093.

Gale, A. S. (1972). Ketamine prevention of penile tumescence. *Journal of the American Medical Association 219*, 1629.

Geissler, A. H., Turnlund, J. R., & Cohen, R. D. (1986). Effect of chlorthalidone on zinc levels, testosterone, and sexual function in man. *Drug–Nutrient Interactions*, *4*, 275–283.

General Practitioners Research Group (1975). A single-dose anti-anxiety drug. *Practitioner*, *25*, 98–101.

Gerstenberg, T. C., Nordling, J., Hald, T., & Wagner, G. (in press). Standardized evaluation of erectile dysfunction in 97 consecutive patients. *Journal of Urology*.

Gifford, L. M., Aeugle, M. E., Myerson, R. M., & Tannenbaum, P. J. (1980). Cimetidine postmarket outpatient surveillance program. *Journal of the American Medical Association*, *243*, 1532–1535.

Girgis, S. M., Etriby, A., & El-Hefnawy, H. (1968). Aspermia: A survey of 49 cases. *Fertility and Sterility*, *19*, 580–588.

Gold, D. P., & Justino, J. D. (1988). Bicycle kickstand phenomenon: Prolonged erections associated with antipsychotic agents. *Southern Medical Journal*, *81*, 792–794.

Goldstein, J. A. (1986). Erectile failure and naltrexone. *Annals of Internal Medicine*, *105*, 799.

Greenberg, H. R. (1971). Inhibition of ejaculation by chlorpromazine. *Journal of Nervous and Mental Disease*, *152*, 364–366.

Greenblatt, D. J., & Koch-Weser, J. (1973). Gynecomastia and impotence complications of spironolactone therapy. *Journal of the American Medical Association*, *223*, 82.

Gross, M. D. (1982). Reversal by bethanechol of sexual dysfunction caused by anticholinergic antidepressants. *American Journal of Psychiatry*, *139*, 1193–1194.

Gwee, M. C. E., & Cheah, L. S. (1986). Actions of cimetidine and ranitidine at some cholinergic sites: Implications in toxicology and anesthesia. *Life Sciences*, *39*, 383–388.

Gwee, M. C. E., Cheah, L. S., & Lee, H. S. (1985). Ganglion blocking activity of cimetidine in the anaesthetized cat. *Clinical and Experimental Pharmacology and Physiology*, *12*, 475–480.

Haider, I. (1966). Thioridazine and sexual dysfunctions. *International Journal of Neuropsychiatry*, *2*, 255–257.

Hall, W. H. (1976). Breast changes in males on cimetidine. *New England Journal of Medicine*, *295*, 841.

Harrison, W. M., Rabkin, J. G., Ehrhardt, A. A., Stewart, J. W., McGrath, P. J., Ross, D., & Quitkin, F. M. (1986). Effects of antidepressant medication on sexual function: A controlled study. *Journal of Clinical Psychopharmacology*, *6*, 144–149.

Harrison, W. M., Stewart, J., Ehrhardt, A. A., Rabkin, J., McGrath, P., Liebowitz, M., & Quitkin, F. M. (1985). A controlled study of the effects of antidepressants on sexual function. *Psychopharmacology Bulletin, 21,* 85–88.

Hedley, D. W., Maroun, J. A., & Espir, M. L. E. (1975). Evaluation of baclofen (Lioresal) for spasticity in multiple sclerosis. *Postgraduate Medical Journal, 51,* 615–618.

Heger, J. J., Solow, E. B., Prystowsky, E. N., & Zipes, D. P. (1984). Plasma and red blood cell concentrations of amiodarone during chronic therapy. *American Journal of Cardiology, 53,* 912–917.

Hegeler, S., & Mortensen, M. M. (1977). Sexual behavior in elderly Danish males. In C. C. Wheeler (Ed.), *Progress in sexology.* New York: Plenum Press.

Hekimian, L. J., Friedhoft, A. T., & Deever, E. (1978). A comparison of the onset of action and therapeutic efficacy of amoxapine and amitriptyline. *Journal of Clinical Psychiatry, 39,* 633–637.

Hennereuser, H. H., Pabst, K., Poeplau, W., & Gerok, W. (1969). Thiabendazole for the treatment of trichinosis in humans. *Texas Reports in Biology and Medicine,* 27(Suppl. 2), 581–596.

Hogan, M. J., Wallin, J. D., & Baer, R. M. (1980). Antihypertensive therapy and male sexual dysfunction. *Psychosomatics, 21,* 234–237.

Hollifield, J. W., Sherman, K., & Vanderzwagg, R. (1976). Proposed mechanisms of propranolol's antihypertensive effect in essential hypertension. *New England Journal of Medicine, 295,* 68–73.

Howard, D. J., & Rees, J. R. (1976). Long-term perhexiline maleate and liver function. *British Medical Journal, i,* 133.

Hughes, J. M. (1964). Failure to ejaculate with chlordiazepoxide. *American Journal of Psychiatry, 121,* 610–611.

Jack, D., Richards, D. A., & Granata, F. (1982). Side-effects of ranitidine. *Lancet, ii,* 264–265.

Jackson, D. A. (1980). Nadolol, a once daily treatment for hypertension: Multicenter clinical evaluation. *British Journal of Clinical Practice, 34,* 211–221.

Jarowenko, M. V., & Bennett, A. H. (1982). Pharmacology of impotence–sexual dysfunction. In A. H. Bennett (Ed.), *Management of male impotence* (pp. 162–171). Baltimore: Williams & Wilkins.

Jensen, R. T., Collen, M. J., McArthur, K. E., Howard, J. M., Maton, P. N., Cherner, A., & Gordner, J. D. (1984). Comparison of the effectiveness of ranitidine and cimetidine in inhibiting acid secretion in patients with gastric hypersecretory states. *American Journal of Medicine, 77,* 90–105.

Jensen, R. T., Collen, M. J., Pandol, S. J., Allende, H. D., Raufman, J. P., Bissonnette, B. M., Duncarr, W. C., Durgin, P. L., Gillin, J. C., & Gardner, J. D. (1983). Cimetidine-induced impotence and breast changes in patients with gastric hypersecretory states. *New England Journal of Medicine, 308,* 883–887.

Johnson, P., Kitchin, A. H., & Lowther, C. P. (1966). Treatment of hypertension with methyldopa. *British Medical Journal, i,* 133–137.

Joint National Committee on Detection, Evaluation and Treatment of High Blood Pressure. (1984). Report of the Joint National Committee on Detection, Evaluation and Treatment of High Blood Pressure. *Archives of Internal Medicine, 144,* 1045–1057.

Kahn, E., & Fisher, C. (1969). REM sleep and sexuality in the aged. *Journal of Geriatric Psychiatry, 2,* 181–199.

Karacan, I., Hursch, C. J., & Williams, R. L. (1972). Some characteristics of nocturnal penile tumescence in elderly males. *Journal of Gerontology, 27,* 39–45.

Karacan, I., Williams, R. I., Thornby, J. I., & Salis, P. J. (1975). Sleep-related tumescence as a function of age. *American Journal of Psychiatry, 132,* 932–937.

Keidan, H. (1976). Impotence during antihypertensive treatment. *Canadian Medical Association Journal, 114,* 874.

King, B. D., Pitchon, R., Stern, E. H., Schweiter, P., Schneider, R. R., & Weiner, I. (1983). Impotence during therapy with verapamil. *Archives of Internal Medicine, 143,* 1248–1249.

Kinsey, A. C., Pomeroy, B., & Martin, C. I. (1948). *Sexual behavior in the human male.* Philadelphia: W. B. Saunders.

Kline, M. D. (1989). Fluoxetine and anorgasmia. *American Journal of Psychiatry, 146,* 804–805.

Knarr, J. W. (1976). Impotence from propranolol. *Annals of Internal Medicine, 85,* 259.

Kolodny, R. C. (1987). Effects of alpha-methyldopa on male sexual function. *Sexuality and Disability, 1,* 223–227.

Kostis, J. B., Rosen, R. C., Holzer, B. C., Randolph, C., Taska, L. S., & Miller, M. H. (1990). CNS side effects of centrally-active antihypertensive agents: A prospective, placebo-controlled study of sleep, mood state, cognitive and sexual function in hypertensive males. *Psychopharmacology, 102,* 163–170.

Kotin, J., Wilbert, D. E., & Verburg, D. (1976). Thioridazine and sexual dysfunction. *American Journal of Psychiatry, 133,* 82–85.

Kowalski, A., Stanley, R. O., Dennerstein, L., Burrows, G., & MacQuire, K. P. (1985). The sexual side-effects of antidepressant medication: A double blind comparison of two antidepressants in a non-psychiatric population. *British Journal of Psychiatry, 147,* 413–418.

Krane, R. J., Goldstein, I., & Saenz de Tejada, I. (1989). Impotence. *New England Journal of Medicine, 321,* 1648–1659.

Labby, D. H. (1985). Aging's effects on sexual function. *Postgraduate Medicine, 78,* 32–34, 39–43.

Lal, S., Ackman, D., Thavundayil, J. X., Kiely, M. E., & Etienne, P. (1984). Effect of apomorphine, a dopamine receptor agonist, on penile tumescence in normal subjects. *Progress in Neuropsychopharmacology and Biological Psychiatry, 8,* 695–699.

Lal, S., Rios, O., & Thavundayil, J. X. (1990). Treatment of impotence with trazodone: A case report. *Journal of Urology, 143,* 819–820.

Laver, M. C. (1974). Sexual behavior patterns in male hypertensives. *Australian and New Zealand Journal of Medicine, 4,* 29–31.

Layzer, R. B. (1978). Myeloneuropathy after prolonged exposure to mitrous oxide. *Lancet, iii,* 1227–1230.

Leiblum, S. R., & Rosen, R. C. (1984). Alcohol and human sexual response. In D. J. Powell (Ed.), *Alcoholism and sexual dysfunction: Issues in clinical management.* New York: Haworth Press.

Leiblum, S. R., & Segraves, R. T. (1989). Sex therapy with aging adults. In S. R. Leiblum

& R. C. Rosen (Eds.), *Principles and practice of sex therapy* (2nd ed.): *Update for the 1990s* (pp. 352-381). New York: Guilford Press.

LeWinn, E. B. (1953). Gynecomastia during digitalis therapy. *New England Journal of Medicine, 248,* 316-320.

Lin, S., Yu, P., Yang, M. C. M., Chang, L. S., Chiang, B. N., & Kuo, J. (1988). Local suppressive effect of clonidine on penile erections in the dog. *Journal of Urology, 139,* 849-852.

Lipson, L. G., Moore, D., Pope, A. M., Todd, F. J., & Avila, S. M. (1981). Sexual dysfunction in diabetic men. *Journal of Cardiovascular Medicine, 43*(Suppl. 1), 30-37.

Lipson, L. G. (1985). Treatment of hypertension in diabetic men: Problems with sexual dysfunction. *American Journal of Cardiology, 53,* 46A-50A.

Long, J. P., Smyth, P. P., Culliton, M., Cunningham, S., O'Donoghue, D. P., Fitzgerald, O., & McKenna, T. J. (1985). Prolactin and the hypothalamic-pituitary-testicular axis in cimetidine-treated men. *Irish Medical Journal, 78,* 48-51.

Loriaux, D. L., Menard, R., Taylor, A., Pita, J. C., & Santen, R. (1976). Spironolactone and endocrine dysfunction. *Annals of Internal Medicine, 85,* 630-636.

Luther, R. R. (1989). New perspectives on selective alpha 1 blockade. *American Journal of Hypertension, 2,* 729-735.

MacCarthy, E. P., & Bloomfield, S. S. (1983). Labetalol: A review of its pharmacology, pharmacokinetics, clinical uses and adverse effects. *Pharmacotherapy, 3,* 193-219.

Magnus, R. V., Dean, B. C., & Curry, S. H. (1977). Clorazepate: Double blind crossover comparison on a single nightly dose with diazepam twice daily in anxiety. *Diseases of the Nervous System, 38,* 317-321.

Marley, J. E. (1989). Safety and efficacy of nifedipine 20 mg. tablets in hypertension using electronic data collection in general practice. *Journal of the Royal Society of Medicine, 82,* 272-275.

Marley, J. E., & Curram, J. B. (1989). General practice data derived tolerability assessment of antihypertensive drugs. *Journal of International Medical Research, 17,* 473-478.

Masters, W. H., & Johnson, V. E. (1966). *Human sexual response.* Boston: Little, Brown.

Masters, W. H., & Johnson, V. E. (1977). Sex after sixty-five. *Reflections, 12,* 31-43.

Materson, B. J., Vlachakis, N. D., Glasser, S. P., Lucas, C., Ramanathan, K. B., Ahmad, S., Morledge, J. H., Saunders, E., Lutz, L. J., Schnaper, H. W., Maxwell, M., & Poland, M. C. (1989). Influence of beta$_2$ antagonism on adverse effects and plasma lipoproteins: Results of a multicenter comparison of dilevalol and metoprolol. *American Journal of Cardiology, 63,* 58-63.

Mattson, R. H., Cramer, J. A., Collins, J. F., Smith, D. B., Delgado-Escueta, A. V., Broune, T. R., Williamson, P. P., Treiman, D. M., McNamara, J. O., & McCutchen, C. B. (1985). Comparison of carbamazepine, phenobarbital, phenytoin, and primidone in partial and secondarily generalized tonic-clonic seizures. *New England Journal of Medicine, 313,* 145-151.

McHaffie, D. J., Guz, A., & Johnson, A. (1977). Impotence in patients on disopyramide. *Lancet, i,* 859.

McMahon, C. D., Shaffer, R. N., & Hoskins, H. D. (1979). Adverse effects experienced by patients taking timolol. *American Journal of Ophthalmology, 88,* 736-738.

McMahon, F. G. (1978). *Management of essential hypertension*. Mount Kisco, NY: Futura.

Meco, G., Falachi, P., Casacchia, M., Rocco, A., Petrini, P., Rosa, M., & Agnoli, A. (1985). Neuroendocrine effects of haloperidol decanoate in patients with chronic schizophrenia. In D. Kemali & G. Ragagni (Eds.), *Chronic treatments in neuropsychiatry* (pp. 89–93). New York: Raven Press.

Medical Research Council Working Party on Mild to Moderate Hypertension. (1981). Adverse reactions to bendrofluozide and propranolol for the treatment of mild hypertension. *Lancet, i*, 539–542.

Melman, A., Fersel, J., & Weinstein, P. (1984). Further studies on the effect of chronic alpha-methyldopa administration upon the central nervous system and sexual function in male rats. *Journal of Urology, 132*, 804–808.

Mendelson, J. H., Ellingboe, J., Keuhnle, J. C., & Mello, N. K. (1979). Effect of naltrexone on mood and neuroendocrine function in adult males. *Psychoneuroendocrinology, 3*, 231–236.

Miller, L. G., Rogers, J. C., & Swee, D. E. (1989). Indomethacin-associated sexual dysfunction. *Journal of Family Practice, 29*, 210–211.

Miller, R. A. (1976). Propranolol and impotence. *Annals of Internal Medicine, 85*, 682.

Modell, J. G. (1989). Repeated observations of yawning, clitoral engorgement and orgasm associated with fluoxetine administration. *Journal of Clinical Psychopharmacology, 9*, 63–65.

Morales, A., Condra, M., Owen, J. A., Surridge, D. H., Fenemore, J., & Harris, C. (1987). Is yohimbine effective in the treatment of organic impotence?: Results of a controlled trial. *Journal of Urology, 137*, 1168–1172.

Moser, M., Prandoni, A. G., & Orison, J. A. (1974). Clinical experience with sympathetic blocking agents in peripheral vascular disease. *Annals of Internal Medicine, 38*, 1245–1246.

Moss, H. B., & Procci, W. R. (1982). Sexual dysfunction associated with oral antihypertensive medication: A critical survey of the literature. *General Hospital Psychiatry, 4*, 121–129.

Mroczek, Q. J., Davidou, M., & Finnerty, F. A. (1972). Prolonged treatment with clonidine: Comparative antihypertensive effects with a diuretic. *American Journal of Cardiology, 30*, 536–541.

Munjack, D. J., & Crocker, B. (1986). Alprazolam-induced ejaculatory inhibition. *Journal of Clinical Psychopharmacology, 6*, 57–58.

Nankin, H. R., & Calkins, J. H. (1986). Decreased bioavailable testosterone in aging normal and impotent men. *Journal of Clinical Endocrinology and Metabolism, 63*, 1418–1420.

Nashan, D., Knuth, V. A., Weidinger, G., & Nieschlag, E. (1989). The antimycotic drug terbinafine in contrast to hetoconazole lacks acute effects on the pituitary-testicular function of healthy men: A placebo controlled double-blind trial. *Acta Endocrinologica, 120*, 677–681.

Neaves, W. B., Johnson, L., Porter, J. C., Parker, C. R., & Petty, C. S. (1984). Leydig cell number, daily sperm production and serum gonadotropin levels in aging males. *Journal of Clinical Endocrinology and Metabolism, 59*, 756–763.

Neri, A., Aygen, M., Zuckerman, Z., & Baharh, C. (1980). Subjective assessment of sexual dysfunction of patients on long-term administration of digoxin. *Archives of Sexual Behavior, 9*, 343–347.

Neri, A., Zuckerman, Z., Aygen, M., Lidor, Y., & Kaufman, H. (1987). The effect of long-term administration of digoxin or plasma androgens and sexual dysfunction. *Journal of Sex and Marital Therapy, 13*, 58–63.

New Zealand Hypertension Study Group. (1977). Initial experience with prazosin in New Zealand. *Medical Journal of Australia, ii*(Special Suppl.), 23–26.

Newman, A. F. (1970). Vibratory sensitivity of the penis. *Fertility and Sterility, 21*, 791–793.

Newman, R. J., & Salerno, H. R. (1974). Sexual dysfunction due to methyldopa. *British Medical Journal, iv*, 106.

Oaks, W. W., & Moyer, J. H. (1972). Sex and hypertension. *Medical Aspects of Human Sexuality, 61*, 128–137.

Ohman, K. P., & Karlberg, B. E. (1984). Enalapril and atenolol in primary hypertension: A comparative study of blood pressure lowering and hormonal effects. *Scandinavian Journal of Urology and Nephrology, 79*(Suppl.), 93–97.

Onesti, G., Bock, K. D., & Heimsoth, U. (1971). Clonidine: A new antihypertensive agent. *American Journal of Cardiology, 28*, 74–83.

Othmer, E., & Othmer, S. C. (1987). Effect of buspirone on sexual dysfunction in patients with generalized anxiety disorder. *Journal of Clinical Psychiatry, 48*, 201–203.

Papadopoulos, C. (1989). *Sexual aspects of cardiovascular disease.* New York: Praeger.

Participating Veterans Administration Medical Centers. (1982). Low doses versus standard dose of reserpine: A randomized, double-blind, multiclinic trial in patients taking chlorthalidone. *Journal of the American Medical Association, 248*, 2471–2472.

Pearlman, C. K., & Kobashi, L. I. (1972). Frequency of intercourse in men. *Journal of Urology, 107*, 298–301.

Peden, N. R., Cargill, J. M., Browning, M. C. K., Saunders, J. H. B., & Wormsley, W. G. (1979). Male sexual dysfunction during treatment with cimetidine. *British Medical Journal, i*, 659.

Pfeiffer, E. (1974). Sexuality in the aging individual. *Journal of the American Geriatrics Society, 22*, 481–484.

Pierini, A. A., & Nusimovich, B. (1981). Male diabetic sexual impotence: Effects of dopaminergic agents. *Archives of Andrology, 6*, 347–350.

Pietras, J. R., Cromie, W. J., & Duckett, J. W. (1979). Ketamine as a detumescence agent during hypospadias repair. *Journal of Urology, 121*, 654.

Pilcher, J., Chandrasekhar, K. P., Rees, J. R., Boyce, M. J., Pierce, T. H., & Ikram, H. (1973). Long-term assessment of perhexiline maleate in angina pectoris. *Postgraduate Medical Journal, 49*(Suppl.), 115–118.

Pillay, V. K. G. (1976). Some side-effects of alpha-methyldopa. *South African Medical Journal, 50*, 625–626.

Pitts, N. E. (1974). The clinical evaluation of prazocin hydrochloride, a new antihypertensive agent. In D. W. K. Cotton (Ed.), *Prazocin—evaluation of a new antihypertensive agent: Proceedings of a symposium* (pp. 149–163). Amsterdam: Excerpta Medica.

Pont, A., Graybill, J. R., Craven, P. C., Galgiani, J. N., Dismukes, W. E., Reitz, R. E., & Stevens, D. A. C. (1984). High-dose hetoconazole therapy and adrenal and testicular function in humans. *Annals of Internal Medicine, 144*, 2150-2153.

Prichard, B. N. C., Johnston, A. W., Hill, I. D., & Rossenheim, M. L. (1968). Bethanidine, guanethidine, and methyldopa in treatment of hypertension: A within-patient comparison. *British Medical Journal, i*, 135-144.

Raftos, J., Bauer, G. E., & Lewis, R. G. (1973). Clonidine in the treatment of severe hypertension. *Medical Journal of Australia, 30*, 786-793.

Reid, K., Morales, A., Harris, C., Surridge, D. H. C., Condra, M., Owen, J., & Fenemore, J. (1987). Double-blind trial of yohimbine in treatment of psychogenic impotence. *Lancet, ii*, 421-423.

Reynolds, C. F., Thase, M. E., Jennings, J. R., Howell, J. R., Frank, E., Berman, S. R., Houck, P. R., & Kupfer, D. J. (1989). Nocturnal penile tumescence in healthy 20- to 59-year olds: A revisit. *Sleep, 12*, 368-373.

Riley, A. J., Goodman, R. E., Kellet, J. M., & Orr, R. (1989). Double-blind trial of yohimbine hydrochloride in the treatment of erection inadequacy. *Sexual and Marital Therapy, 4*, 17-26.

Riley, A. J., & Riley, E. J. (1986). The effect of single dose diazepam on female sexual response induced by masturbation. *Sexual and Marital Therapy, 1*, 49-53.

Rosen, R. C., Kostis, J. B., & Jekelis, A. W. (1989). Beta-blocker effects on sexual function in normal males. *Archives of Sexual Behavior, 17*, 241-255.

Rosenthal, J. (1979). Treatment of hypertension with a beta-adrenoceptor blocker: A multicenter trial with pindolol. *British Journal of Clinical Practice, 33*, 165-181.

Rubin, S. O. (1968). Priapism as a possible sequel to medication. *Scandinavian Journal of Urology and Nephrology, 2*, 81-86.

Ruskin, D. B., & Goldner, R. D. (1959). Treatment of depression in private practice with imipramine. *Diseases of the Nervous System, 20*, 391-399.

Sandison, R. A., Whitelaw, E., & Currie, J. D. C. (1960). Clinical trials with Mellaril (TPZI) in the treatment of schizophrenia. *Journal of Mental Science, 106*, 732-741.

Sangal, R. (1985). Inhibited female orgasm as a side-effect of alprazolam. *American Journal of Psychiatry, 142*, 1223-1224.

Saunders, E., & Kong, B. (1980). Sexual activity in male hypertensive patients while taking clonidine. *Urban Health, 9*, 22-26.

Scheithauer, W., Ludwig, H., & Maida, E. (1985). Acute encephalopathy associated with continuous vircristine sulfate combination therapy: Case report. *Investigational New Drugs, 3*, 315-318.

Schiavi, R. C. (1990a). Chronic alcoholism and male sexual dysfunction. *Journal of Sex and Marital Therapy, 16*, 23-33.

Schiavi, R. C. (1990b, March 17). *Male sexual function and aging.* Paper presented at the annual meeting of the Society for Sex Therapy and Research, Baltimore.

Schiavi, R. C., & Schreiner-Engel, P. (1988). Nocturnal penile tumescence in healthy aging men. *Journal of Gerontology, 43*, 146-150.

Schiavi, R. C., Schreiner-Engel, P., Mandeli, J., Schanzer, H., & Cohen, E. (1990). Healthy aging and male sexual function. *American Journal of Psychiatry, 147*, 766-771.

Schimert, G., & Buschbeck, K. (1981). Multicentre study with nadolol in hypertension. In F. Gross (Ed.), *International experience with nadolol* (pp. 197–205). London: Academic Press.

Schinger, A., & Gifford, R. W. (1962). Guanethidine, a new antihypertensive agent: Experience in the treatment of 36 patients with severe hypertension. *Mayo Clinic Proceedings, 37,* 100–108.

Schlatter, E. K. E., & Lal, S. (1972). Treatment of alcoholism with Dent's oral apomorphine method. *Quarterly Journal of Studies on Alcohol, 33,* 430–436.

Schneider, J., & Kaffarnik, H. (1975). Impotence in patients treated with clofibrate. *Atherosclerosis, 21,* 455–475.

Schover, L. R., & Jensen, S. B. (1988). *Sexuality and chronic illness.* New York: Guilford Press.

Schwartz, N. H., & Robinson, B. D. (1952). Impotence due to methantheline bromide. *New York State Journal of Medicine, 52,* 165–167.

Segraves, R. T. (1987). Treatment of premature ejaculation with lorazepam. *American Journal of Psychiatry, 144,* 1240.

Segraves, R. T. (1988a). Drugs and desire. In S. R. Leiblum & R. C. Rosen (Eds.), *Sexual desire disorders* (pp. 313–347). New York: Guilford Press.

Segraves, R. T. (1988b). Hormones and libido. In S. R. Leiblum & R. C. Rosen (Eds.), *Sexual desire disorders* (pp. 271–312). New York: Guilford Press.

Segraves, R. T. (1988c). Sexual side-effects of psychiatric drugs. *International Journal of Psychiatry in Medicine, 18,* 243–252.

Segraves, R. T. (1989). Effects of psychotropic drugs on human erection and ejaculation. *Archives of General Psychiatry, 46,* 275–284.

Segraves, R. T., Bari, M., Segraves, K. B., & Spirnak, P. (1991). Effect of apomorphine on penile tumescence in men with psychogenic impotence. *Journal of Urology, 145,* 1174–1175.

Segraves, R. T., Madsen, R., Carter, S. C., & Davis, J. M. (1985). Erectile dysfunction associated with pharmacological agents. In R. T. Segraves & H. W. Schoenberg (Eds.), *Diagnosis and treatment of erectile disturbances* (pp. 23–64). New York: Plenum.

Shalet, S. M. (1980). Effect of cancer chemotherapy on gonadal function of patients. *Cancer Treatment Reviews, 7,* 141–152.

Shantha, T. R., Finnerty, D. P., & Rodriquez, A. P. (1989). Treatment of persistent penile erection and priapism using terbutaline. *Journal of Urology, 141,* 1427–1429.

Sharifi, R. (1982). More on drug-induced sexual dysfunction. *Clinical Pharmacology, 1,* 397.

Simpson, G. M., Blair, J. H., & Amvso, D. (1965). Effects of antidepressants on genitourinary function. *Diseases of the Nervous System, 26,* 787–789.

Simpson, W. T. (1977). Nature and incidence of unwanted effects with atenolol. *Postgraduate Medical Journal, 53*(Suppl.), 162–167.

Smith, R. N., & Elsdon-Dew, R. W. (1983). Alleged impotence with ranitidine. *Lancet, ii,* 798.

Snyder, S., Karacan, I., & Salis, P. J. (1981). Disulfiram and nocturnal penile tumescence in the chronic alcoholic. *Biological Psychiatry, 16,* 399–406.

Sondra, L. P., Mazo, R., & Chancellor, M. B. (1990). The role of yohimbine for the treatment of erectile impotence. *Journal of Sex and Marital Therapy, 16*, 15-21.

Spark, R. F., & Melby, J. C. (1968). Aldosteronism in hypertension. *Annals of Internal Medicine, 69*, 685-691.

Stevenson, J. G., & Umsted, G. S. (1984). Sexual dysfunction due to antihypertensive agents. *Drug Intelligence and Clinical Pharmacy, 18*, 113-121.

Stevenson, R. W. D., & Solyom, L. (1990). The aphrodisiac effect of fenfluramine: Two case reports of a possible side effect to the use of fenfluramine in the treatment of bulimia. *Journal of Clinical Psychopharmacology, 10*, 69-71.

Stokes, G. S., Mennie, B. A., Gellatly, R., & Hill, A. (1983). On the combination of alpha- and beta-adrenoceptor blockade in hypertension. *Clinical Pharmacology and Therapeutics, 34*, 576-582.

Stokes, G. S., & Oates, H. F. (1978). Prazosin: New alpha-adrenergic blocking agent in treatment of hypertension. *Cardiovascular Medicine, 3*, 41-57.

Stressman, J., & Ben-Ishay, D. (1980). Chlorthalidone induced impotence. *British Medical Journal, 281*, 714.

Strum, W. B. (1983). Epigastric pain and HBP after biliary disease. *Hospital Practice, 18*, 98N, 98T.

Suskind, R. R., & Hertzberg, V. S. (1984). Human health effects of 2,4,5-T and its toxic contaminants. *Journal of the American Medical Association, 251*, 2372-2380.

Susset, J. G., Tessier, C. D., Wincze, J., Bansal, S., Malhotra, C., & Schwacha, M. G. (1989). Effect of yohimbine hydrochloride on erectile impotence: A double-blind study. *Journal of Urology, 141*, 1360-1363.

Suzuki, H., Tominaga, T., Kumagai, H., & Saruta, T. (1988). Effects of first line antihypertensive agents on sexual function and sex hormones. *Journal of Hypertension, 6*(Suppl. 4), S649-S651.

Tcherdakoff, P. (1983). Side-effects with long-term labetalol: An open study of 251 patients in a single center. *Pharmatherapeutica, 3*, 342-348.

Tennett, G., Bancroft, J., & Cass, J. (1974). The control of deviant sexual behavior by drugs: A double-blind controlled study of benperidol, chlorpromazine, and placebo. *Archives of Sexual Behavior, 3*, 261-271.

Tosi, S., & Cagnoli, M. (1982). Painful gynaecomastia with ranitidine. *Lancet, ii*, 160.

Tsitouras, P. D., Martin, C. E., & Harman, E. M. (1982). Relationship of serum testosterone to sexual activity in healthy elderly men. *Journal of Gerontology, 37*, 288-293.

Tuchman, H., & Crumpton, C. W. (1955). A comparison of rauwolfia serpentia compounds cruderoot, alseroxylon derivatives and single alkaloid in the treatment of hypertension. *American Heart Journal, 49*, 742-750.

Uhde, T. W., Tancer, M. E., & Shea, C. A. (1988). Sexual dysfunction related to alprazolam treatment of social phobia. *American Journal of Psychiatry, 145*, 531-532.

Vermeulen, A. (1986). The effects of aging on the male reproductive system. In G. E. Striker & C. H. Rodgers (Eds.), *Conference on the Scientific Basis of Sexual Dysfunction: Abstracts* (pp. 1-7). Baltimore: National Institutes of Health.

Vermeulen, A., Rubens, A., & Verdonck, L. (1971). Testosterone secretion and metabolism in male senescence. *Journal of Clinical Endocrinology and Metabolism, 34*, 730-735.

Verwoerdt, A., Pfeiffer, E., & Wang, H. (1969). Sexual behavior in senescence: Changes in sexual activity and interest of aging men and women. *Journal of Geriatric Psychiatry*, 2, 163–180.

Veterans Administration Study Group on Antihypertensive Drugs. (1983). Efficacy of nadolol alone and combined with bendroflumethiazide and hydralazine for systemic hypertension. *American Journal of Cardiology*, 52, 1230–1237.

Veterans Administration Cooperative Study Group on Antihypertensive Agents. (1977). Propranolol in the treatment of essential hypertension. *Journal of the American Medical Association*, 237, 2303–2310.

Veterans Administration Cooperative Study Group on Antihypertensive Agents. (1981). Comparison of prazosin with hydralazine in patients receiving hydrochlorothiazide: A randomized, double-blind clinical trial. *Circulation*, 64, 722–729.

Veterans Administration Cooperative Study Group on Antihypertensive Agents. (1982). Comparison of propranolol and hydrochlorothiazide for the initial treatment of hypertension. *Journal of the American Medical Association*, 248, 2004–2011.

Viana, L. (1983). Probable case of impotence due to ranitidine. *Lancet*, i, 635–636.

Vinarova, E., Uhlir, O., & Stika, L. (1972). Side-effects of lithium administration. *Activitas Nervosa Superior* (Praha), 14, 105–107.

Wagar, G., Tolonen, M., Stenman, U., & Helpio, E. (1981). Endocrinological studies in men exposed occupationally to carbon disulfide. *Journal of Toxicology and Environmental Health*, 7, 363–371.

Wahl, B. N., Turlapaty, P., & Singh, B. (1985). Comparison of acebutolol and propranolol in essential hypertension. *American Heart Journal*, 109, 313–321.

Wallace, T. R., Fraunfelder, F. T., & Petursson, G. L. (1979). Decreased libido—a side-effect of carbonic anhydrase inhibitor. *Annals of Ophthalmology*, 11, 1563–1566.

Warren, S. C., & Warren, S. G. (1977). Propranolol and sexual impotence. *Annals of International Medicine*, 86, 112.

Warren, S. G., Brewer, D. L., & Orgain, E. S. (1976). Long-term propranolol therapy for angina pectoris. *American Journal of Cardiology*, 37, 420–426.

Weizman, A., Maoz, B., Treves, I., Asher, I., & Ben-David, M. (1985). Sulpiride-induced hyperprolactinemia and impotence in male psychiatric outpatients. *Progress in Neuropsychopharmacology and Biological Psychiatry*, 9, 193–198.

Welti, R. S., & Brodsky, J. B. (1980). Treatment of intraoperative penile tumescence. *Journal of Urology*, 124, 925–926.

Williams, G. H., Croog, S. H., Levine, S., Testa, M. A., & Sudilovsky, A. (1987). Impact of antihypertensive therapy on quality of life: Effect of hydrochlorothiazide. *Journal of Hypertension*, 5(Suppl. 1), 529–535.

Wilson, G. T. (1981). The effects of alcohol on human sexual behavior. *Advances in Substance Abuse*, 2, 1–40.

Witton, K. (1962). Sexual dysfunction secondary to Mellaril. *Diseases of the Nervous System*, 23, 175.

Wolfe, M. M. (1979). Impotence on cimetidine treatment. *New England Journal of Medicine*, 300, 94.

Wootten, L. W., & Bailey, R. I. (1975). Experiences with clomipramine (Anafranil) in the treatment of the phobic anxiety states in general practice. *Journal of International Medical Research*, 3(Suppl. 1), 1001–1007.

Yassa, R. (1982). Sexual disorders in the course of clomipramine treatment: A report of three cases. *Canadian Journal of Psychiatry*, 27, 148–149.

Zacharias, F. J. (1980). Comparison of the side-effects of different beta-blockers in the treatment of hypertension. *Primary Cardiology*, 6, 86–89.

Zacharias, F. J., Cowan, K. J., & Cuthbertson, P. J. R. (1977). Atenolol in hypertension: A study of long-term therapy. *Postgraduate Medical Journal*, 53, 102.

Zarren, H. S., & Black, P. M. (1975). Unilateral gynecomastia and impotence during low-dose spironolactone administration in men. *Military Medicine*, 140, 417–419.

Zimmerman, T. W. (1984). Problems associated with medical treatment of peptic ulcer disease. *American Journal of Medicine*, 77, 51–56.

Current Assessment
and Treatment Approaches
III

6

Laboratory Methods for Evaluating Erectile Dysfunction

Raul C. Schiavi

Diagnostic procedures for the assessment of erectile dysfunction have become increasingly complex and sophisticated in the past decade. As noted in Chapter 1 of this book, both patients and clinicians are currently faced with a potentially bewildering array of testing options. Most of these procedures are costly, are intrusive, and in some instances may involve significant medical risk for the patient. Moreover, there is little standardization in assessment protocols from one center to another, and conflicting reports have been published regarding the specificity, sensitivity, and reliability of currently used diagnostic procedures. Clearly, there is a pressing need for a comprehensive and critical evaluation of this important area.

In the present chapter, Schiavi provides a "state-of-the-art" review of laboratory procedures for evaluation of erectile dysfunction. Given the historical importance and continued use of nocturnal penile tumescence (NPT) testing as the "reference standard" in many centers, this procedure is considered in depth. Although NPT testing was initially viewed as a straightforward means for differentiating organic and psychogenic dysfunction, evidence has accumulated of the confounding effects of several factors, including aging, hypoactive desire, sleep disorders, and depression, on NPT. Interpretation of NPT findings requires considerable sophistication nowadays, as illustrated in both the research findings and case vignettes presented. Nonlaboratory methods for assessment of NPT (i.e., snap gauges, portable monitors) are especially controversial, and Schiavi offers a thoughtful critique of these widely used procedures.

Current alternatives to NPT include the use of visual sexual stimulation and intracorporal injection of vasoactive drugs for assessment of erectile function. Despite the potential value of visual sexual stimulation procedures, this approach is only suitable for patients who are comfortable with viewing explicit sexual materials in a laboratory setting. Nevertheless, several studies have indicated that the procedure provides a valuable adjunct to conventional NPT testing. Intracavernosal injections are frequently used to evaluate vasculogenic erectile dysfunction, despite *the potential lack of sensitivity or specificity of this approach. When combined with duplex ultrasonography, intracavernosal injections may be useful in assessing arterial inflow, or pharmacocavernosometry and cavernosography can be used to assess venous outflow. Given the relative invasiveness and potential difficulties in interpretation, Schiavi recommends these latter procedures only in special instances (e.g., when vascular surgery is being considered).*

Less progress has been made in the assessment of neurogenic dysfunction. Although several procedures are available for testing afferent innervation (e.g., biothesiometry, somatosensory evoked potentials), these methods have not been sufficiently evaluated to date. Furthermore, there are no currently available procedures for assessing autonomic control of genital vasocongestion. This is clearly an important area for further research.

Overall, this chapter provides a thoughtful and balanced discussion of current laboratory testing procedures for erectile dysfunction. On the basis of his extensive research and clinical experience in the field, Schiavi has carefully evaluated the pros and cons of each approach. Although considerable advances have clearly taken place in the past decade, this chapter also outlines the limitations and deficiencies in our current assessment approaches.

Raul C. Schiavi, M.D., is Professor of Psychiatry at the Mount Sinai School of Medicine in New York City. He has made major contributions to both basic research and clinical practice in the field of sex therapy, and has received numerous grants and awards for his work in this area. He has published widely on such topics as sex and aging, hypoactive sexual desire, and alcohol effects on sexual response. Dr. Schiavi is a recent recipient of the Masters and Johnson Award from the Society of Sex Therapy and Research.

––––––––––

Correct assessment of the nature and extent of erectile failure is of critical significance for effective therapeutic intervention. The importance of diagnostic accuracy is emphasized by the wide range of therapeutic modalities available, from sexual counseling to vascular surgery and prosthetic implantation. The coexistence of psychological and organic determinants in the development and maintenance of erectile disorders frequently creates considerable problems in differential diagnosis and in the selection of appropriate treatment strategies. An adequate diagnostic workup of erectile dysfunction is based on a multidisciplinary approach that considers organic and psychological factors within an integrative framework. Central to this process is a comprehensive medical, psychosexual, and relationship evaluation. However, this information, although essential, is at times not sufficient, and several laboratory methods are presently available to improve diagnostic accuracy. The development of these new approaches has been facilitated by, and in turn has contributed to, increasing psychobiological knowledge about male sexual function.

The assessment of nocturnal penile tumescence (NPT) was among the first and probably is still the most widely utilized laboratory method to evaluate organic impairment in erectile capacity. It has served as a "reference standard" against which the accuracy of other diagnostic procedures has frequently been compared. NPT recordings assess erectile capacity and the overall integrity of mediating psychobiological systems, but do not provide direct information about vascular, neurological, and hormonal mechanisms. Several specific techniques, varying in degree of physical invasiveness, have been recently developed to evaluate neurovascular competence in erectile function; they have added an important complementary dimension as well as a new level of complexity to the evaluation process.

The purpose of this chapter is to review critically the laboratory procedures most frequently employed in the evaluation of erectile disorders, with specific emphasis on the NPT method. The review considers validity data as well as information about diagnostic accuracy and clinical utility. Hormonal methods of evaluation are not discussed, since they are covered in another chapter of this book.

THE NOCTURNAL PENILE
TUMESCENCE DIAGNOSTIC METHOD

The phenomenon of erection cycles during sleep in adult males was first described in 1944 by Ohlmeyer, Brilmayer, and Hullstrung on the basis of kymographic penile recordings. Approximately 10 years later, the observation by Aserinsky (1953) of periodic conjugate rapid eye movements (REMs) in sleeping infants led to the discovery of what is now well known as REM sleep cyclicity. The close correspondence between the periodicity of erectile episodes and REM sleep was noted by Aserinsky and Kleitman (1955) and demonstrated experimentally by Fisher, Gross, and Zuch (1965) and by Karacan, Goodenough, Shapiro, and Starker (1966). Since then, a considerable body of normative data has been gathered in different age groups. The pervasive nature of NPT and its apparent individual stability in healthy men led Karacan (1970) to speculate that the recording of NPT might provide a useful diagnostic and prognostic tool in erectile impotence.

Normative Studies

The evaluation of diagnostic tests for the differential diagnosis of erectile impotence requires age-related normative data in sexually nondysfunctional individuals. Karacan, Salis, Thornby, and Williams (1976) conducted a series of studies on 125 healthy subjects 3 to 79 years of age, who were assessed in the sleep laboratory during at least three nights under standardized conditions. The investigators found a significant decrease in duration and frequency of nocturnal episodes in relation to aging. These changes were observed even after the age-related decreases in sleep time were controlled for. Duration of total tumescence diminished progressively from an average of 191 minutes per night at ages 13–15 to 96 minutes at ages 70–79. This change represented a decrease in tumescence duration from 37% to 22% of sleep period time. Duration of REM sleep remained relatively constant following adolescence and did not account for the age-related variations in tumescence. The number of erectile episodes also decreased from an average of more than 6 per night during early adolescence to 3.4 in men above age 70. There was a close association between REM sleep and erectile episodes, but older men, as compared to younger adults, showed a reduction in the duration of tumescence during REM sleep and more frequent erections during non-REM sleep. The overall evidence of ontogenic changes in NPT reported by Karacan et al. (1976) was consistent with earlier reports by Jovanovic and Tan-Eli (1969) and by Kahn and Fisher (1969).

The assessment of degree of tumescence in these investigations was based on the measurement of penile circumferential changes; maximum episodes were defined by Karacan et al. (1976) as penile circumference increases between 81% and 100% of the greatest circumference recorded for the subject. The importance of not relying solely on circumferential measures for the assessment of erectile capacity has become increasingly recognized in recent years. None of the studies mentioned above reported systematic awakenings during tumescent episodes for estimation of degree of penile rigidity. In view of the significance of this information for the diagnostic interpretation of NPT, a colleague and I conducted a normative study in 40 healthy sexually nondysfunctional men aged 23 to 73 (Schiavi & Schreiner-Engel, 1988). Sleep and NPT recordings were made under standard conditions during three nights; during the third night, visual checks were carried out during tumescent episodes to ascertain degree of erection relative to the recorded increase in penile circumference. The subject and the investigator separately rated the degree of erection on a 1–10 scale; the investigator also noted the angle of the erection from the horizontal plane and then obtained a photographic record. Lack of stable penile rigidity in older subjects prevented the systematic application of the buckling pressure method to quantify rigidity across all age groups.

As previously reported, frequency and duration of NPT decreased progressively with age, independently of variations in sleep (Figure 6.1). Among the 31 men less than 60 years of age, 96% had full erections verified by observation. In contrast, 5 of the 9 subjects above age 60 did not have full

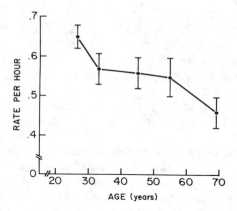

FIGURE 6.1. Age-related changes in tumescent time as percentage of total sleep time. Data points (mean ± *SEM*) are plotted at the average age per group. From "Nocturnal Penile Tumescence in Healthy Aging Men" by R. C. Schiavi and P. Schreiner-Engel, 1988, *Journal of Gerontology, 43*, M146–M150. Copyright 1988 by the Gerontological Society of America. Reprinted by permission.

erections, even though they and their partners indicated (independently of each other) that they were having regular intercourse. These observations, replicated in a larger subject sample of older, healthy volunteers (Schiavi, Schreiner-Engel, Mandeli, Schanzer, & Cohen, 1990), emphasize the importance of ontogenetic investigations of penile rigidity. Reynolds et al. (1989) also provided electroencephalographic (EEG) and rigidity data in 48 healthy, sexually nondysfunctional men aged 20 to 59 years. There were modest but significant decreases in frequency and duration of NPT, but between these age limits there were no differences in estimates of erectile rigidity by visual inspection or buckling force. The relevance of normative findings of penile rigidity for the use of NPT as a diagnostic tool is discussed in a latter section.

Psychobiology of Nocturnal Penile Tumescence

The role of central processes in NPT activity has been emphasized by recent psychophysiological, hormonal, and psychological evidence. We continue to know relatively little about the brain mechanisms that control sleep erections, although it is likely that they involve limbic and pontine structures that mediate REM cyclicity and erectile activity. Differences in the ontogenetic development of REM sleep and NPT (Karacan et al., 1976) and their differential response to psychoactive drugs (Fisher, Kahn, & Edwards, 1972) suggest, however, that the processes may be dissociated, although they are closely related. Research conducted by Rosen, Goldstein, Scoles, and Lazarus (1986) showed activation of the nondominant cerebral hemisphere during NPT in normal volunteers, but the overlapping between REM sleep and NPT did not allow determination of the extent to which the pattern of hemispheric asymmetry was specifically related to REM activity or to NPT. These investigators noted that the nondominant-hemispheric activation during the NPT phase was consistent with the changes in cerebral laterality that they had previously observed during waking studies of sexual arousal in normal men (Cohen, Rosen, & Goldstein, 1985).

Hormonal studies have supported the distinction between erotic and sleep-related erections. Studies on hypogonadal men have shown that their sleep erections are impaired prior to treatment, and that these are significantly enhanced by androgen administration (Davidson, Camargo, & Smith, 1979; Kwan, Greenleaf, Mann, Crapo, & Davidson, 1983). O'Carroll, Shaprio, and Bancroft (1985) further noted that the androgen effect on NPT is not secondary to changes in total sleep time or REM time. In contrast, erections induced in response to erotic stimuli in nontreated hypogonadal men do not appear to differ from those of normal subjects and are not affected by androgen replacement (Bancroft & Wu, 1983). These findings have led some authors to propose that NPT is androgen-dependent and that androgens are more important in sustaining sexual interest and sleep-related erections than they are in maintaining erectile responses to external stimuli. We have hypothesized (Schiavi & Schreiner-Engel, 1988) that the lack of rigid sleep erections in some healthy older men, who report continued ability to have intercourse, may be due to age-related changes in central neurobiological processes that mediate internally generated sexual arousal. These individuals may compensate by increased reliance on the synergistic effect of direct penile stimulation for the development of reflexogenic erections and maintenance of intercourse capacity. The role of age-related declines in androgen secretion on NPT activity in older individuals remains to be investigated.

Several investigators have noted an association between erectile impotence on the one hand, and sleep apneas and periodic leg movement disorders on the other (Foreman, Stahl, Hobbins, Paskewitz, & Gross, 1986; Guilleminault, Eldridge, Tilkian, Simmons, & Dement, 1977; Schmidt & Wise, 1981). Schmidt and Wise speculated that abnormal central nervous system activity may be etiologically responsible for the NPT abnormalities of patients with sleep disorders in whom an organic cause cannot be identified. We have recently examined the possible role of sleep disorders in age-related variations in sexual function and NPT among healthy, nonobese married men aged 45 to 75 years (Schiavi, Mandeli, Schreiner-Engel, & Chambers, 1991). The results corroborated previous reports of age-related increases in sleep-disordered breathing, but did not demonstrate changes in periodic leg movements with age. There was no evidence that sleep disorders are involved in the increased prevalence of erectile impotence, or in the decrease in NPT activity observed in healthy older men. It is possible, however, that sleep disorders are more closely associated with disturbances in sexual function in seniors unselected for health status.

NPT is more responsive to psychological phenomena than was once thought. The earliest information stems from Karacan et al. (1966) and Fisher (1966), who noted an inhibition of NPT in normal subjects during REM periods associated with dreams of high anxiety content. NPT may be decreased during the first study night, presumably because of the stressful aspects of the experimental situation (Jovanovic, 1969). There is compelling evidence that clinical depression may be associated with marked NPT abnormalities that are independent of alterations in sleep architecture; recovery from depression is followed by restoration of sexual drive, erectile capacity, and normalization of NPT (Roose, Glassman, Walsh, & Cullen, 1982; Thase et al., 1987, 1988). We have also observed that healthy, non-depressed men with a primary diagnosis of hypoactive sexual desire and secondary erectile difficulties (*Diagnostic and Statistical Manual of Mental Disorders,* third edition, revised; DSM-III-R) have marked abnormalities in degree, frequency, and duration of nocturnal erections (Schiavi, Schreiner-Engel, White, & Mandeli, 1988). The influence of affective disorders and low sexual drive on NPT suggests that the central neurobiological substrates of affect and sexual motivation are involved in the modulation of sleep erections.

The possibility that sleep erections reflect central processes associated with sexual desire, pleasure, or satisfaction was recently investigated in our laboratories in healthy volunteers (Schiavi et al., 1990). Sexual desire, defined as the maximum time a subject reported feeling comfortable without sex, was significantly related (after age adjustment) to an NPT variable: frequency of erectile episodes during REM sleep. Sexual pleasure and satisfaction were not associated with any NPT measure. Information about central physiological mechanisms that subserve sleep erections, and about the role of psychological processes in NPT activity, is of considerable relevance for the diagnostic interpretation of the method.

Clinical Application of the Method

Jovanovic and Tan-Eli (1969) found that a preparation containing methyltestosterone and yohimbine, among other pharmacological agents, restored sexual function and normalized NPT in men with erectile disorders. This study was followed by a monograph (Jovanovic, 1972) reporting the investigation of a large number of normal men and patients with psychiatric or medical illnesses. Of particular interest was the observation that men with either erectile impotence or psychopathological conditions, including mood disorders, showed abnormal sleep-erection patterns. Jovanovic concluded from the parallelism between erectile abnormalities during wakefulness and sleep that the recording of sleep erections may permit the objective verification of sexual potency.

Empirical evidence on the value of NPT monitoring for the differential diagnosis of erectile disorders was first provided by our research group (Fisher, Schiavi, Lear, Davis, & Witkin, 1975) and by Karacan, Williams, Thornby, and Salis (1975). On the basis of a systematic, clinical, and NPT evaluation of a small number of impotent men, we (Fisher et al., 1975) proposed:

> In psychologic impotence, nocturnal REM erections may be normal in amount and degree and an excellent indication of erectile potential. In these cases, a marked discrepancy exists between the amount and degree of nocturnal erection and the patient's daytime performance level attained during attempted coitus or masturbation. In the organic patients, on the contrary, such a discrepancy does not exist; instead, the maximal nocturnal erection attained corresponds closely to and mirrors the patient's impaired waking performance. (p. 277)

Karacan et al. (1975), in the context of an article in which they summarized their normative data on healthy men, also emphasized the diagnostic value of NPT for differentiating organogenic from psychogenic impotence.

These two reports marked the beginning of a long series of studies that have employed NPT recordings for diagnostic assessments (Karacan et al., 1977; Karacan, 1978; Karacan, Salis, & Williams, 1978; Fisher et al., 1979; Hosking et al., 1979; Wasserman, Pollak, Spielman, & Weitzman, 1980a; Zuckerman et al., 1985). However, despite the wide utilization of this method, relatively few investigations have evaluated its diagnostic accuracy (Marshall, Morales, & Surridge, 1982; Marshall, Surridge, & Delva, 1981). We have reported a validation study of NPT on 52 young men divided into four age-matched groups: diabetic men with and without erectile problems, men with psychogenic erectile difficulties, and normal controls (Schiavi, Fisher, Quadland, & Glover, 1985). The groups were formed on the basis of extensive medical and psychological evidence that was independent of NPT data. Quantitative comparisons of degree, frequency, and duration of NPT over three study nights were made across groups. Diabetic impotent men exhibited a significantly decreased number of erectile episodes, episodes during REM, and episodes of maximum tumescence per night. They also spent significantly less time in tumescence and in simultaneous REM sleep and tumescence. Diabetic men without sexual problems, psychogenically impotent men, and normal subjects did not differ on the frequency and duration variables. However, nonimpotent diabetic men showed circumferential increases during erection that were significantly lower than those of the psychogenic and normal control groups and similar in degree to those of the impotent diabetic patients. The diagnostic efficiency of the method (capacity of the test to identify men both with and without organic pathology, minimizing false positives and false negatives) ranged form 77.8% to 88.9% (Schiavi, 1988). It should be emphasized that these results require replication and may not be generalizable to other causes of organic impotence or to older patients.

The procedures for NPT testing are usually carried out during two to three recording nights. EEG activity, eye movements, muscle tone, and penile tumescence (measured by two strain gauge loops placed at the base of the penis and behind the corona of the glans) are monitored continuously. Penile rigidity is assessed by visual ratings and photographic recordings during systematic awakenings on the last study night. Penile rigidity may also be assessed by a special device that applies a known pressure to the erected penis and measures the force required to make it buckle.

Sleep records are scored according to standardized criteria, and the amount and distribution of sleep stages are determined. Frequency and duration of erectile episodes during the night are quantified; the penile strain gauges are calibrated so that the degree of circumferential increases of the penis are also measured. NPT evaluations in the sleep laboratory are labor-intensive; this is reflected in the cost of the procedure, which ranges from $300 to $600 per study night.

Considerations Relevant to Diagnostic Accuracy

The diagnostic accuracy of NPT measurement may be severely compromised if findings from the research discussed above are not taken into account. Some of these issues have been discussed in more detail in a recent review article (Schiavi, 1988).

Effect of Aging

The distinction between normal and pathological aging, which has been frequently discussed in gerontological research (Rowe & Kahn, 1987), has not been adequately considered in the assessment of sexual function in older individuals. The paucity of NPT norms for men above age 65 raises a note of caution about the significance of NPT findings in this age group, since these may not indicate pathology, but instead may reflect physiological variations associated with aging. Age should be always taken into account in the diagnostic interpretation of apparently atypical observations in older subjects.

Effect of Emotional States

As mentioned above, there is evidence that anxiety, clinical depression, and hypoactive sexual desire may be associated with abnormalities in NPT in physically healthy individuals. It is possible that other psychopathological states also may affect NPT, although these have not been investigated, with the exception of the monograph by Jovanovic (1972). Anxiety should be considered when there is evidence of sleep fragmentation, frequent arousals, or diminished REM sleep associated with depressed NPT activity. Although individual responses are highly variable, some subjects have inhibited erections during the first study night or when they are aware that awakenings will take place for rigidity verification. It is important for diagnostic purposes to rely on more than one recording night, as well as for clinicians to be aware of the psychological context in which the recordings take place. The existence of a mood disorder or inhibited sexual desire also needs to be clinically assessed and taken into account in the interpretation of abnormal NPT findings.

Case Vignette

Mr. S., a 39-year-old married man, stated that he had had a problem-free sexual life until 6 years ago, when his sexual desire gradually declined. Two years ago, he "lost all interest in sex" and began having erectile difficulties. His wife became increasingly angry and self-incriminating, and in response to her demands, the couple was referred to our program to be evaluated as part of a study on hypoactive sexual desire. Both partners were unable to identify a specific event or problem as being related to his decrease in sexual desire. Mr. S.'s medical and psychiatric histories were noncontributory, and a comprehensive medical and endocrine evaluation was essentially negative. Mr. S. was studied in the sleep laboratory during four nights. Although the sleep architecture was within normal limits, the NPT was markedly decreased in frequency, duration, and degree. These findings were characteristic of a group of healthy men with hypoactive sexual desire and secondary erectile problems (Schiavi et al., 1988).

Recording Variables

The importance of assessing sleep parameters for the interpretation of NPT cannot be underestimated. Any illness, pharmacological agent, or psychological state associated with abnormalities in sleep and REM activity is likely to disrupt NPT patterns and to lead to false diagnostic conclusions. Although we have not obtained evidence that sleep disorders affect sexual function and NPT recordings in healthy individuals, they may have a deleterious influence on erectile capacity in obese men or patients with associated medical conditions or sleep complaints. Identification of sleep apnea or periodic leg movement disorders require the monitoring of respiration and tibial electromyographic (EMG) activity during sleep. In addition, the presence of unrecognized sleep disorders may result in NPT monitoring artifacts that may be overlooked in the absence of respiratory and EMG measures (Pressman, DiPhillipo, Kendrick, Conroy, & Fry, 1986).

Assessment of Rigidity

Early in the development of NPT diagnostic monitoring, it became apparent that there were considerable variations in penile circumference increases associated with rigid erections (Fisher et al., 1979). The discrepancy between penile tumescence and rigidity led to systematic observations of penile firmness and to the use of a device developed by Karacan (1978) that measures the axial force required for the bending of the penis (buckling pressure). Penile buckling at pressures of less than 100 mm Hg is interpreted as an indication of insufficient rigidity for vaginal penetration (Wabrek, 1986). My colleagues and I have found this approach useful in younger individuals but impractical in older subjects because of rapid detumescence at the time of testing. There is, to our knowledge, no information on validity and reliability of buckling pressure determinations, and only one study that has assessed the reliability of visual estimates of penile rigidity (Campbell et al., 1987). Male technologists' visual estimates of rigidity correlated more highly with the subjects' own estimates and with measures of buckling force than did female technologists' estimates.

The technical difficulties of carrying out observations at the optimum time of maximum erection, as well as the problem of sleep disruption, have fostered procedures for continuous monitoring of penile rigidity. One of these methods is based on periodic and automatic checks of radial loading by means of a loop transducer placed around the penis (Bradley, Timm, Gallagher, & Johnson, 1985). With a similar device (Rigiscan, Dacomed Corp., Mineapolis, MN), Kaneko and Bradley (1986) observed several recording patterns, including a dissociation of rigidity between the tip and base of the penis; they concluded that the approach could improve the distinction between organic and psychogenic impotence. However, Wein, Malloy, Hannon, Barrett, and Furlow (1988) have challenged the diagnostic value of this approach, in part because of the lack of independent information about the accuracy of rigidity determinations, and the limitation inherent in not assessing sleep variables. The development and validation of a method for the simultaneous monitoring of rigidity and tumescence are likely not only to enhance diagnostic accuracy, but also to permit the investigation of the mechanisms involved in the uncoupling of rigidity and tumescence and the study of the role of perineal muscles on penile rigidity (Karacan, Hirshkowitz, Salis, Narter, & Safi, 1987). At present, however, rigidity data obtained with current methodologies should be interpreted with caution.

Criteria for Diagnostic Assignments

Diagnostic categorizations are usually based on criteria that have apparent face validity—that is, the presence or absence of sleep erections that are adequate for vaginal penetration and of sufficient duration to permit satisfactory completion of intercourse (Wasserman, Pollak, Spielman, & Weitzman, 1980b). These criteria may be sufficient to permit distinctions between nonoverlapping conditions, but are less than adequate when psychogenic and organic causative factors coexist or when there are gradual changes in NPT associated with illness or aging. There is a need to formulate decision rules based on empirically derived quantitative observations, and to assess objectively the accuracy of diagnostic discriminations. The idiosyncratic interpretation of NPT recordings limits the meaningful comparison of results across laboratories.

Case Vignette

A 61-year-old married diabetic man suffering from erectile impotence, in the context of considerable marital distress, came to our program requesting a second opinion concerning his sexual problem. The patient had had an NPT evaluation at another center, where prosthetic surgery had been recommended on the basis of lack of evidence of erections with circumferential increases greater than 16 mm at the base of the penis. The patient was studied in our sleep laboratories with systematic awakenings for verification of rigidity during the third study night. Although the patient's penile circumferential increases were indeed less than 16 mm, the results were not consistent with our clinical criteria for organogenic impotence (an average of less than one full erection per study night, lasting a minimum of 5 minutes). Marital counseling was recommended, and this resulted in a significant amelioration of his sexual function.

Nocturnal Penile Tumescence Screening Devices

Lack of technical expertise, scarcity of laboratory facilities, and economic considerations have fostered the development of devices that facilitate the screening of patients with erectile disorders. Three approaches have evolved: the stamp and snap gauge techniques, and the use of portable equipment for monitoring NPT. The stamp technique consists of the placement of a ring of stamps around the shaft of the penis; the breaking of the ring signifies that an erection has taken place (Barry, Blank, & Boileau, 1980). Results of studies on erotically induced erections (Marshall, Earls, Morales, & Surridge, 1982) and sleep erections (Marshall, Morales, Phillips, & Fenemore, 1983) have questioned the validity of this technique.

Another approach based on the same principle is the use of snap gauges, consisting of bands placed around the penis that incorporate three plastic elements designed to rupture sequentially at increasing degrees of expansive pressure (Ek, Bradley, & Krane, 1983). Ellis, Doghramji, and Bagley (1988) have assessed the reliability of the snap gauge band by comparing the breakage of the strips with direct technician evaluation of erectile rigidity during NPT testing. The snap gauge correctly predicted 77.5% of patients with rigid or nonrigid erections, with a sensitivity of 70% and specificity of 80%. Factors contributing to inaccurate diagnosis are improper use due to excessively loose or tight placement of the band around the penis, or accidental breakage due to body movements during sleep. The snap gauge technique also does not obtain information on frequency and duration of erections, and may lead to incorrect diagnosis in organically impotent men who have brief periods of rigidity sufficient to break the strip but of insufficient duration for intercourse.

Portable NPT monitoring instruments have the advantage of recording frequency, duration, and degree of sleep erections at home (Bohlen, 1981). Some commercial monitors contain a sound signaling system that is triggered at a predetermined increase in penile circumference for direct estimation of rigidity. The difficulty that a patient or his bed partner may have in obtaining reliable observations of rigidity during sudden awakenings may be obviated by recently developed instrumentation such as the Rigiscan, aimed at monitoring penile rigidity during uninterrupted sleep (see above). Lack of electrophysiological information to assess sleep architecture and REM activity, to identify sleep disorders, and to rule out movement artifacts seriously limits the diagnostic accuracy of portable monitoring equipment, however. The snap gauge technique and portable monitors should be used only as screening tools in the context of a comprehensive medical and psychological evaluation, with full appreciation of the potential for artifacts.

THE VISUAL SEXUAL STIMULATION METHOD

Several investigators have evaluated arousal responses to controlled visual presentation of erotic stimuli as a diagnostic test, either alone or in conjunction with the NPT method. The value of the visual stimulation method rests on theoretical and practical grounds. Erotically induced erections may reflect more closely the processes involved in dysfunctional sexual behavior, and may be mediated by physiological mechanisms different from those involved in sleep erections. The evaluation of sexual arousal during wakefulness not only records penile circumferential changes, as does the NPT method, but also assesses subjective responses. The visual stimulation method has the further advantage of being simpler and less costly than NPT recording.

The diagnostic value of this method has not yet been clearly established, however. An important limiting factor is the difficulty that a substantial proportion of physically normal men have in becoming aroused under laboratory conditions (Earls, Morales, & Marshall, 1988; Wincze et al., 1988). Some investigators have attempted to enhance erectile responses by permitting self-stimulation following erotic videotape exposure (Fisher et al., 1979; Sakheim, Barlow, Abrahamson, & Beck, 1987). Obviously, the subjects' attitudes toward visual erotica and masturbation are important factors in the applicability of this method—a consideration particularly relevant to older individuals.

Zuckerman et al. (1985) and Wincze et al. (1988) reported a discrepancy between low erectile responses in the laboratory and normal NPT activity in cases where there was a psychological inhibition regarding the experimental induction of sexual arousal. Of greater interest is the occasional reverse observation of abnormal sleep erections and adequate penile responses to erotica during wakefulness (Melman, Kaplan, & Redfield, 1984; Wincze et al., 1988). It has been suggested that the combined evaluation of penile circumferential changes during presentation of erotic stimuli and during sleep may enhance diagnostic accuracy and permit differentiation of subgroups of men with erectile dysfunction (Melman, Tiefer, & Pedersen, 1988; Wincze et al., 1988).

More research is required to determine the significance of divergent erectile responses to visual erotica and to REM sleep in normal subjects and in different diagnostic groups. Because of the low correlation between individuals' perceptions of degree of penile rigidity and polygraphic recordings of erections during laboratory-induced arousal (Sakheim et al., 1987; Earls et al., 1988), these studies may be enhanced by the continuous monitoring of penile rigidity. The results would be relevant to the elucidation of central mechanisms of sexual arousal and to the determination of the accuracy of NPT and visual sexual stimulation methods.

VASCULAR ASSESSMENT

New evidence on the vascular mechanisms of penile erection and on the high prevalence of vasculogenic factors in erectile impotence has fostered the development of diagnostic tests for vascular competency. It is presently thought that the hemodynamic processes responsible for erection involve relaxation of the smooth muscles of the sinusoidal system and the penile arterioles, resulting in decreased vascular resistance and a corresponding increase in arterial inflow into the corpora cavernosa. The passive occlusion of the emissary veins, compressed between the expanding cavernosal sinusoids and the inellastic tunica albuginea, contributes to the development of intracorporal pressure and the maintenance of erections (Krane, Goldstein, & Saenz de Tejada, 1989). It is still unclear whether active physiological mechanisms also paticipate in the restriction of penile venous outflow (Aboseif & Lue, 1988). Several noninvasive as well as invasive tests now permit clinicians to evaluate the arterial and venous physiological components of penile rigidity. These tests provide complementary information on possible pathogenic mechanisms of erectile failure, but do not directly assess erectile capacity, as do the NPT or visual sexual stimulation methods.

Noninvasive Tests

Penile Blood Pressure

One of the techniques most often used for diagnosing vasculogenic impotence is the measurement of penile blood pressure with a pneumatic cuff applied to the base of the penis and a Doppler ultrasound flow detector to record systolic occlusion pressures in the six penile arteries (Abelson, 1975). The penile–brachial index (PBI) is defined as the ratio between the penile systolic blood pressure and the brachial systolic blood pressure. It is commonly accepted that PBI values below 0.6 are diagnostic of vasculogenic impotence and that values between 0.6 and 0.75 suggest arterial insufficiency (Queral et al., 1979). The accurate determination of penile blood pressure is time-consuming because of the difficulty in obtaining reliable recordings of the cavernosal arteries, which are more directly responsible for erection.

Several laboratories have used strain gauge plethysmography, which does not require Doppler measurements of individual penile arteries, as an alternative noninvasive measurement of penile blood flow. In this procedure, a silicone mercury strain gauge is placed around the penis distal to the pneumatic cuff, and the systolic pressure readings are obtained when the cuff is deflated and pulsatile changes are first recorded. Strain gauge measures have shown good agreement with Doppler penile pressure determinations (Doyle & Yu, 1986; R. C. Schiavi, H. Schanzer, & E. Cohen, manuscript in preparation). With the combined use of strain gauge plethysmography and Doppler blood pressure measurements, Metz and Bengtsson (1981) found that a PBI of 0.6 or less was predictive of 91% of impotent men with peripheral arteriosclerotic disease. Inaccurate classifications (i.e., nondysfunctional men with a PBI less than 0.6 or dysfunctional men with a higher PBI) was 22% in a group of 45 patients.

Goldstein et al. (1982) called attention to the existence of pathological vascular conditions that may lead to decreased penile blood flow and erectile failure following exercise. Monitoring of penile blood pressures before and after exercise of the lower limbs improved the sensitivity of the penile blood pressure test and facilitated the identification of previously unrecognized vascular pathology, mainly in patients with borderline PBI values between 0.6 and 0.75. A decrease in PBI of 0.15 or more following exercise is considered a positive "pelvic steal" test, indicative of vascular abnormalities in the internal iliac or internal pudendal arterial system. (For further discussion of the pelvic steal syndrome, see Melman & Tiefer, Chapter 10, this volume.)

Case Vignette

A 56-year-old married man reported the gradual development of erectile problems during intercourse. Occasionally he was able to achieve vaginal penetration, but lost the erection during thrusting. His sexual desire and ejaculatory capacity were not impaired. There was a history of moderate hypertension that subsided following weight loss. NPT and endocrine evaluations were within normal limits. His PBI, which was 0.73 at rest, decreased to 0.49 following exercise. Pelvic arteriography revealed bilateral pathology in the pudendal arteries.

Pulse Wave Assessment of Penile Blood Flow

With the pulse wave technique, variations in penile arterial blood velocity are detected with a Doppler flow meter, and the pulse waves are recorded on a chart. Analysis of the waveforms may provide a measure of penile arterial function. A penile flow index, defined as the radial arterial acceleration (peak velocity over pulse rise time) divided by average penile artery acceleration, is calculated. Impotent men with angiographic demonstration of vascular disease were found to have a penile flow index significantly elevated over the values measured in nondysfunctional individuals (Velcek, Sniderman, Vaughan, Sos, & Muecke, 1980). The application of this technique is complicated by the difficulty in distinguishing superficial from deep penile artery pulse signals and in obtaining reliable recordings of the cavernosal arteries.

All noninvasive diagnostic tests of vascular competency assess the hemodynamics of the penis in the flaccid state, but do *not* evaluate the functional capacity of the cavernosal arteries or the venous system during the acquisition and maintenance of penile rigidity. This important limitation prompted the development of invasive procedures, which are summarized below.

Invasive Tests

Intracorporal Pharmacological Testing

Virag, Frydman, Legman, and Virag (1984) first reported that the response to intracavernosal injection of papaverine, which relaxes the sinusoidal smooth muscles in the corpora cavernosa, could serve as a diagnostic test. They observed that intracorporal papaverine administration induces rigid erections in normal subjects and in psychologically impotent men, but only partial or delayed erections in patients with vasculogenic impotence. Abber, Lue, Orvis, McClure, and Williams (1986) confirmed the diagnostic value of the papaverine injection test for vasculogenic impotence, but found a low correlation with PBI measures and the results of snap gauge testing. Research findings since then have shown that severe vasculogenic impotence can be ruled out by the timely development of full erections in response to papaverine. Conversely, the observation of only partial erections following papaverine administration has limited diagnostic value, since these responses have been observed in men with psychogenic impotence (Buvat, Buvat-Herbaut, Dehaene, & Lemaire, 1986; Allen & Brendler, 1988). Men with neurogenic impotence show normal erectile responses to intracorporal pharmacological testing (Sidi, Cameron, Duffy, & Lange, 1986; Nellans, Ellis, & Kramer-Levien, 1987). There is insufficient information to permit conclusions about pharmacological erections in men with endocrine causes of erectile dysfunction.

There are differences of opinion on the relative value of NPT and intracorporal pharmacological evaluation for the differential diagnosis of erectile disorders. Allen and Brendler (1988), who compared intracavernosal testing with extensive electrophysiological assessments of penile tumescence and rigidity in the sleep laboratory, found that the response to pharmacological testing did not accurately distinguish psychogenic from organic impotence. In vasculogenically impotent men, the degree of erectile change ranged from no erection in instances of severe vascular pathology to 90% of full erection in milder cases—a response rate that could be predicted accurately by NPT measurements. The patients with neurogenic impotence had abnormal NPT recordings, but normal erectile responses to papaverine. The authors concluded that NPT assessments should be carried out before intracorporal pharmacological erection testing, to help distinguish among the various causes of erectile impotence. Lue (1988) agrees with the value of NPT testing to differentiate psychogenic from organic impotence, but believes that in patients with suspected vascular difficulties, functional tests of arterial insufficiency and venous incompetence are more strongly indicated.

The use of intracavernosal pharmacological testing as a diagnostic procedure is presently carried out in highly variable ways across laboratories (Shengh-Hwang et al., 1989). Patients are usually injected with 30-60 mg of papaverine (alone or in combination with phentolamine, an alpha-adrenergic blocking agent) into the lateral side of one corpus cavernosum. More recently, prostaglandin E_1 (20 μg) has been used as an alternative drug for the diagnosis of impotence. The size and rigidity of the penis are then assessed repeatedly at various intervals before the patient's departure from the clinic. The onset of the response, the angle of the erection, the degree of tumescence, and the degree of rigidity are recorded. Patients are instructed to monitor the duration of the erection and to inform the clinician if an erection lasts longer than 4-6 hours. There is a need for standardization of the technique in terms of drug, dosage, and response criteria, in order to determine the accuracy of this approach across different patient groups.

Case Vignette

A 52-year-old widowed diabetic man sought help for his erectile problems, which had begun after his wife's death of uterine cancer 3 years before. He had been free from sexual difficulties until that time. His grief at her death was intense, and for a period of 1 year he lost his sexual desire and did not attempt sexual experiences. His first attempt at intercourse was characterized by marked erectile difficulties. At the time of the evaluation, he was able to achieve penetration with a partial erection in 30% of his attempts. He did not masturbate, but reported occasional early morning erections. His diabetes was under unstable metabolic control, and there was some evidence of peripheral neuropathy; otherwise, his medical evaluation was unremarkable. Assessment of NPT demonstrated a pattern of tumescent episodes of normal frequency and duration, but no evidence of rigidity. Intracorporal testing on two occasions with 60 mg papaverine and 0.83 mg phentolamine revealed a markedly diminished erectile response consistent with vasculogenic impotence. Angiographic studies of the pudendal arteries confirmed the diagnosis.

Duplex Ultrasonography

Duplex ultrasonography permits the visualization of the corpora cavernosa and cavernosal arteries, as well as the determination of blood flow in the penile vessels during flaccidity and in response to erections induced by intracorporal administration of vasoactive substances. The duplex system includes an ultrasound transducer that measures changes in the inner diame-

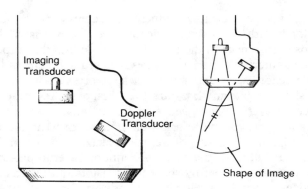

FIGURE 6.2. Schematic drawing of duplex probe with two transducer elements in same plane, with one mechanical transducer element used for real-time imaging and one used for pulse Doppler. From "Evaluation of Vasculogenic Erectile Impotence Using Penile Duplex Ultrasonography" by R. Shabsigh, I. J. Fishman, E. T. Quesada, C. K. Seale-Hawkins, and J. K. Dunn, 1989, *Journal of Urology*, 142, 1469-1474. Copyright 1989 by the American Urological Association. Reprinted by permission.

ter of the cavernosal arteries, and a pulsed Doppler transducer that can be focused on a predetermined artery to measure blood flow (Figure 6.2). A defective arterial dilatation and minimal changes in mean peak flow velocity following intracavernosal pharmacological challenge are suggestive of arteriogenic impotence (Lue, Hricak, Marich, & Tanagho, 1985; Shabsigh, Fishman, Quesada, Seale-Hawkins, & Dunn, 1989). Using the technique of duplex ultrasonography, Nelson and Lue (1989) have recently measured changes in total penile blood volume following papaverine injection; this approach may provide valuable data for the diagnosis of venous insufficiency and the understanding of the uncoupling between penile tumescence and rigidity. Duplex ultrasonography and pulsed Doppler analysis are sensitive procedures that require considerable time and experience for reliable use. Diagnostic interpretations are based on the combined evaluation of several parameters, and determination of the accuracy of these judgments necessitates the development of a normative data base and explicit criteria.

Cavernosometry and Cavernosography

An impaired response to intracavernosal pharmacological testing may be due not only to inadequate arterial inflow, but also to venous insufficiency. The techniques of cavernosometry and cavernosography assess cavernosal venous outflow resistance; they add another level of invasiveness to the evaluation

procedure, and it is advisable to carry these procedures out only after intracavernosal testing in order to clarify the significance of abnormal findings.

Cavernosometry involves the infusion of saline into the corpora cavernosa and the monitoring of perfusion rates required to obtain and maintain
an artificial erection while the intracavernosal pressure is measured. An
elevated infusion flow rate and low intracavernosal pressures indicate venous
incompetence (Buvat, Lemaire, Dehaene, Buvat-Herbaut, & Guien, 1986).
Cavernosography involves the infusion of contrast media into the corpora
cavernosa to visualize the site of venous leakage and identify possible
anatomical abnormalities for surgical intervention. Cavernosometry and cavernosography are carried out by some investigators during pharmacologically induced erections (Lue, Hricak, Schmidt, & Tanagho, 1986). These
techniques have not been standardized yet, and there is no agreement about
the physiopathological significance of venous leakage as diagnosed by these
methods, particularly in instances of moderately elevated maintenance flow
rates.

In sum, among the tests for evaluation of vasculogenic impotence,
intracorporal pharmacological testing appears the most useful diagnostic
procedure. Although invasive, it is well tolerated and simple to perform, and
provides information on erectile function that is unobtainable with noninvasive measures such as the PBI. Doppler ultrasonography and cavernosome-
try/cavernosography, because of their technological complexity and greater
degree of invasiveness, may be considered in instances when there is
evidence of vascular pathology and finer diagnostic discriminations are
required.

NEUROLOGICAL ASSESSMENT

Genital vasocongestion is under the control of sympathetic and parasympathetic pathways arising in the sacral and thoracolumbar spinal cord. The
spinal mechanisms are activated by genital stimulation with afferent input
via the pudendal nerves, and by psychological or sensory processes mediated through supraspinal centers (deGroat, 1980). There are no techniques
that assess the integrity of the autonomic components of erection. Some
investigators have developed noninvasive cardiovascular tests to evaluate
autonomic status (Ewing, Campbell, & Clarke, 1980), but the results have
limited diagnostic and prognostic specificity concerning erectile function
(Robinson, Woodcock, & Stephenson, 1987). Most of the tests currently used
to investigate neurogenic erectile disorders assess the afferent, pudendally
mediated components of the erectile reflex.

Penile Biothesiometry

Penile biothesiometry measures the threshold of vibratory perception in the glans and penile shaft by means of an electromagnetic vibration device. Since there is an age-related decrease in penile sensitivity, abnormal results need to be interpreted in relation to results for age-appropriate controls (Newman, 1970). Approximately 50% of patients with abnormal biothesiometric results were found also to have abnormal somatosensory evoked potentials (Padma-Nathan & Levine, 1987). Biothesiometry has been proposed as a useful, noninvasive screening test of penile sensory afferent pathways, but more empirical information is needed to determine its diagnostic value.

Dorsal Nerve Conduction Velocity

Bradley, Lin, and Johnson (1984) have described an electrophysiological technique to measure conduction of the dorsal nerve of the penis, which is a terminal branch of the pudendal nerve. This technique may permit the direct evaluation of penile neuropathy in men with erectile disorders. Few data have been accumulated with this procedure, however, and its practical use will require further standardization and validation.

Bulbocavernosus Reflex Latency

Bulbocavernosus reflex latency was one of the earliest tests employed to diagnose neurogenic impotence, and is still probably the most frequently used. It consists of recording the latency of the EMG response of the bulbocavernosus muscles to electric stimulation of the dorsal nerve of the penis (Rushworth, 1967; Ertekin & Reel, 1976). Absent or prolonged reflex latency is interpreted as indicative of neuropathic changes within the reflex arc, which includes the afferent and efferent components of the pudendal nerve and sacral segments S_2, S_3, and S_4 of the spinal cord. Variations of this test include measurement of the conduction latency from the dorsal nerve to the distal urethral sphincter, measurement of the latency from stimulation of the urethral sphincter to the anal sphincter, and determination of sensory perception thresholds of the dorsal nerve and the posterior urethra (Desai, Dembny, Morgan, Gingell, & Prothero, 1988; Parys, Evans, & Parsons, 1988).

There is conflicting evidence about the diagnostic value of this test. Some investigators have described it as a sensitive and useful diagnostic procedure (Parys et al., 1988), whereas others have found it of doubtful validity and of limited predictive value in discriminating between neurogenic (diabetic) and nonorganic impotence (Desai et al., 1988; Lavoisier, Proulx, Courtois, & deCarufel, 1989).

Somatosensory Evoked Potential

The somatosensory evoked potential test records the evoked potential waveforms of the cerebral cortex (EEG) elicited by electric stimulation of the dorsal nerve of the penis. The total conduction time is thought to be a measure of peripheral as well as central pudendal afferent pathways (Ertekin, Akyüreli, Gürses, & Turgut, 1985; Oposomer, Guerit, & Wese, 1986; Tackmann, Vogel, & Porst, 1987). Padma-Nathan (1988) has recently reported that this test permits the further evaluation of patients with sensory deficit erectile dysfunction identified by abnormal biothesiometric responses. In some individuals, the erectile dysfunction may be due to defective sensory input from the penis to cerebral structures that activate efferent lumbosacral erectile reflexes. These patients are described as having normal NPT patterns and difficulty in sustaining (but not in gaining) erections. More information is required to define this syndrome further, and to evaluate the significance of somatosensory evoked potential testing for diagnosis of erectile disorders.

SUMMARY AND CONCLUSIONS

Most ancillary diagnostic tests that contribute to the evaluation of specific pathogenic mechanisms in erectile failure have been developed during the last decade. The recency of their clinical application has not yet permitted a full assessment of their diagnostic accuracy. Lacking objective information, the algorithms suggested by investigators to guide the sequence of testing procedures have varied considerably, depending on individual orientation, expertise, and test availability.

The choice of diagnostic tests should be determined by (1) an informed opinion of likely causal determinants, based on the psychosexual history and medical evaluation; (2) data on validity, reliability, and predictive value of individual tests; and (3) practical considerations, such as degree of methodological complexity, patient's acceptance, and cost. A comprehensive psychosexual evaluation involving the patient and his partner, a psychological and medical history, and a physical examination (with particular focus on the neurological, vascular, and endocrine systems) provide the cornerstone of a sound diagnostic approach. Several psychological tests and questionnaires have been proposed, but their value for differential diagnosis of erectile disorders has not been confirmed (Beutler et al., 1975; Staples,

Ficher, Shapiro, Martin, & Gonick, 1980; Derogatis, Meyer, & Dupkin, 1976; Melman & Redfield, 1981).

NPT monitoring conducted in the sleep laboratory is the best procedure to differentiate psychogenic from organic forms of impotence. Interpretation of abnormal NPT findings should be made in the context of age-related normative information and should take into account the presence of (1) emotional states such as clinical depression or excessive anxiety, (2) hypoactive sexual desire disorders, and (3) sleep disorders. Rigidity monitoring without sleep disruption is a methodological development that, once fully validated, will enhance the application of the NPT method. The use of snap gauges or portable NPT monitoring equipment provides a less costly approach, but should be used as screening devices with considerable caution because of the high rate of false-positive and false-negative results.

When the NPT results indicate organic impairment, or the clinical history and medical evaluation suggest vascular compromise, noninvasive tests for the assessment of penile blood pressure may be carried out first. The diagnostic value of penile blood pressure determinations with a Doppler probe or strain gauge plethysmography is limited, however, and intracavernosal administration of vasoactive substances may be required as a functional test of vascular capacity. The pharmacological induction of a firm and lasting erection rules out vascular pathogenesis, but does not discriminate between psychogenic and neurogenic impotence, because in both cases the erectile responses are normal. Lack of erections following intracavernosal testing strongly suggests vascular compromise, whereas a partial response may be indicative of either vascular pathology or the result of test anxiety. The significance of partial or absent erectile responses to intracavernosal vasoactive administration may be further assessed with duplex ultrasonography to evaluate arterial inflow, or with pharmacavernosometry and cavernosography to assess venous outflow. Several articles proposing algorithms of vascular evaluation of erectile disorders, beginning with intracavernosal papaverine testing, have recently been published (DePalma et al., 1987; Wespes, Delcour, Rondeux, Struyven, & Schulman, 1987; Shabsigh et al., 1989; Gerstenberg, Wardling, Hald, & Wagner, 1989).

Methods for the assessment of neurogenic impotence are limited to the afferent somatic pathway of the pudendal nerve and includes biothesiometry, bulbocavernosus reflex latency, and somatosensory evoked potential measurements. Their diagnostic value is presently uncertain because they do not evaluate the autonomic control of genital vasocongestion, but they may be considered when the erectile disorder is associated with clinical evidence of neurological impairment.

Considerable advances in laboratory methods for the assessment of erectile failure have recently taken place. Additional information on test validity and accuracy, age-related norms, and further clinical experience will be needed to clarify the diagnostic utility of the wide range of tests presently available.

Acknowledgments. Research in the NPT method conducted in the Human Sexuality Program, Department of Psychiatry, Mount Sinai School of Medicine, has been carried out with the support of the following grants from the U.S. Public Health Service: No. MH 27513, No. AM 20845, and No. AG 06895. I thank Ms. Natalie Weinstein for her assistance in the preparation of the manuscript.

REFERENCES

Abber, J. C., Lue, T. F., Orvis, B. R., McClure, R. D., & Williams, R. D. (1986). Diagnostic tests for impotence: A comparison of papaverine injection with the penile–brachial index and nocturnal penile tumescence monitoring. *Journal of Urology, 135*, 923–925.

Abelson, D. (1975). Diagnostic value of the penile pulse and blood pressure: A Doppler study of impotence in diabetes. *Journal of Urology, 113*, 636–639.

Aboseif, S. R., & Lue, T. F. (1988). Hemodynamics of penile erection. *Urologic Clinics of North America, 15*, 1–7.

Allen, R. P., & Brendler, C. B. (1988). Nocturnal penile tumescence predicting response to intracorporeal pharmacological erection testing. *Journal of Urology, 140*, 518–522.

Aserinsky, E. (1953). *Ocular motility during sleep and its application to the study of rest-activity cycles and dreaming.* Unpublished doctoral dissertation, University of Chicago.

Aserinksy, E., & Kleitman, N. A. (1955). A motility cycle in sleeping infants as manifested by ocular and gross bodily activity. *Journal of Applied Physiology, 8*, 11–18.

Bancroft, J., & Wu, F. C. W. (1983). Changes in erectile responsiveness during androgen replacement therapy. *Archives of Sexual Behavior, 12*, 59–66.

Barry, J. M., Blank, B., & Boileau, M. (1980). Nocturnal penile tumescence monitoring with stamps. *Urology, 15*, 171–172.

Beutler, L. E., Karacan, I., Anch, A. M., Salis, P., Scott, F. B., & Williams R. L. (1975). MMPI and MIT discriminations of biogenic and psychogenic impotence. *Journal of Consulting and Clinical Psychology, 43*, 899–903.

Bohlen, J. G. (1981). Sleep erection monitoring in the evaluation of male erectile failure. *Urologic Clinics of North America, 8*, 119–134.

Bradley, W. E., Lin, J. T. Y., & Johnson, B. (1984). Measurement of the conduction velocity of the dorsal nerve of the penis. *Journal of Urology, 131*, 1127–1129.

Bradley, W. E., Timm, G. W., Gallagher, J. M., & Johnson, B. K. (1985). New methods for continuous measurement of nocturnal penile tumescence and rigidity. *Urology, 16*, 4–9.

Buvat, J. J., Buvat-Herbaut, M., Dehaene, J. L., & Lemaire, A. (1986). Is intracavernosus injection of papaverine a reliable screening test for vascular impotence? *Journal of Urology, 135,* 476–478.

Buvat, J. J., Lemaire, A., Dehaene, J. L., Buvat-Herbaut, M., & Guien, J. D. (1986). Venous incompetence: Critical study of the organic basis of high maintenance flow rates during artificial erection test. *Journal of Urology, 135,* 926–928.

Campbell, P. I., Reynolds, C. F., Jennings, J. R., Thase, M., Frank, E., Howell, J., & Kupfer, D. J. (1987). Reliability of NPT scoring and visual estimates of erectile fullness. *Sleep, 10,* 480–485.

Cohen, A. S., Rosen, R. C., & Goldstein, L. (1985). EEG hemispheric asymmetry during sexual arousal: Psychophysiologic patterns in responsive, unresponsive and dysfunctional men. *Journal of Abnormal Psychology, 94,* 580–590.

Davidson, J. M., Camargo, C., & Smith, E. R. (1979). Effects of androgen on sexual behavior in hypogonadal men. *Journal of Clinical Endocrinology and Metabolism, 48,* 955–958.

de Groat, W. C. (1980). Physiology of male sexual function. *Annals of Internal Medicine, 92,* 329–331.

DePalma, R. G., Emsellem, H. A., Edwards, C. M., Druy, E. M., Shultz, S. W. Miller, H. C., & Bergsrud, D. (1987). A screening sequence for vasculogenic impotence. *Journal of Vascular Surgery, 5,* 228–236.

Derogatis, L. R., Meyer, J. K., & Dupkin, C. N. (1976). Discrimination of organic versus psychogenic impotence with the DSFI. *Journal of Sex and Marital Therapy, 2,* 229–240.

Desai, K. M., Dembny, K., Morgan, H., Gingell, J. C., & Prothero, D. (1988). Neurophysiologic investigation of diabetic impotence: Are sacral response studies of value? *British Journal of Urology, 61,* 68–73.

Doyle, D. L., & Yu, J. (1986). Comparison of Doppler and strain gauge plethysmography to detect vasculogenic impotence. *Canadian Journal of Surgery, 29,* 338–339.

Earls, C. M., Morales, A., & Marshall, W. L. (1988). Penile sufficiency: An operational definition. *Journal of Urology, 139,* 536–538.

Ek, A., Bradley, W. E., & Krane, R. J. (1983). Snap-gauge band: New concept in measuring penile rigidity. *Urology, 21,* 63–67.

Ellis, D. J., Doghramji, K., & Bagley, D. H. (1988). Snap-gauge band versus penile rigidity in impotence assessment. *Journal of Urology, 140,* 61–63.

Ertekin, C., Akyüreli, D., Gürses, A. N., & Turgut, H. (1985). The value of somatosensory-evoked potentials and bulbocavernosus reflex in patients with impotence. *Acta Neurologica Scandinavica, 71,* 48–53.

Ertekin, C., & Reel, F. (1976). Bulbocavernosus reflex in normal men and in patients with neurogenic bladder and/or impotence. *Journal of Neurological Science, 28,* 1–15.

Ewing, D. J., Campbell, I. W., & Clarke, B. F. (1980). Assessment of cardiovascular effects in diabetic autonomic neuropathy and prognostic implications. *Annals of Internal Medicine, 92,* 308–311.

Fisher, C. (1966). Dreaming and sexuality. In R. M. Loewenstein, L. M. Newman, & M. Schur (Eds.), *Psychoanalysis: A general psychology. Essays in honor of Heinz Hartman* (pp. 537–569). New York: International Universities Press.

Fisher, C., Gross, J., & Zuch, T. (1965). Cycle of penile erection synchronous with dreaming (REM) sleep. *Archives of General Psychiatry*, *12*, 29–45.

Fisher, C., Kahn, E., & Edwards, A. (1972). Total suppression of REM sleep with the MAO inhibitor Nardil in a subject with painful nocturnal REMP erection. *Psychophysiology*, *9*, 91.

Fisher, C., Schiavi, R. C., Edwards, A., Davis, D., Reitman, M., & Fine, J. (1979). Evaluation of nocturnal penile tumescence in the differential diagnosis of sexual impotence: A quantitative study. *Archives of General Psychiatry*, *36*, 431–437.

Fisher, C., Schiavi, R. C., Lear, H., Davis, D. M., & Witkin, A. P. (1975). The assessment of nocturnal REM erections in the differential diagnosis of sexual impotence. *Journal of Sex and Marital Therapy*, *1*, 277–289.

Foreman, P. J., Stahl, J., Hobbins, T. E., Paskewitz, D. A., & Gross, H. S. (1986). Sleep apnea in five patients evaluated for nocturnal penile tumescence. *Maryland Medical Journal*, *35*, 46–48.

Gerstenberg, T. C., Nordling, J., Hald, T., & Wagner, G. (1989). Standard evaluation of erectile dysfunction in 95 consecutive patients. *Journal of Urology*, *141*, 857–862.

Goldstein, I., Siroky, M. B., Nath, R. L., McMillian, T. N., Menzoian, J. O., & Krane, R. J. (1982). Vasculogenic impotence: Role of the pelvic steal test. *Journal of Urology*, *128*, 300–306.

Guilleninault, C., Eldridge, F. L., Tilkian, A., Simmons, F., & Dement, W. C. (1977). Sleep apnea syndrome due to upper airway obstruction: A review of 25 cases. *Archives of Internal Medicine*, *137*, 296–300.

Hosking, D. J., Bennet, T., Hampton, J. R., Evans, D. F., Clark, A. J., & Robertson, G. (1979). Diabetic impotence: Studies of nocturnal erection during REM sleep. *British Medical Journal*, *ii*, 1394–1396.

Jovanovic, V. J. (1969). Der effekt der ersten untersuchungsnacht auf die erektionen im schlaf. *Psychotherapy and Psychosomatics*, *17*, 295–308.

Jovanovic, V. J. (1972). Sexuelle reaktionen und schlafperiodik bei menschen: Ergebnisse experimenteller untersuchungen. *Beitrage für Sexualforschung*, *51*, 1–292.

Jovanovic, V. J., & Tan-Eli, B. (1969). Penile erections during sleep. *Arzneimittel-Forschung*, *19*, 966–974.

Kahn, E., & Fisher, C. (1969). REM sleep and sexuality in the aged. *Journal of Geriatric Psychiatry*, *2*, 181–199.

Kaneko, S., & Bradley, W. E. (1986). Evaluation of erectile dysfunction with continuous monitoring of penile rigidity. *Journal of Urology*, *136*, 1026–1029.

Karacan, I. (1970, April). Clinical value of nocturnal erection in the prognosis and diagnosis of impotence. *Medical Aspects of Human Sexuality*, pp. 27–34.

Karacan, I. (1978). Assessment of nocturnal penile tumescence as an objective method for evaluating sexual functioning in ESRD patients. *Dialysis and Transplantation*, *7*, 872–876.

Karacan, I., Scott, F. B., Salis, P. J., Attia, S. L., Ware, J. C., Actinel, A., & Williams, R. L. (1977). Nocturnal erections, differential diagnosis of impotence and diabetes. *Biology and Psychiatry*, *12*, 373–380.

Karacan, I., Goodenough, D. R., Shapiro, A., & Starker, S. (1966). Erection cycle during sleep in relation to dream anxiety. *Archives of General Psychiatry*, *15*, 183–189.

Karacan, I., Hirshkowitz, M., Salis, P. J., Narter, E., & Safi, M. F. (1987). Penile blood flow and musculovascular events during sleep-related erections of middle-aged men. *Journal of Urology, 138*, 177-181.

Karacan, I., Salis, P. J., Thornby, J. I., & Williams, R. L. (1976). The ontogeny of nocturnal penile tumescence. *Waking and Sleeping, 1*, 27-44.

Karacan, I., Salis, P. J., & Williams, R. L. (1978). The role of the sleep laboratory in the diagnosis and treatment of impotence. In R. L. Williams, I. Karacan, & S. H. Frazier (Eds.), *Sleep disorders: Diagnosis and treatment* (pp. 353-382). New York: Wiley.

Karacan, I., Williams, R. L., Thornby, J. I., & Salis, P. J. (1975). Sleep-related penile tumescence as a function of age. *American Journal of Psychiatry, 132*, 932-937.

Krane, R. J., Goldstein, I., & Saenz de Tejada, I. (1989). Impotence. *New England Journal of Medicine, 321*, 1648-1659.

Kwan, M., Greenleaf, W. J., Mann, J., Crapo, L., & Davidson, J. (1983). The nature of androgen action on male sexuality: A combined laboratory/self-report study on hypogonadal men. *Journal of Clinical Endocrinology and Metabolism, 57*, 557-562.

Lavoisier, P., Proulx, J., Courtois, F., & deCarufel, F. (1989). Bulbocavernosus reflex: Its validity as a diagnostic test for neurogenic impotence. *Journal of Urology, 141*, 311-314.

Lue, T. F. (1988). [Editorial comment to Allan, R. P., & Brendler, C. B., Nocturnal penile tumescence predicting response to intracorporeal pharmacologic erection testing]. *Journal of Urology, 140*, 522.

Lue, T. F., Hricak, H., Marich, K. W., & Tanagho, E. A. (1985). Evaluation of vasculogenic impotence with high-resolution ultrasonography and pulse Doppler spectrum analysis. *Radiology, 155*, 777-781.

Lue, T. F., Hricak, H., Schmidt, R. A., & Tanagho, E. A. (1986). Functional evaluation of penile veins by cavernosography in papaverine-induced erection. *Journal of Urology, 135*, 479-482.

Marshall, P., Earls, C., Morales, A., & Surridge, D. (1982). Nocturnal penile tumescence recording with stamps: A validity study. *Journal of Urology, 128*, 946-947.

Marshall, P., Morales, A., Phillips, P., & Fenemore, J. (1983). Nocturnal penile tumescence with stamps: A comparative study under sleep laboratory conditions. *Journal of Urology, 130*, 88-89.

Marshall, P., Morales, A., & Surridge, D. (1982). Diagnostic significance of penile erections during sleep. *Urology, 20*, 1-6.

Marshall, P., Surridge, D., & Delva, N. (1981). The role of nocturnal penile tumescence in differentiating between organic and psychogenic impotence: The first stage of validation. *Archives of Sexual Behavior, 10*, 1-10.

Melman, A., Kaplan, D., & Redfield, J. (1984). Evaluation of the first 70 patients in the Center for Male Sexual Dysfunction of Beth Israel Medical Center. *Journal of Urology, 131*, 53-55.

Melman, A., & Redfield, J. (1981). Evaluation of the DSFI as a test of organic impotence. *Sexuality and Disability, 4*, 108-112.

Melman, A., Tiefer, L., & Pedersen, R. (1988). Evaluation of first 406 patients in urology department based center for male sexual dysfunction. *Urology, 32*, 6-10.

Metz, P., & Bengtsson, J. (1981). Penile blood pressure. *Scandinavian Journal of Urology and Nephrology, 15,* 161–164.

Nellans, R. E., Ellis, L. R., & Kramer-Levien, D. (1987). Pharmacological erection: Diagnosis and treatment applications in 69 patients. *Journal of Urology, 138,* 52–54.

Nelson, R. P., & Lue, T. F. (1989). Determination of erectile penile volume by ultrasonography. *Journal of Urology, 141,* 1123–1126.

Newman, A. F. (1970). Vibratory sensitivity of the penis. *Fertility and Sterility, 21,* 791–795.

O'Carroll, R., Shapiro, C., & Bancroft, J. (1985). Androgens, behavior and nocturnal erection in hypogonadal men: The effect of varying the replacement dose. *Clinical Endocrinology, 23,* 527–538.

Ohlmeyer, P., Brilmayer, H., & Hullstrung, H. (1944). Periodische vorgange im schlaf. *Pfluegers Archives, 248,* 559–560.

Oposomer, R. J., Guerit, J. M., & Wese, T. X. (1986). Pudendal cortical somatosensory evoked potentials. *Journal of Urology, 135,* 1216.

Padma-Nathan, H. (1988). Neurologic evaluation of erectile dysfunction. *Urologic Clinics of North America, 15,* 77–80.

Padma-Nathan, H., & Levine, F. (1987). Vibrating testing of the penis. *Journal of Urology, 137,* 201A.

Parys, B. T., Evans, C. M., & Parsons, K. F. (1988). Bulbocavernosus reflex latency in the investigation of diabetic impotence. *British Journal of Urology, 61,* 59–62.

Pressman, M. R., DiPhillipo, M. A., Kendrick, J. I., Conroy, K., & Fry, J. M. (1986). Problems in the interpretation of nocturnal penile tumescence studies: Disruption of sleep by occult sleep disorders. *Journal of Urology, 136,* 595–598.

Queral, L. A., Whitehouse, W. M., Flinn, W. R., Zarins, C. K., Bergan, J. J., & Yao, J. S. T. (1979). Pelvic hemodynamics after aortoliac reconstruction. *Surgery, 86,* 799–804.

Reynolds, C. F., III, Thase, M. E., Jennings, J. R., Howell, J. R., Frank, E., Bermann, S. R., Hovck, P. R., & Kupfer, D. J. (1989). Nocturnal penile tumescence in healthy 20- to 59-year-olds: A revisit. *Sleep, 12,* 368–373.

Robinson, L. Q., Woodcock, J. P., & Stephenson, T. P. (1987). Results of investigation of impotence in patients with overt or probable neuropathy. *British Journal of Urology, 60,* 583–587.

Roose, S. P., Glassman, A. H., Walsh, T., & Cullen, K. (1982). Reversible loss of nocturnal penile tumescence during depression: A preliminary report. *Neuropsychobiology, 8,* 284–288.

Rosen, R. C., Goldstein, L., Scoles, V., & Lazarus, C. (1986). Psychophysiologic correlates of nocturnal penile tumescence in normal males. *Psychosomatic Medicine, 48,* 423–429.

Rowe, J. W., & Kahn, R. L. (1987). Human aging: Usual and successful. *Science, 237,* 143–149.

Rushworth, G. (1967). Diagnostic value of the electromyographic study of reflex activity in man. *Electroencephalography and Clinical Neurophysiology, 25*(Suppl.), 65–73.

Sakheim, D. K., Barlow, D. H., Abrahamson, D. J., & Beck, J. G. (1987). Distinguishing between organogenic and psychogenic erectile dysfunction. *Behaviour Research and Therapy, 25,* 379–400.

Schiavi, R. C. (1988). Nocturnal penile tumescence in the evaluation of erectile disorders: A critical review. *Journal of Sex and Marital Therapy, 14,* 83–96.

Schiavi, R. C., Fisher, C., Quadland, M., & Glover, A. (1985). Nocturnal penile tumescent evaluation of erectile function in insulin-dependent diabetic men. *Diabetologia, 28,* 90–94.

Schiavi, R. C., Mandeli, J., Schreiner-Engel, J., & Chambers, A. (1991). Aging, sleep disorders and male sexual function. *Biological Psychiatry, 30,* 15–24.

Schiavi, R. C., & Schreiner-Engel, P. (1988). Nocturnal penile tumescence in healthy aging men. *Journal of Gerontology, 43,* M146–M150.

Schiavi, R. C., Schreiner-Engel, P., Mandeli, J., Schanzer, H., & Cohen, E. (1990). Healthy aging and male sexual function. *American Journal of Psychiatry, 147,* 766–771.

Schiavi, R. C., Schreiner-Engel, P., White, D., & Mandeli, J. (1988). Pituitary–gonadal function during sleep in men with hypoactive sexual desire and normal controls. *Psychosomatic Medicine, 50,* 304–318.

Schmidt, H. S., & Wise, H. A. (1981). Significance of impaired penile tumescence and associated polysomnographic abnormalities in the impotent patient. *Journal of Urology, 126,* 348–352.

Shabsigh, R., Fishman, I. J., Quesada, E. T., Seale-Hawkins, C. K., & Dunn, J. K. (1989). Evaluation of vasculogenic erectile impotence using penile duplex ultrasonography. *Journal of Urology, 142,* 1469–1474.

Shengh-Hwang, T. I., Yang, C. R., Wang, S. J., Chang, C. L., Tzai, T. S., Chang, C. H., & Wu, H. C. (1989). Impotence evaluated by the use of prostaglandin E_1. *Journal of Urology, 141,* 1357–1359.

Sidi, A. A., Cameron, J. S., Duffy, L. M., & Lange, P. H. (1986). Intracavernosus drug-induced erections in the management of male erectile dysfunction: Experience with 100 patients. *Journal of Urology, 135,* 704–706.

Staples, R. B., Ficher, I. V., Shapiro, M., Martin, K., & Gonick, P. (1980). A reevaluation of MMPI discriminations of biogenic and psychogenic impotence. *Journal of Consulting and Clinical Psychology, 48,* 543–554.

Tackmann, W., Vogel, P., & Porst, H. (1987). Somatosensory evoked potentials after stimulation of the dorsal nerve: Normative data and results from 145 patients with erectile dysfunction. *European Neurology, 27,* 245–250.

Thase, M. E., Reynolds, C. F., Glanz, L. M., Jennings, J. R., Sewitch, D. E., Kupfer, D. J., & Frank, E. (1987). Nocturnal penile tumescence in depressed men. *American Journal of Psychiatry, 144,* 89–92.

Thase, M. E., Reynolds, C. F., Jennings, J. R., Frank, E., Howell, J. R., Hovck, P. R., Berman, S., & Kupfer, D. J. (1988). Nocturnal penile tumescence is diminished in depressed men. *Biological Psychiatry, 24,* 33–46.

Velcek, D., Sniderman, K. W., Vaughan, E. D., Sos, T. A., & Muecke, E. C. (1980). Penile flow index utilizing a Doppler pulse wave analysis to identify penile vascular insufficiency. *Journal of Urology, 123,* 669–673.

Virag, R., Frydman, D., Legman, M., & Virag, H. (1984). Intracavernosis injection of papaverine as a diagnostic and therapeutic method in erectile failure. *Angiology, 35*, 79–83.

Wabrek, A. J. (1986). In-hospital nocturnal penile tumescence (NPT) monitoring and penile-rigidity determination in the differential diagnosis of erectile dysfunction. *Journal of Psychosomatic Obstetrics and Gynecology, 5*, 137–145.

Wasserman, M. D., Pollak, C. P., Spielman, A. J., & Weitzman, E. D. (1980). The differential diagnosis of impotence: The measurement of nocturnal penile tumescence. *Journal of the American Medical Association, 243*, 2038–2042.

Wasserman, M. D., Pollak, C. P., Spielman, A. J., & Weitzman, E. D. (1980b). Theoretical and technical problems in the measurement of nocturnal penile tumescence for the differential diagnosis of impotence. *Psychosomatic Medicine, 42*, 575–585.

Wein, A. J., Malloy, T. R., Hanno, P. M., Barrett, D. M., & Furlow, W. L. (1988). Re: Evaluation of erectile dysfunction with continuous monitoring of penile rigidity [Letter]. *Journal of Urology, 139*, 1072.

Wespes, E., Delcour, C., Rondeux, C., Struyven, J., & Schulman, C. C. (1987). The erectile angle: Objective criterion to evaluate the papaverine test in impotence. *Journal of Urology, 138*, 1171–1173.

Wincze, J. P., Bansal, S., Malhotra, C., Balko, A., Susset, J. G., & Malamud, M. (1988). A comparison of nocturnal penile tumescence and penile response to erotic stimulation during waking states in comprehensively diagnosed groups of males experiencing erectile difficulties. *Archives of Sexual Behavior, 17*, 333–347.

Zuckerman, M., Neeb, M., Ficher, M., Fishkin, R. E., Goldman, A., Fink, P., Cohen, S. N., Jacobs, J. A., & Weisberg, M. (1985). Nocturnal penile tumescence and penile responses in the waking state in diabetic and non-diabetic sexual dysfunctionals. *Archives of Sexual Behavior, 14*, 109–129.

7

Postmodern Sex Therapy for Erectile Failure

JOSEPH LOPICCOLO

Joseph LoPiccolo is one of the major scholars and innovators in the field of sex therapy. He has been especially influential in promulgating a cognitive–behavioral approach for the treatment of both female and male sexual disorders, and has conducted numerous studies documenting the efficacy of his approach. In recent years, LoPiccolo has expanded his theoretical vision to include a greater emphasis on systemic interventions. In part, his embracing of a "postmodern" approach to sex therapy can be traced to a growing awareness that the basic anxiety reduction/skills training model espoused by Masters and Johnson was inadequate for resolving the more complex and heterogeneous cases currently presenting in sex therapy clinics.

In this chapter, LoPiccolo notes that three elements are particularly involved in the postmodern approach to erectile failure: the functional analysis of the positive value that the erectile problem may have for the couple and the individual partners; the diagnosis of both physiological and psychological contributions to erectile impairment; and, finally, the actual sexual behavior patterns engaged in by the couple.

With respect to the functional value of the symptom, LoPiccolo notes that it is crucially important to assess the role played by the sexual dysfunction in the maintenance of homeostasis in the couple's relationship and the partners' individual dynamics. In fact, he suggests that the "symptom" of erectile failure may play an adaptive role in maintaining the couple's equilibrium, as well as in warding off individual intrapsychic conflict or unresolved family-of-origin issues; moreover, the dysfunction may be reinforced by the external environment. LoPiccolo believes that a fundamental principle of postmodern sex therapy is that patient "resistance" is due to the therapist's conceptual error in failing to make a functional analysis of the positive value of sexual dysfunction for an individual or couple.

In making a diagnosis, LoPiccolo notes that assessment should focus not only on quantifying the degrees of psychological and physiological causality of the problem, but on identifying, through a functional analysis, the issues to be targeted in treatment, and on determining the prognosis for response to physical interventions (e.g., vasoactive injections, vacuum erection devices, or penile prostheses).

Finally, LoPiccolo notes that among the behavioral exercises recommended in sex therapy, sensate focus represents a paradoxical intervention at times. Although the therapist assigns sensate focus in the hopes of relieving performance anxiety, most patients do not experience a reduction in such anxiety; rather, they experience "metaperformance anxiety," or anxiety about not performing despite the injunction not to feel pressure to perform. Moreover, sensate focus may not be effective in cases where systemic issues or severe physiological impairments are involved. Instead of sensate focus exercises, LoPiccolo suggests that patients be reassured that sexual gratification does not depend on the male's having a firm erection. Rather, oral and manual stimulation techniques are equally effective ways of providing and receiving sexual pleasure.

LoPiccolo presents a truly integrated model for the treatment of erectile difficulties, and one that appears to work well with a wide variety of patients. In his introduction of the postmodern sex therapy approach, LoPiccolo has made a major contribution to our therapeutic armamentarium.

Joseph LoPiccolo, Ph.D., is a professor in the Department of Psychology at the University of Missouri–Columbia. He has written and lectured widely about sex therapy and has conducted several large-scale outcome studies in the field. He is coauthor (with Julia R. Heiman) of Becoming Orgasmic: Personal Growth and Sexual Health for Women (second edition), and coeditor (with Leslie LoPiccolo) of the Handbook of Sex Therapy.

———

This chapter reviews a current conceptualization of the causes and treatment of erectile failure. The evolution of professional views of the causes of erectile failure is presented, culminating in the postmodern view that cases of erectile failure involve complex psychological and physiological etiology. A functional-analysis-based model for diagnosis and treatment is then offered, with emphasis on techniques useful for our postmodern era's complex cases, which often do not respond to standard sex therapy.

HISTORICAL CONCEPTUALIZATIONS OF ERECTILE FAILURE

The Victorians

Erectile failure first became a concern of psychologists and psychiatrists in the late 19th and early 20th centuries. During this period, Richard von Krafft-Ebing (1902) and Havelock Ellis (1910) published their monumental books on sexual disorders. In addition, a number of popular books were published in the United States and England, including August Forel's *The Sexual Question* (in 1906), Bernard MacFadden's *The Virile Powers of Superb Manhood* (in 1900), and the noted phrenologist Orson Fowler's *Amativeness, or Evils and Remedies of Excessive and Perverted Sexuality, Including Warnings and Advice to the Married and Single* (in 1875).

The themes in the works of Krafft-Ebing, Ellis, and the popular writers were similar. Erectile failure was held to result largely from "moral degeneracy." Childhood masturbation was held to be the link between moral degeneracy and adult sexual dysfunction: Krafft-Ebing and Ellis both suggested that excessive childhood masturbation damages the sexual organs and exhausts some reservoir of sexual energy in the body, resulting in inability to function sexually as an adult. Krafft-Ebing wrote that masturbation causes "neuroses of the sexual apparatus" and "weakness of the center governing erection" (pp. 188–189). Excessively frequent sexual actitivy in adulthood was also considered to cause erectile failure, as a commonly cited dictum was that "the loss of one drop of semen is equivalent to the loss of seven drops of blood." During this period, assessment of erection problems was focused on identifying the character flaws in patients that made it impossible for them to control and restrain their dangerous sexual appetites. Treatment consisted of encouraging continence in a variety of ways. These methods included restraint devices, such as metal mittens to prevent childhood masturbation. For adults, plenty of healthful outdoor exercise and a bland, vegetarian diet to avoid stimulation of the senses was recommended. As John Money (1985) has noted, this focus on continence led to the development of Kellogg's corn flakes and graham crackers as antiaphrodisiacs of a sort.

Freudian Theory

The movement away from viewing erectile failure as a symptom of moral degeneracy began with the work of Freud (1905/1962) and his followers at about the turn of the century. Although Freudian theory is both too complex and too well known to be reviewed here in detail, it can be said that Freudian theory stressed that adult sexual dysfunction results from failure to resolve the Oedipal complex and to progress through the stages of psychosexual development to true genital (mature) sexuality. Adult sexual dysfunction, then, was thought to represent immaturity or arrested development. Treatment of sexual dysfunction was not directly undertaken, as any adult difficulties with sexual functioning were seen as symptoms of an underlying defect in psychic development. Assessment consisted of examining the patient's dreams, fantasies, real and screen memories of childhood events, and so forth, in order to gain an insight into just how the patient's defense mechanisms were dealing with this arrested sexual development. Treatment occurred through the attainment of insight, as well as the working through of developmental blockages via the transference relationship with the analyst.

Although this Freudian view of immaturity, arrested development, and an unresolved Oedipal complex was certainly a great advance over the moral degeneracy view advocated by Ellis and Krafft-Ebing, Freud's views did not lead to the development of effective assessment strategies or treatment interventions. Focusing on the Oedipal problems of a man who has developed erectile failure at age 60, after a lifetime of adequate functioning, has not been found to be a productive approach.

Behaviorism

Freudian views of the causes of erectile failure remained dominant in American psychology and psychiatry through the first half of the 20th century, despite, as has been noted, there being remarkably little evidence for the therapeutic utility of Freudian theory (Sherfey, 1973). The first major challenges to Freudian views of sexual dysfunction were advanced by early behavioristic writings, notably those of Wolpe (1958), Salter (1949), and Lazarus (1965).

Early behaviorists believed that anxiety is the major cause of erectile failure. Anxiety was posited to be incompatible with, or reciprocally inhibitory to, sexual arousal. The basic treatment strategies were progressive relaxation and systematic desensitization. Within this early behavioral framework, assessment was focused on identifying a hierarchy of sexual activity, graded in terms of the amount of anxiety each activity produced in the client. Treatment then consisted of teaching the patient deep muscle relaxation (to inhibit anxiety) and having the patient visualize the hierarchy items while relaxed. Following this visualization, the hierarchy items were actually engaged in by the patient, again during relaxation, as a form of in vivo desensitization.

Modern Sex Therapy: Masters and Johnson

Although the behavioral movement gained considerable force within American psychology (and, to a lesser degree, psychiatry), it had no real impact on how the average educated person thought about erectile failure. The primary cultural view of sexual dysfunction remained a psychoanalytic one until the landmark publication of Masters and Johnson's (1966, 1970) works. Masters and Johnson proposed a relatively atheoretical scheme for treatment of sexual dysfunction. In their discussion of the causes of sexual dysfunctions, they stressed a type of informal social learning theory approach. They posited that exposure to certain critical constellations of events in childhood, adolescence, and adulthood results in adult erectile failure. Masters and Johnson stressed the role of religious, cultural, and familial negative messages about sex and anxiety induced by traumatic first sexual experiences, and they introduced the idea that sexual dysfunctions are examples of self-maintaining vicious cycles mediated by anxiety (Masters & Johnson, 1970). They basically proposed that although a variety of early life experiences may result in the first occasion of sexual dysfunction, the anxiety attendant upon sexual failure and the development of an anxious, self-evaluative, "spectator" role maintain the occurrence of erectile failure.

In the Masters and Johnson schema for sexual dysfunction, assessment focuses on two issues. First, an extensive and detailed sex history is taken to identify the original pathogenic life experiences. Second, a careful assessment is made of the patient's actual sexual behavior, so that new sexual techniques that disrupt the vicious cycle of performance anxiety and the spectator role can be implemented. Thus, Masters and Johnson presented the relatively revolutionary notion of "sex as a learned skill."

Treatment by the Masters and Johnson method involves forbidding further anxiety-laden attempts at intercourse, and instead focusing on the process of arousal through nongenital body massage, called "sensate focus." Only when erections are already occurring spontaneously may the couple advance to genital caressing. Caressing is interrupted when good erections occur in the "tease technique," so that the couple learns that an erection can be regained if lost. Anxiety about coitus is reduced by teaching the "stuffing" technique, in which the flaccid penis is inserted in the vagina.

The Masters and Johnson technique is remarkably similar to what the behaviorists earlier described as *in vivo* desensitization. However, the notion of forbidding anxiety-laden attempts at intercourse and focusing on body caressing did not originate with the behaviorists. Sir John Hunter, an 18th-century British physician, described a very similar treatment approach long ago (Comfort, 1965).

The Beginnings of Postmodernism in Cognitive-Behavioral Therapy

The next major change in our thinking about erectile failure occurred with the development of cognitive-behavioral therapy. In the late 1970s, within the field of behavioral therapy, there came to be renewed interest in cognition as well as overt behavior. Within the field of sex therapy, the cognitive-behavioral approach led to an emphasis on the patient's *thinking* about sex.

Assessment of erectile failure came to include evaluation of the patient's cognitions regarding sexual issues. Unrealistic expectations, negative self-images, distorted views of the opposite sex's needs and requirements, and tendencies toward catastrophic thinking became major foci of treatment. Although these changes developed as part of the cognitive revolution in psychotherapy, they were also a response to treatment failures when using the Masters and Johnson model. The Masters and Johnson (1970) approach of anxiety reduction plus skill training does not work well when the patient's distorted cognitions about sexual functioning are paramount factors. In such cases, instructions to relax and enjoy sensate focus exercises are as ineffective as advising an obsessive–compulsive neurotic to relax and stop worrying, or advising a drug addict to "just say no."

THE POSTMODERN VIEW OF ERECTILE FAILURE:
A THREE-PART THEORY

The postmodern view of erectile failure emphasizes three elements: systems theory; physiological as well as psychological impairment; and sexual technique.

The First Component: Systems Theory

Although systems theory approaches were developed initially in working with schizophrenic patients, they quickly became a mainstay of the family therapist and, to a somewhat lesser degree, of the marital therapist (Gurman & Kniskern, 1981). However, it is only in the last few years that systems theorists have begun to apply their ideas to sexual dysfunction. In the earlier years of family systems work, sexual dysfunctions were seen merely as symptoms of underlying family dynamics and were not focused upon in their own right. There was an underlying assumption that sexual dysfunctions would disappear when the family issues were resolved.

In more recent years, systems theorists have begun to look more closely at sexual dysfunctions. The focus now is upon assessing the role that sexual dysfunction plays in the maintenance of homeostasis in the emotional relationship between the partners (LoPiccolo & Friedman, 1985). Systemic and strategic issues often maintain erectile failure. For example, a wife who is dominated by her husband may gain power if he develops erectile failure. In cases where there is major systemic value associated with erectile failure, patients often "resist" standard sex therapy procedures by not performing the sensate focus exercises, breaking the initial prohibition on further attempts at intercourse, and so forth. These so-called "resistant" cases often fail in modern sex therapy. Kaplan (1974), for example, suggested that when patients resist standard techniques, sex therapy must be discontinued, and individual analytic therapy should be conducted to attain insight into underlying psychoanalytic issues that are blocking progress. We (Heiman, LoPiccolo, & LoPiccolo, 1981) first offered the alternative view that, rather than focusing only on individual dynamic issues, a clinician should undertake a more broadly focused assessment of the total functional and adaptive value of the sexual dysfunction for the patient couple, and should help the patients to find adaptive mechanisms to meet the needs currently being met in a maladaptive way by the sexual dysfunction. The postmodern view suggests that instead of beginning with standard sex therapy and moving to a consideration of cognitive, dynamic, and systemic factors only when resistance occurs, the clinician must consider these issues from the first session and prevent resistance by dealing with such factors in a proactive fashion. In postmodern sex therapy, then, patient "resistance" is viewed as actually caused by the therapist's conceptual error in failing to make a functional analysis of the sexual dysfunction's positive value for the patients.

In making a functional analysis, four factors involved in erectile failure need to be carefully assessed, and a treatment plan must be developed to address each of the factors.

Maintenance of Homeostasis in the Couple's Relationship

The first factor to be considered, as noted above, is the value that erectile failure may have in maintenance of emotional homeostasis in the patient couple's relationship. Erectile failure may have an impact on such issues as intimacy, closeness, trust, power sharing, conflict resolution, time spent together, and so forth. Sometimes the erectile failure develops as a result of problems in these areas, but an erectile problem that develops entirely for other reasons can come to have systemtic adaptive value in these areas, as a sort of positive side effect of the erectile failure.

In broaching the systems theory notions, the therapist must be very careful. Stated improperly, a systems theory interpretation can sound as if the therapist is accusing a patient of having the symptom "on purpose," to punish the partner or to gain something from the partner. It must always be stressed the systems function to maintain homeostasis, and do not develop unless there is a positive value for *both* partners in the system.

One way to keep a systems theory interpretation from sounding accusatory is to present the notion of "secondary gain." My colleagues and I explain to our patients that it is very apparent that each partner is suffering greatly from the sexual dysfunction, and it is causing each of them great pain. We tell them that there are two victims and no villains involved in their difficulties. We then go on to explain, however, that because humans are adaptable, people come to adjust to having a sexual dysfunction. The dysfunction then comes to have some effects on how their relationship is structured. We then ask the couple what effect the sexual dysfunction has had on their relationship.

As might be expected, virtually all couples indicate some negative effects on their emotional relationship. We then ask whether they have seen any positive effects on their relationship. That is, we ask whether the sexual dysfunction has any positive side effects for each of them. Not too surprisingly, virtually 100% of patients say "No." However, by the time a therapist asks this question (toward the end of the assessment), the therapist should have a very good idea of just what the functional value of the symptom may be.

We typically offer the patients an example of the adaptive value of sexual dysfunction, focusing on a presenting complaint other than their erectile failure. Doing this prevents activation of the patients' defenses, and they can more easily hear the notion of functional value of a sexual dysfunction. Therefore, in erectile failure cases, we give an example of female dysfunction. This might be an explanation that in the case of a wife's lack of arousal, while the husband is frustrated and upset, he also has the positive gain of not worrying about his wife having sex with other men, or of worrying whether or not he will be able to satisfy a high level of her sexual needs.

Following explanation of an opposite-sex example, we then again ask the partners whether they are now aware of any positive effects of their sexual problem. At this point, many couples will be able to offer a systemic value. For those who cannot as yet see such an issue, an alternative approach is to ask the clients to speculate about any possible negative effects on their marital stability of recovering erectile functioning, to raise awareness of systemic value of erectile failure (LoPiccolo & Daiss, 1987). For example, might a husband feel more powerful and revert to a more authoritarian role with the wife if he became "potent" again? Might the wife find his sexual needs burdensome if the husband regained erectile function?

Ideally, the patients will attain insight into the systemic value of their problem during initial assessment, so therapy can begin immediately to address the needs that are now being served by the erectile failure. However, if the clients still cannot see that the problem has any systemic value (even though this may be obvious to the therapist), the therapist should not attempt to convince them, but should merely drop the subject. After all, there are only two possibilities: If the therapist is incorrect, and there is no homeostatic value attached to the sexual dysfunction, the issue will never arise again in therapy. If, as is more likely, the therapist is correct and there is homeostatic value, at some point the patients will begin to show "resistance" to therapeutic manipulations. At this point, the therapist can interpret the resistance in terms of the homeostatic value of the symptom, and can point out that fears of disrupting homeostasis are motivating the "resistant" behavior. "Resistance," in this systems theory approach, is not conceptualized as patients' lack of motivation, recalcitrance, or expression of intrapsychic defense mechanisms. Rather, "resistance" means that the therapist needs to intervene in the system, which is involved in maintenance of the sexual dysfunction. Of course, it is preferable to avoid "resistance" by identifying and addressing systemic issues early in therapy, if the patients are amenable to this approach.

A wide variety of couple relationship issues may be involved in the systemic etiology of erectile failure. Elsewhere (LoPiccolo, 1988), I list the following as commonly occurring systemic issues: lack of attraction to the partner; poor sexual skills of the partner; general marital unhappiness; fear of closeness; differences between the couple in degree of "personal space" desired in the relationship; passive–aggressive solutions to a power imbalance; poor conflict resolution skills; inability to blend feelings of love and sexual desire; and reaction to the problems caused by lack of knowledge about normal age-related changes in male erectile functioning.

Examination of Individual Psychodynamics

The second issue to be assessed in a functional analysis concerns the value that the erectile failure has for the patients' individual psychodynamics. Erectile failure may be valuable to a patient in avoiding anxiety about what it would mean to be a sexually functional man. For some such men, erectile failure is a way of resolving negative feelings about their sexuality. These negative feelings may be moralistically based, or may result from negative cultural messages about sexuality. Similarly, erectile failure may ward off depression about some highly distressing life situation by simply giving the man another problem upon which to focus. A man who is very unhappy in his marriage, but who finds divorce too threatening an idea to process, exemplifies this issue. Erectile failure may also be an adaptive dynamic mechanism for avoiding repressed homosexual urges. Some men with ego-dystonic homosexual impulses experience a breakdown of repression during intercourse with their wives, and have intrusive mental images or fantasies of sex with a man. Other men may find that during erection and intercourse, deviant fantasies such as sex with a child occur. In such cases, erectile failure fosters repression of unacceptable sexual impulses, and allows maintenance of a self-image as a decent, moral person. Similarly, for patients with an image of themselves as hard-working, serious, non-self-indulgent persons, erectile failure may almost be a psychic necessity to maintain self-esteem.

Elsewhere (LoPiccolo, 1988), I cite the following as common individual factors in erectile failure: religious orthodoxy; gender identity conflicts; homosexual orientation or conflict; anhedonic or obsessive–compulsive personality; sexual phobias or aversions; fear of loss of control over sexual urges; masked sexual deviation; fears of having children; the "widower's syndrome" (unresolved feelings about death of the first wife); underlying depression; aging concerns; and attempting sex in a context or situation that is not psychologically comfortable for the patient.

Impact of Unresolved Family-of-Origin Issues

The third issue to be assessed in a functional analysis is the impact of unresolved family-of-origin issues on erectile functioning. For example, a patient raised in a family in which the mother was emotionally erratic or abusive may have difficulty in letting himself feel sexual pleasure and desire for his partner. Men raised in families in which physical affection—let alone overt sexuality—was taboo may be re-enacting these parental messages in their own relationships. Of course, men who were sexually abused by parents or other adults are very vulnerable to sexual dysfunction in adulthood.

Case Vignette

One recent case illustrates these mechanisms. Fred, an only child, was raised in a family in which he and not his father was the focus of his mother's emotional needs. The mother was overtly hostile and demeaning to the father with Fred present. In addition, she would privately confide to Fred her latest unhappiness and disappointment in his father. These complaints centered around his father's lack of financial success (despite the solid middle-class status of the family), emotional insensitivity, and "crudeness." Fred, on the other hand, was told that he himself was "sweet, loving, good, gentlemanly, smart, ambitious," and so forth. Although the mother was not overtly sexual with Fred, their relationship was very romanticized, and included a degree of physical intimacy and physical affection that began to make him very uncomfortable as an adolescent. For example, Fred and his mother would exchange back and leg rubs, and he was embarrassed to experience sexual stirring and some erection as an early teenager when he was massaging his mother's legs. As might be expected, Fred's father was not close to Fred (although he was overtly a good parent), and Fred was aware that his father resented him.

In this family constellation, Fred learned several things that contributed to his erectile failure: Women are emotionally intrusive; women are hostile and judgmental; sexual feelings are shameful; other men are dangerous rivals; sex is beneath someone of Fred's refined sensibilities; and so forth. Obviously, attempts to deal with Fred's erectile failure through the sensate focus and anxiety reduction techniques of modern sex therapy would have met with little success or with overt resistance, if these underlying unresolved family-of-origin issues had not been dealt with in therapy.

Operant Value of the Dysfunction

The fourth area to be considered in a functional analysis of erectile failure concerns the possible operant value the dysfunction may have for either partner. "Operant value" here refers to reinforcing consequences of the erectile failure that come not from the relationship with the partner or from the patient's own psyche, but from the external world. For example, the patient's erectile failure may lead him to devote long hours to his business or profession, resulting in great financial reward. Similarly, the wife of a man with erectile failure may be rewarded for her attention to her career or her focus on her role as mother/homemaker. In one recent case, the wife informed all her friends and relatives of her husband's history of total erectile failure in their 20-year marriage, and received admiration and praise for her loyalty, self-sacrifice, and fidelity.

In summary, the first element of postmodernism holds that erectile failure is not just a function of performance anxiety and lack of sexual skills, as was proposed in modern sex therapy (Masters & Johnson, 1970; Kaplan, 1974). While acknowledging that erectile failure is a painfully distressing condition, postmodernism stresses that erectile failure has positive value for the patient and his partner in terms of maintaining homeostasis in their emotional relationship system, warding off individual intrapsychic conflicts or unresolved family-of-origin issues, and producing reinforcing consequences from the external environment.

Postmodern sex therapy arose partly out of the movement of general psychotherapy toward an integrated cognitive–behavioral–systemic approach. However, postmodern sex therapy also arose in response to treatment failures. That is, the basic anxiety reduction/skill training approach called "sensate focus" by Masters and Johnson (1970) has been widely publicized in the popular media, and effective self-help books using this approach are widely available (e.g., Zilbergeld, 1978). Many of the cases seen by professionals today are failures of such "bibliotherapy" or guided self-treatment. Often, the reason the patient has not been able to follow a self-help program, or to succeed if the program was followed, involves the functionally useful nature of erectile failure. The first element of a postmodern therapy for erectile failure thus consists of making a functional analysis of the positive value of the problem, and helping the patient find more adaptive mechanisms for dealing with systemic, psychodynamic, family-of-origin, and environmentally reinforcing issues related to the maintenance of erectile failure. However, just as the modern approach of anxiety reduction/skill training proved inadequate with today's more complex cases, there is now another issue that needs to be addressed if a postmodern approach is to succeed with today's cases. This issue involves the fact that erectile failure very commonly involves both complex psychological factors *and* coexisting physiological impairment of erectile capability.

The Second Component: Integrated Prognostic Planning

In 1970, Masters and Johnson stated that 95% of all cases of erectile failure were purely psychogenic. More recently, new diagnostic procedures have revealed that neurological, vascular, and hormonal abnormalities are involved in a considerable percentage of cases of erectile failure (Mohr & Beutler, 1990; Tanagho, Lue, & McClure, 1988). Indeed, some studies (e.g., Spark, White, & Connolly, 1980) have reported very high rates of physiological pathology in cases of erectile failure, but selective referral seems to account for these extremely high rates. Spark et al. (1980) found that almost one-half of erectile failure cases had hormonal abnormalities. More typical hormonal abnormality rates for unselected patients in various studies are 5–10% (Bancroft, 1984; Segraves, Schoenberg, Zarins, Knopf, & Carnic, 1981). However, vascular and neurological impairments are much more common, and recent studies indicate that between one-third and two-thirds of unselected erectile failure patients have some degree of organic impairment of erectile ability (LoPiccolo, in press; Melman, Tiefer, & Pedersen, 1988; Mohr & Beutler, 1990).

The high incidence of physical pathology has led to the argument that sex therapy is no longer a viable treatment for erectile failure. One has only to look in the sports pages of any major newspaper to see advertisements with headings such as this: "Impotence Is a Medical Problem—Effective Medical Treatment Available." These advertisements are usually from urological centers that offer a treatment array of penile prostheses, vasoactive injections, revascularization surgery, and vacuum devices for inducing erection. Although such centers usually offer some assessment prior to intervention, this assessment is typically aimed at making a differential diagnosis of erectile failure as organic *or* psychogenic, with the latter presumably a rare phenomenon.

A postmodern view of erectile failure rejects differential diagnosis as a clinically useful approach, and offers an alternative model. Serious conceptual and methodological flaws are evident in virtually all of the currently published research. Conceptually, most of the research suffers from the flaw of attempting to place patients into discrete, nonoverlapping categories of organic *or* psychogenic erectile failure. However, in many cases, *both* organic *and* psychogenic factors are involved. Recognizing this combined causality, Melman et al. (1988) diagnosed patients with erectile failure along a bipolar scale, from "exclusively psychogenic" through "mixed etiology" to "exclusively organic" in origin. Melman et al. (1988) reported that of 406 patients evaluated, 39.7% had purely psychogenic erectile failure, 25.1% had both organic and psychological problems, and 28.9% had problems that were purely organic in origin. Although this bipolar scale is an advance over a simplistic two-category typology, there is a logical problem. As Bem (1974) has pointed out in regard to the concepts of "masculinity" and "feminity," the dimensions of "organic" and "psychogenic" are not the opposite ends of a unidimensional bipolar scale, but rather represent two separate and independently varying dimensions. That is, a man may have a high degree of *both* organic and psychogenic causes of erectile failure, or a low degree of both factors, or any combination of high and low degrees of impairment on each separate dimension. This fact may seem obvious; however, there are statements in the clinical literature that if one finds a clear psychological cause of the erection problem, one need not conduct any physiological evaluation. This point of view suggests, for example, that having a serious problem in a marital relationship prevents a man from developing atherosclerotic disease processes in the arteries leading to the penis.

Similarly, many physicians currently will perform surgery to implant a penile prosthesis if *any* degree of organic abnormality is found. In many such cases, the patient has only a mild organic impairment, which then makes his erection extremely vulnerable to being disrupted by psychological, behavioral, and sexual technique factors. Many times, cases with such partial organic impairment can be treated successfully by sex therapy. If psychological and behavioral difficulties are eliminated, the patient's mildly impaired physiological capacity may be sufficient to easily produce good erection.

In a recently completed study of etiology of erectile failure (LoPiccolo, in press), 63 men were independently rated for degree of psychological impairment (scored 0–4) and degree of organic impairment (also scored 0–4), following complete psychological, vascular, hormonal, neurological, and nocturnal penile tumescence (NPT) evaluations. These ratings were determined by having three separate clinicians review the patient's evaluation report, which contained all the raw data from the vascular, neurological, hormonal, and NPT assessments. The three raters also reviewed the written psychological evaluation report, which was based on formal testing and extensive interviewing with both patient and spouse (LoPiccolo, in press). These ratings were not completely subjective judgments; whenever possible, scores were anchored to objective criteria. For example, a score of 4 on organic impairment required either a complete absence of NPT, or markedly impaired NPT *plus* abnormality in at least one of the other systems assessed. Initial interrater reliability scores were good (ranging from the .70s to .90s between individual raters on each dimension). In cases where there were disagreements, the raters jointly reviewed the evaluation data and arrived at a consensus score.

The results of these evaluations are shown in Figure 7.1, with each circle representing one patient. The distribution in Figure 7.1 indicates that there

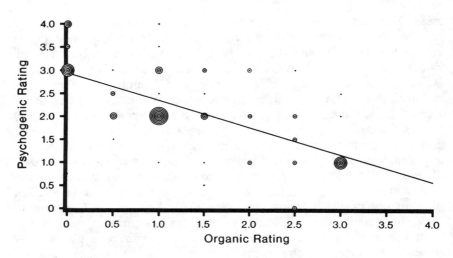

FIGURE 7.1.   Relationship between degrees of organic and psychogenic impairment for 63 patients. Each circle represents one patient. From "Psychological Evaluation of Erectile Failure" by J. LoPiccolo, in press, in R. Kirby, C. Carson, and G. Webster (Eds.), *Diagnosis and Management of Male Erectile Dysfunction*. London: Butterworth Scientific. Copyright by Butterworth Scientific Ltd. Reprinted by permission.

was only a moderate negative correlation (−.58) between degrees of organic and psychological impairment, so a unidimensional, bipolar scale is not an accurate representation of clinical reality. Furthermore, Figure 7.1 shows that of these 63 patients, the erectile problems of only 10 men were found to be purely psychogenic in etiology, and those of only 3 men were found to be purely organic, so an "either–or" two-category typology is even more inappropriate. Figure 7.1 also indicates that a considerable number of men (19 of 63, or 30%) had mild organic impairments (0.5 to 1.0 on this scale) but significant psychological problems (2.0 or greater on this scale). These men might, in a two-part typology, be considered to be "organic" cases of erectile failure, because there was some demonstrated physiological impairment. However, the greater degree of psychological etiology seen in these cases argues against this categorization, and suggest that a physical intervention would probably not be necessary to restore normal erectile functioning for these men.

Diagnostic classification into a two-dimensional schema also offers a comment on the long-term adjustment to implantation of a prosthesis. Consider, in Figure 7.1, the 16 men who scored at least 2.5 on the organic impairment scale, and for whom a prosthesis might therefore be an appropriate treatment. Of these 16 men, 5 (31%) received a rating of 2.0, 2.5, or 3.0 for presence of concurrent psychological problems. It might be anticipated that with this degree of psychological disturbance, long-term adjustment to the prosthesis would be poor. Although patients are typically very eager to have prostheses implanted, and report being very happy with them at short-term surgical follow-up, longer-term follow-up indicates poor sexual adjustment in a significant percentage of cases (Tiefer, Pedersen, & Melman, 1988). It seems reasonable that if a number of psychological problems are involved in a man's erectile failure, the implantation of the prosthetic device will only result in his now having these same difficulties, but with an artificially rigid penis. Although erection is now present, one would not expect the frequency or quality of sexual activity to be high in such cases, and this result is what Tiefer et al. (1988) found. A thorough psychological evaluation is therefore indicated for all cases of erectile failure, even when an organic etiology is clearly established and a surgical treatment is planned. A postmodern view of erectile failure argues that psychotherapy will often be needed when a prosthesis is implanted, because of the functional adaptive value of erectile failure, even when there is an organic impairment involved in causality.

The focus in much of the clinical literature in making a differential diagnosis into mutually exclusive categories of organic or psychogenic etiology is often pursued at the expense of formulating the best treatment plan, which is ultimately the purpose of diagnostic assessment. An effective assessment not only should quantify the degrees of psychological and physiological causality of the erection problem, but should identify (through the four-element functional analysis discussed previously) issues to be focused upon in treatment, and should determine the prognosis for response to physical interventions (e.g., vasoactive injections, vacuum devices, or prostheses). Because it seems to be true that most erectile failure cases involve major psychological etiology, regardless of degree of organic impairment present, assessment should focus on which psychological and/or somatic interventions are most likely to help each particular patient. As Mohr and Beutler (1990) have noted, prognosis, not diagnosis, must be the deciding factor in choice of treatment, and psychological evaluation is critical in making prognostic evaluations for physical interventions.

Prognosis is assessed with information gathered by semistructured interviews, psychometric testing, and symptom-focused questionnaires (see, e.g., LoPiccolo & Daiss, 1988, for a detailed assessment protocol). A typical protocol includes 2–3 hours of interviews and psychometric screening for psychopathology with the patient and sexual partner (LoPiccolo & Daiss, 1988); a general sex history questionnaire (Schover, Friedman, Weiler, Heiman, & LoPiccolo, 1982); an assessment of the marital relationship with a psychometric instrument such as the Locke–Wallace Marital Adjustment Test (Kimmel & VanderVeen, 1974); and an analysis of the detailed nature of the couple's actual sexual behavior with the Sexual Interaction Inventory (LoPiccolo & Steger, 1974).

Prognostic Indicators and Choice of Treatment

Based on the information gathered from the interview and questionnaire materials discussed above, the clinician can now make a prognostic decision about which type of treatment will best suit the individual patient couple. What follows is a brief review of prognostic indicators for psychotherapeutic treatment and for medical interventions (e.g., implantation of a prosthesis, use of a vacuum device, or vasoactive injections).

Good and Poor Prognostic Indicators for Psychotherapy

The best prognosis for successful psychotherapy occurs in cases in which clear behavioral deficits or maladaptive thinking patterns that contribute to lack of erection can be identified. The most common behavioral, cognitive, dynamic, and systemic problems that respond well to postmodern sex therapy are listed below.

   1. *There is a lack of adequate sexual stimulation.* If the woman does not engage in any manual or oral stimulation of her partner's penis, but expects him to have an erection because he is kissing and caressing her, relatively simple behavioral directions for increasing physical stimulation have a good chance of success. These behavioral deficits can be identified clearly with the Sexual Interaction Inventory (LoPiccolo & Steger, 1974). This intervention is indicated in cases of partial organic impairment or in aging males, where the erection response requires a high intensity of physical stimulation of the penis (LoPiccolo, 1991).

   2. *The woman's sexual gratification is currently dependent upon the man's obtaining an erection.* If the woman only has orgasm during coitus, and does not consider an orgasm produced by her partner's manual, oral, or electric vibrator stimulation to be "normal," there is a good prognosis for sex therapy. If the man can be reassured that he is providing full sexual satisfaction for his partner through manual, oral, or electric vibrator stimulation of her genitals, the pressure on him to perform for her by getting an erection will be greatly reduced.

   3. *There is a lack of knowledge about age-related changes in sexual functioning.* Erectile failure is most commonly seen in men aged 50 or older. In aging men, the slowing down of the erection response, the greater dependence upon physical as opposed to psychological stimulation to produce an erection, the longer duration of the refractory period, and the inability to ejaculate on every occasion of intercourse are normal changes with aging (Schover, 1984). However, many couples overreact to these changes with anxiety and distress, which can lead to erectile failure in the male (LoPiccolo, 1991). Simple education about normal aging changes in sexuality, and behavioral techniques for dealing with these changes, can resolve the erectile failure.

4. *Cognitive distortions regarding the male sex-role stereotype are leading to unrealistic demands upon the male for sexual performance.* Many men and women labor under a "macho" set of unrealistic role demands for male sexual performance (Zilbergeld, 1978). Education to promote a realistic view of male sex roles and sexual performance can be very helpful.

5. *Individual dynamic, relationship system, unresolved family-of-origin, or operant reinforcement issues are making it functionally adaptive for the erectile failure to continue to occur* (see discussion above). Although long-term therapy in such cases is often indicated, the prognosis is good if such functional issues can be identified.

Having mentioned some positive prognostic indicators for successful psychotherapy, I now offer a comment on poor prognostic indicators:

1. *Either the patient or his partner is unwilling to reconsider one of the issues noted above* (e.g., male sex-role demands, the role of the female in providing adequate stimulation for the male, or the means of stimulation by which the female reaches her orgasm).

2. *The patient has a sexual deviation.* Obviously, if the male is aroused by an inappropriate sexual object (such as children) or has a paraphilia (such as transvestism), therapy becomes much more difficult.

3. *The patient's religious beliefs about sex are interfering with sexual performance.* These cases are best referred to a pastoral counselor, who may have some credibility in changing or at least helping the patient re-examine these beliefs.

4. *The patient has severe clinical depression.* Sex therapy is routinely unsuccessful in cases of severe clinical depression. However, mild to moderate depression, which may be a reaction to erectile and marital distress, may respond well to sex therapy.

Good and Poor Prognostic Indicators for Medical Treatments

Positive prognostic indicators for a prosthesis, use of a vacuum device, or vasoactive injections include the following:

1. *A presently adequate range of sexual stimulation is provided to the male by the female* (in terms of manual and oral stimulation of the penis during foreplay). However, this stimulation is ineffective in producing an erection.

2. *Both partners are well informed and adaptable.* That is, they have a clear understanding of exactly what sexual behavior can be expected following the medical treatment, and a willingness to adjust to the marked changes in sexual behavior patterns that are necessitated by any of these medical procedures (Tiefer et al., 1988).

3. *The female does enjoy penile–vaginal intercourse, but reports that size of the penis is not important to her.* Because a prosthesis does not increase the size of the penis, as occurs when a man gets a physiological erection, some

women do report disappointment with the prosthesis if they previously enjoyed the sensation of containment of the larger, normally erect penis. These cases are routinely dissatisfied with the prosthetic implant (Tiefer et al., 1988). Very recently, a new version of the inflatable prosthesis has been developed that does increase both diameter and length of the penis. It is possible that a woman's satisfaction in this type of case will be increased with this device.

There are also some indicators of poor prognosis for long-term adjustment to a medical intervention. The more commonly seen factors are as follows:

1. *There is strong positive functional value for either partner in the continuance of the erectile failure.* If either the man or the woman is invested in maintenance of the erectile failure because it helps that partner deal with issues in the relationship or has other functional value, adjustment to a prosthesis or medical procedure will be poor, unless psychotherapy is also provided (preferably prior to any surgery).

2. *The woman is essentially uninterested in resuming an active sex life.* In a recent case, the patient's wife stated, "I've always done my wifely duty, but it's been a great relief not to have to do it these last 5 years, since he's been impotent." The husband in this case was given a penile prosthesis. As might be expected, the results were psychologically disastrous—severe marital distress and ultimately divorce.

3. *A medical solution is seen as a cure-all.* For example, one or both partners may have unrealistic expectations that an artificial erection will resolve conflicts about desired frequency of intercourse, willingness to engage in other forms of sexual activity (such as manual or oral stimulation), and general dissatisfaction with the partner's sexual techniques.

4. *Significant psychopathology is indicated on the psychometric instruments discussed previously.*

The Third Component: Sexual Behavior Patterns

Thus far, it has been stressed that a postmodern view of erectile failure involves a highly complex interaction of psychological and physiological factors. There is, however, a third element in the postmodern view—a less complex but no less important element in the treatment of erectile failure. This is the actual sexual behavior pattern of the couple, which has been briefly alluded to in the preceding section on prognosis.

Modern sex therapy, as developed by Masters and Johnson (1970), suggests that if performance anxiety and the spectator role are eliminated by substituting sensate focus (nongenital body massage) for further attempts at intercourse, erections will spontaneously occur. Although systemic issues can defeat sensate focus, there are two other reasons why sensate focus often fails with today's cases.

First, sensate focus is, in some fashion, a form of paradoxical treatment. The therapist instructs the patient to relax, not to be sexual, not to expect an erection, and only to enjoy the sensual body massage. Of course, a nude massage by a nude partner, even without direct genital caressing, is a highly sexual (not just sensual) situation; with performance anxiety eliminated, erection therefore should occur. The paradox is in labeling for the patient a sexual situation as nonsexual, so that he is not expecting an erection, and neither he nor his partner is placing any performance demands on him. Like most paradoxical procedures, sensate focus only works if the patient is unaware of the underlying paradox. (By analogy, a parent's telling a negativistic adolescent to do the opposite of what the parent actually wants him or her to do will not work if the adolescent is aware that the parent is using "reverse psychology.") Of course, with modern sex therapy procedures widely explicated in books, magazines, newspaper columns, and television talk shows, it is a rare patient today who is unaware that the therapeutic effect of sensate focus lies in reduction of performance pressure. Many patients who are aware of this linkage do *not* experience a reduction in performance anxiety in response to sensate focus; rather, they suffer from what might be called "metaperformance anxiety." Metaperformance anxiety refers to a type of higher order anxiety, nicely explained by a patient as follows:

> I found myself lying there, thinking, "I'm now free of pressure to perform. I'm not supposed to get an erection, and we're not allowed to have intercourse even if I do get one. So now that all the pressure is off, why am I not getting an erection? I'm relaxed, I'm enjoying this, so where's the erection?"

What this patient described is typical for men who understand the role of sensate focus in reducing performance anxiety and eliminating the self-evaluative spectator role (Masters & Johnson, 1970). For these men, simple performance anxiety is replaced by meta-anxiety about why eliminating performance anxiety does not lead to erection during sensate focus body massage.

The second reason why sensate focus often fails is that, as noted earlier, one-third to two-thirds of men with erectile failure have some degree of organic impairment of their erectile capability. For these men, it is unrealistic to expect that physiological arousal (erection) will occur without direct, intense genital stimulation, regardless of the absence of performance anxiety and the degree of sensual pleasure and subjective arousal experienced in sensate focus. Furthermore, erectile failure is much more common in aging men, and even healthy aging men require direct and intense physical stimulation of the penis for erection to occur (Schover, 1984; LoPiccolo, 1991).

Because sensate focus is often ineffective in reducing performance anxiety in today's sophisticated patients, and because the typical erectile failure patient needs intense stimulation for erection, the actual behavior patterns of the patient couple have become crucial in a postmodern therapeutic approach. Far more effective than sensate focus in reducing performance anxiety is the patient's knowledge that his partner's sexual gratification does not depend on his achieving an erection. If the patient can be reassured that his partner finds their lovemaking highly pleasurable, and that she is sexually fulfilled by the orgasms he gives her through manual and oral stimulation, his performance anxiety will be greatly reduced. If these options have never been discussed or tried, therapy may be relatively simple. However, if the sexual partner finds alternative routes to orgasm unacceptable, the therapist may find it more difficult to introduce these activities as a vehicle for therapeutic progress. A recent patient's partner, in response to the suggestion that they discontinue attempts at intercourse and rather focus on bringing her to orgasm by manual or oral stimulation, replied, "If he can't give me the real thing, I don't want him to get me all hot and bothered." In such cases, the therapist must realize that the wife of the typical elderly erectile failure patient was raised in a culture that was very sex-negative for women, and she will need support and encouragement to re-examine her sexual attitudes (Heiman & LoPiccolo, 1988; LoPiccolo & Heiman, 1978; LoPiccolo, 1991).

The couple's acceptance of manual and oral stimulation of the female's genitals as a route to sexual satisfaction for her is important in most erectile failure cases. However, at least as important is the female's direct manual and oral stimulation of the patient's penis. Although the importance of adequate direct penile stimulation is obvious in cases with major organic pathology, it is also important because of normal aging changes in sexual response in healthy men, as previously noted in this chapter and discussed in more detail by Segraves and Segraves in Chapter 5 of this volume.

One especially important normal change that can cause problems is that the erection response slows down, and it takes longer for men to get an erection as they age. Similarly, with aging, the erection response becomes more dependent on direct physical stimulation of the penis, and less responsive to visual, psychological, or nongenital physical stimulation. Rigidity of the penis and angle of erection both decline somewhat, but typically not enough to interfere with intercourse (Masters & Johnson, 1966). All of these changes are minor, and need not interfere with a full sexual life. However, for patients who are unaware of the normality of these changes, there may be great anxiety and distress about them. The partners begin to make love, and they notice that the man doesn't immediately obtain an erection; they therefore cease all sexual activity, assuming that he is "impotent," perhaps because of his age. If the couple simply continued with direct physical stimulation of his penis for a while longer, the man would probably obtain an erection. Such a couple typically does not profit from therapy based on sensate focus.

The need for more direct physical stimulation of the penis is especially problematic in the older couple for whom direct physical stimulation of the penis has not previously been a major component of their sexual activity. A couple who are in their 70s or 80s grew up in a culture in which a decent woman was not encouraged to be sexually active, and did not necessarily engage in touching the man's penis. Their sexual repertoire may have consisted of hugging and kissing, some breast caressing, and intercourse. As the male ages, this repertoire will often not be sufficient to produce erection for the male, even though he feels psychologically aroused. In such cases of insufficient stimulation, and demands for coital performance by either the woman's or the man's own unrealistic expectations, several therapeutic tactics are indicated. The therapist should instruct the couple that erection is not subject to voluntary control and is neither spontaneous nor instantaneous (especially in older men); however, it should automatically occur, *given sufficient stimulation in an anxiety-free setting*. Both performance demands on the man and the woman's frustration can be reduced through instructing the couple to insure the woman's orgasm by means of manual, oral, or electric vibrator stimulation of her genitals, none of which requires the man to have an erect penis. Explicit films and books can be used to train the woman in effective stimulation techniques.

If the woman makes demanding or derogatory statements about the man's sexual abilities, the therapist should emphasize that such demands or criticisms are counterproductive and may increase the anxiety that causes the man's erectile failure. The clinician, however, should not simplistically assume that all such women are hostile, demanding, or deriving secondary benefits from their partners' dysfunction. It should be remembered that it is personally very threatening to all but the most secure women for their partners to have erectile failure. A woman commonly interprets a man's erectile failure as an indication that he does not love her, is having an affair, is no longer sexually attracted to her, and so forth. The critical and demanding behavior these women show may be a reflection of inner anxiety, despair, and depression rather than one of hostility. In such cases, reassurance on these issues by the clinician—and, more importantly, by the man—will be much more effective in insuring the woman's therapeutic cooperation than will any confrontive "resistance interpretations."

A COURT OF LAST RESORT

I have had some success with the therapeutic use of NPT in cases of global, lifelong erectile failure. This diagnostic label refers to the patient who has never been able to achieve an erection, in any way, in his entire life.

Masters and Johnson (1970) noted that their sex therapy procedures often failed with such cases, and postmodern techniques also have less than optimal success with this difficult group. For these patients, it is worthwhile to consider the therapeutic use of naturally occurring NPT. In this procedure, the couple is instructed that the man is to retire to bed and go to sleep. The woman is to remain in another room. After an or hour or two has passed, she should begin to check on him every 15 minutes or so. At some point, she will observe that he has an erection while he sleeps. The couple is instructed that at this point she is to begin caressing his penis very gently. The result is that he gradually awakens to an absolutely unique experience for him—an erection during sexual activity with his partner. This milestone experience has led to remarkable treatment progress in deadlocked and unsuccessful cases. In one case, the wife was even able to accomplish vaginal intromission while her husband was awakening, thus achieving intercourse for the first time in an unconsummated marriage of 7 years' duration. However, it should be noted that this technique is highly stressful for some couples, in whom there has been major adaptive value for both partners in the man's *never* having an erection. This intervention is contraindicated in such cases until these issues are addressed in psychotherapy.

A CASE EXAMPLE

This case is presented because it illustrates, in an unusually clear way, many of the postmodern issues discussed in this chapter.

Bill and Emily, both in their 70s, presented for treatment of his erectile failure. They had been together for only a few months. She had been widowed many years ago, and he had been divorced some 15 years ago. They had only had sex on a few occasions, and Bill was completely unable to achieve an erection.

History revealed that Bill had begun having erectile failure in his 50s, and this problem had been a factor in his divorce. Shamed and humiliated by his "impotence," he and his wife had never sought sex therapy. He had tried sex with a few different women after his divorce, with uniform occurrence of erectile failure. He also experienced erectile failure in masturbation. Consequently, he had been celibate for the last several years, until meeting Emily. When erectile failure also occurred with her, he responded to an ad in the sports section of the local newspaper for "medical treatment of impotence." However, to his great disappointment, he was turned down for prosthetic surgery because of his medical condition and history. He was told he should be thankful he was alive, and should just "not worry" about sex any more at his age.

History revealed that Bill had suffered two heart attacks and a stroke. He was also an insulin-dependent diabetic, and was under treatment for an unidentified "Parkinson-like" disorder. When asked about his medications, he produced 11 different pill bottles from the pockets of his suit! He was on several coronary medications, insulin, medication for the Parkinson-like condition, an antidepressant, an antianxiety drug, and sleeping medications. At least 8 of these 11 medications are commonly considered to cause sexual dysfunction (for a discussion of medication effects, see Segraves & Segraves, Chapter 5, this volume).

Bill was informed that his erectile problems almost certainly resulted from his disease processes and from the side effects of his medications. I suggested that it was not necessary for him to go through our complete erectile failure evaluation, which includes vascular, neurological, hormonal, and NPT studies; I felt that we could predict the results, based on his history. I suggested that counseling to help the two of them discover a rewarding sex life that did *not* require an erect penis was perhaps the best course of action.

However, Bill indicated that he *would* like the complete workup. Because he was a financially comfortable retiree, time and money were not issues for him, and he indicated that he would prefer a definitive answer as to the cause of his erectile problems. Accordingly, I proceeded to question them further about their current sexual difficulties.

When Emily was asked about her reaction to Bill's erectile failure, her reply was "Frankly, except for him feeling bad about it, I don't care." This type of response is typical of many elderly women, raised in a repressive culture, who have no interest in sex. However, this ageist stereotype was not true in Emily's case. Rather, she reported that she enjoyed sex greatly and had a high sex drive. Emily was not disturbed by Bill's erectile failure because she had not enjoyed penile–vaginal intercourse very much in her marriage, and had always wished her husband would spend more time in caressing her genitals, which was how she was able to reach orgasm. Emily thought that Bill was "willing" to spend time in caressing her genitals because he "felt guilty" about his erection problems. With some embarrassment, she stated that she considered him a "fantastic lover," as he had provided oral–genital stimulation for her on the last time they made love, and she had been multiply orgasmic. Emily even expressed some concern that if Bill should regain his erection, he might stop doing the manual and oral genital caressing that she enjoyed. She was surprised and delighted to hear that Bill did these things not just because he felt guilty, but because he genuinely enjoyed caressing her and bringing her to orgasm. Bill was also amazed to hear that she considered him a "great lover" and that she was unconcerned about his erectile failure. The topics of erectile failure, and sex in general, were too embarrassing for them to have discussed these issues previously.

I then asked Emily if she spent as much time in manually and orally stimulating Bill's penis as he did in caressing her genitals. Bill interjected that he wouldn't ask her "to service me like a prostitute," and was surprised when Emily indicated that she would *enjoy* manually and orally caressing him. She had been too inhibited to attempt these activities, sensing that he was humiliated by what he saw as her futile attempts to stimulate him. Emily reported that she did not care whether he got an erection; she just *liked* touching and kissing his penis.

Some further discussion centered on the role of intense and sustained physical stimulation in producing erection for older men, especially when physiological or medication factors contribute to the erectile failure. I suggested that although Bill was almost certainly not capable of achieving an erection, and probably would not ejaculate, they were well on their way to a wonderful sex life centered on mutual manual and oral genital caressing.

Bill and Emily were scheduled for a physiological evaluation in about 3 weeks, on the first available date for our NPT laboratory. When they returned for this session, they reported that he had had an erection in one of their lovemaking sessions, and they had had intercourse. They reported that the erection came as a surprise to both of them. The erection occurred after much oral and manual stimulation of his genitals, and after she had had several orgasms during his oral stimulation of her. The penis never became fully rigid, but it was firm enough for intromission and thrusting to occur, and he had even reached orgasm and ejaculation.

Our complete physical evaluation did reveal marked vascular and neurological abnormalities, with minimal sleep erections. There was no question that Bill had major physiological and pharmacological damage to his erectile system. However, in their relationship, he knew that Emily was sexually satisfied and had no investment in his having an erection as the source of her sexual gratification. Furthermore, she provided high levels of physical stimulation of his penis for long periods of time. In this ideal psychological and physical context, the slight degree of his erectile capacity that remained intact despite his illnesses and medications was fully expressed, and was sufficient for functional intercourse on occasion.

However, after this initial success at intercourse, Bill and Emily went through a difficult period of several months. His erectile functioning was erratic, but this in itself was not very distressing to Emily, as her pleasure and orgasms did not depend on his erection. Similarly, Bill was regularly achieving orgasm, whether during intercourse with an erection, or in oral or manual stimulation with a flaccid or only partially erect penis. What was more problematic for the couple was some mutual avoidance of sexual activity, as well as some lovemaking sessions that, although sexually satisfying, left them feeling emotionally uncomfortable. At this point in therapy, the notion that Bill's erectile failure might have been in some way functional for them was

presented. The thorough, four-element functional analysis previously discussed was conducted, and one major issue emerged: Both Bill and Emily
had some reservations about getting married or making a long-term commitment to each other. The issues included the fact that each of them owned a
home, the question of where they would live, the problems of merging their
finances, their adult children's reactions, questions of inheritance, and so
forth. At some level, however, they both felt that if they were having intercourse they should be married. Erectile failure was functional for them in
dealing with the conflict between their moral values about nonmarital intercourse and their ambivalence about getting married. With further therapy,
they resolved that they did not need to be married to enjoy sex together, and
did not need erectile failure as a mechanism to avoid rushing into a more
committed relationship than felt comfortable for them.

Because Bill and Emily had been together for only a short time, and were
not married or living together, I erred in not making a postmodern functional
analysis of the value of erectile failure for them. This error occurred primarily
because—given the short duration of their relationship, as well as the
obviousness of the organic impairment and behavioral deficits—it was easy
to assume that systemic issues would not be a relevant factor. This case nicely
illustrates that all three elements of postmodern theory always need to be
considered, and that an individualized treatment plan needs to be developed
for each unique case.

CONCLUSION

This chapter has reviewed historical and current conceptions of the etiology
and treatment of erectile failure. Early theories were based primarily on
Victorian cultural values, and then on psychoanalytic theory, with a lack of
an empirical base of knowledge in each of these approaches. More recently,
erectile failure has been cast in the framework of mainstream cognitive-
behavioral psychotherapy. Following Masters and Johnson's emphasis on a
purely psychogenic model, we have seen an increase in purely medical
approaches to erectile failure. Coexistent with this medical trend, however,
the systemic therapists have begun to see erectile failure as an issue to be
integrated into their therapeutic approach. A postmodern view argues that
erectile failure represents a complex, overdetermined psychophysiological
problem. In a sense, erectile failure is a sexual representation of the old
mind–body problem that first philosophers, and now neuroscientists and
psychologists, debate with great passion. Like many "either–or" debates, this
one ignores the reality of complex, multiple causality in seeking a single
unifying principle. Perhaps we should cease speaking of "erectile failure" in
the singular, and instead refer to a plurality of "erectile failures.'" Erectile

failure is a form of "final common pathway" to which many tributary factors contribute. Although unitary approaches may make for elegantly simple theory, they are also likely to result in ineffective clinical practice with many of our patients who struggle with erectile failure. We owe each patient and his partner a thorough assessment of the factors involved in their unique case, and a treatment plan individualized for maximum possibility of therapeutic success.

REFERENCES

Bancroft, J. (1984). Testosterone therapy for low sexual interest and erectile dysfunctions in man: A controlled study. *British Journal of Psychiatry, 14,* 146–151.

Bem, S. (1974). The measurement of psychological androgyny. *Journal of Consulting and Clinical Psychology, 42,* 155–162.

Comfort, A. (1965). *The anxiety makers.* Camden, NJ: Nelson.

Ellis, H. (1910). *Studies in the psychology of sex* (7 vols.). Philadelphia: F. A. Davis.

Freud, S. (1962). *Three essays on the theory of female sexuality* (E. Jones, Trans.). New York: Avon. (Original work published 1905)

Gurman, A., & Kniskern, D. (Eds.). (1981). *Handbook of family therapy.* New York: Brunner/Mazel.

Heiman, J. R., & LoPiccolo, J. (1988). *Becoming orgasmic: A personal and sexual growth program for women* (2nd ed.). Englewood Cliffs, NJ: Prentice-Hall.

Heiman, J., LoPiccolo, L., & LoPiccolo, J. (1981). Treatment of sexual dysfunction. In A. S. Gurman & D. P. Kniskern (Eds.), *Handbook of family therapy.* New York: Brunner/Mazel.

Kaplan, H. S. (1974). *The new sex therapy.* New York: Brunner/Mazel.

Kimmel, D., & VanderVeen, F. (1974). Factors of marital adjustment in Locke's Adjustment Test. *Journal of Marriage and the Family, 29,* 57–63.

Krafft-Ebing, R. von. (1902). *Psychopathia sexualis.* Brooklyn, NY: Physicians and Surgeons Books.

Lazarus, A. A. (1965). The treatment of a sexually inadequate man. In L. P. Ullmann & L. Krasner (Eds.), *Case studies in behavior modification* (pp. 243–240). New York: Holt, Rinehart & Winston.

LoPiccolo, J. (1988). Management of psychogenic erectile failure. In E. Tanagho, T. Lue, & R. McClure (Eds.), *Contemporary management of impotence and infertility.* Baltimore: Williams & Wilkins.

LoPiccolo, J. (1991). Counseling and therapy of sexual problems in the elderly. In L. K. Dial (Ed.), *Clinics in geriatric medicine: Vol. 7. Sexuality in the elderly* (pp. 161–179). Philadelphia: W. B. Saunders.

LoPiccolo, J. (in press). Psychological evaluation of erectile failure. In R. Kirby, C. Carson, & G. Webster (Eds.), *Diagnosis and management of male erectile dysfunction.* London: Butterworth Scientific.

LoPiccolo, J., & Daiss, S. (1987). The assessment of sexual dysfunction. In K. D. O'Leary (Ed.), *Assessment of marital discord.* Hillsdale, NJ: Erlbaum.

LoPiccolo, J., & Daiss, S. (1988). Psychological issues in the evaluation of erectile failure. In E. Tanagho, T. Lue, & R. McClure (Eds.), *Contemporary management of impotence and infertility*. Baltimore: Williams & Wilkins.

LoPiccolo, J., & Friedman, J. (1985). Sex therapy: An integrative model. In S. Lynn & J. Garske (Eds.), *Contemporary psychotherapies: Models and methods*. Columbus, OH: Charles E. Merrill.

LoPiccolo, J., & Heiman, J. R. (1978). The role of cultural values in the prevention of sexual problems. In C. B. Qualls, J. P. Wincze, & D. H. Barlow (Eds.), *The prevention of sexual disorders* (pp. 43–74). New York: Plenum Press.

LoPiccolo, J., & Steger, J. (1974). The Sexual Interaction Inventory: A new instrument for assessment of sexual dysfunction. *Archives of Sexual Behavior*, 3, 585–595.

Masters, W. H., & Johnson, V. E. (1966). *Human sexual response*. Boston: Little, Brown.

Masters, W. H., & Johnson, V. E. (1970). *Human sexual inadequacy*. Boston: Little, Brown.

Melman, A., Tiefer, L., & Pedersen, R. (1988). Evaluation of the first 406 patients in urology department based center for male sexual dysfunction. *Urology*, 32, 6–10.

Mohr, D. C., & Beutler, L. E. (1990). Erectile dysfunction: A review of diagnostic and treatment procedures. *Clinical Psychology Review*, 10(1), 123–150.

Money, J. (1985). *The destroying angel: Sex, fitness, and food in the legacy of graham crackers, Kellogg's corn flakes, and American health history*. Buffalo, NY: Prometheus Books.

Salter, A. (1949). *Conditioned reflex therapy*. New York: Creative Age Press.

Schover, L. R. (1984). *Prime time: Sexual health for men over fifty*. New York: Holt, Rinehart & Winston.

Schover, L. R., Friedman, J., Weiler, S., Heiman, J. R., & LoPiccolo, J. (1982). A multiaxial diagnostic system for sexual dysfunctions: An alternative to DSM-III. *Archives of General Psychiatry*, 39, 614–619.

Segraves, R. T., Schoenberg, H. W., Zarins, C. K., Knopf, J., & Carnic, P. (1981). Discrimination of organic versus psychological impotence with the DSFI: A failure to replicate. *Journal of Sex and Marital Therapy*, 7(3), 230–238.

Sherfey, M. (1973). *The nature and evolution of female sexuality*. New York: Vintage.

Spark, R. F., White, R. A., & Connolly, P. B. (1980). Impotence is not always psychogenic: Newer insights into hypothalamic–pituitary–gonadal dysfunction. *Journal of the American Medical Association*, 243, 750–755.

Tanagho, E. A., Lue, T. F., & McClure, R. D. (Eds.). (1988). *Contemporary management of impotence and infertility*. Baltimore: Williams & Wilkins.

Tiefer, L., Pedersen, B., & Melman, A. (1988). Psychosocial follow-up of penile prosthesis implant patients and partners. *Journal of Sex and Marital Therapy*, 14, 184–201.

Wolpe, J. (1958). *Psychotherapy by reciprocal inhibition*. Stanford, CA: Stanford University Press.

Zilbergeld, B. (1978). *Male sexuality*. New York: Bantam Books.

8

Intrapsychic and Interpersonal Aspects of Impotence: Psychogenic Erectile Dysfunction

Stephen B. Levine

In his traditionally provocative and thoughtful way, Stephen Levine presents a comprehensive model for exploring and treating the intrapsychic and interpersonal aspects of psychogenic erectile dysfunction. Levine suggests that erectile failure represents an enigma for both the professional and the patient, but one that may be better understood through a careful assessment of three underlying spheres of causality that derive from different phases of time: the present, the recent past, and childhood/adolescence. These three spheres of causality are performance anxiety, antecedent life events, and developmental vulnerabilities, all of which interact in certain situations to produce the complaint of an "uncooperative penis."

Secondary psychogenic impotence is quite common, and may be related to common life stresses such as deterioration of a man's nonsexual relationship with a partner, divorce, death of a spouse, vocational failure, or loss of health; by contrast, primary psychogenic impotence is rarer. Nevertheless, using a liberal definition of "primary impotence"—which includes men who have occasionally been able to have intercourse, but cannot do so with any regularity—Levine suggests that approximately 5% of men may fall into this category. In these cases, the pathogenesis of the disorder often stems from early childhood and adolescent developmental processes, which leave the male frightened by or uninterested in intercourse. Often, basic problems with gender identity, homoeroticism, paraphilias, or a sexual abuse history are instrumental in creating an impossible conflict between wanting to be sexually adequate, but feeling profoundly threatened by closeness with a woman.

Levine suggests that erectile dysfunction usually falls into one of four basic categories: psychogenic, organic, mixed, and idiopathic (i.e., those cases in which the therapist is unable to classify the cause of the problem with any degree of certainty). He notes that all men experience changes in erectile capacity during their late 50s and early 60s, and that a partner's response to these normal age-related changes may be instrumental in disrupting a couple's sexual equilibrium. He reminds clinicians that "erectile unreliability" is a preferable way of viewing these age-related changes in sexual performance, rather than the term "impotence," which implies that the capacity for erectile response is permanently lost.

In conceptualizing male erectile problems, Levine notes that one must understand the larger psychological context of male sexuality. He draws upon three of Freud's observations about male sexual response: namely, that for many men some form of degradation enhances potency; that maturity requires the difficult task of uniting affection with sexual excitement; and that sex and aggression are often inextricably linked. Although most men are unaware of these dynamics, they are likely to contribute in various ways to male sexual problems.

Finally, Levine suggests that treatment with men experiencing psychogenic erectile difficulty depends upon the clinician's ability to accurately formulate the psychodynamic forces that are operative within the three spheres of causality. The clinician assists a patient not only by dealing sensitively with the psychodynamic forces underlying the present difficulty, but also by reassuring the patient and providing a stance of optimism regarding outcome. Nevertheless, even with skilled therapeutic intervention and a highly motivated patient, treatment is not always successful—or, if it is successful in the short term, results are not always stable and long-lasting. Levine is realistic about less than perfect resolution of erectile difficulties; he suggests that some men never entirely resolve such problems. Treatment, however, can still be of considerable value to such individuals, since it may help them to achieve improvements in their overall level of psychological and interpersonal functioning.

Stephen B. Levine, M.D., is Professor of Psychiatry at Case Western Reserve University School of Medicine, and Medical Director of the Center for Human Sexuality at the University Hospitals of Cleveland. He is one of the most innovative and original contributors to the field of sex therapy and has published widely. His most recent book is entitled Sex Is Not Simple.

The idea that personal and interpersonal psychological states can disrupt erectile capacity is so basic to the practice of medicine, psychiatry, and psychology that the age-old affliction of psychogenic impotence no longer receives in-depth consideration. This is ironic because it is a common condition, and clinicians in all disciplines need to be updated on evolving concepts of its pathogenesis and treatment. The progress made during the 1980s in treating organic impotence has generated a new paradox for the treatment of psychogenic impotence: Therapists can now recommend more therapy options to patients than ever before, some of which may harm the patients.

WHAT IS PSYCHOGENIC IMPOTENCE?

"Psychogenic impotence" is one of four diagnostic labels that clinicians place on a man's inability to have intercourse because of a soft or absent erection, when he believes a firm, lasting erection is reasonable. This label is applied when the professional recognizes that the man's basic neurological, vascular, and endocrine capacities to generate adequate erections are intact, yet the physiological sequences of initiating or maintaining penile blood flow do not occur reliably with a partner. Psychogenic impotence is almost always a partial mystery to the man. The man's befuddlement signals the clinician that the patient is not fully aware of how his social or psychological dilemmas affect his potency. A metaphor illuminates the psychodynamic essence of this diagnosis: Psychogenic impotence is a message that tells the man's body not to cooperate with what he is attempting to do.

The correct diagnosis of psychogenic impotence requires a patient who possesses an uncooperative penis and a professional who understands that some personal enigma underlies the man's selective impairment in erectile physiology. The nature of the enigma is a professional issue that has never been completely resolved.

THE THREE SPHERES OF CAUSALITY

It is a fundamental error to assume that all men with psychogenic impotence have a similar underlying enigma. It is also erroneous to assume that any one man's psychodynamics can be simply stated. Concepts about the pathogenesis of psychogenic impotence derive from clinical work with men who have the problem. These concepts consist of a set of working hypotheses about the causes of impotence. They also, however, reflect one clinician's assumptions about how minds work.

What follows is a reordering of many old concepts into a scheme of causality. The symptom of psychogenic impotence is usually generated by the interaction of forces from three spheres of causality: performance anxiety, antecedent life events, and developmental vulnerabilities. These three resonating forces derive from different phases of time: the here-and-now of love-making, the recent past, and childhood/adolescence, respectively (Figure 8.1).

Sphere 1: Performance Anxiety

When Masters and Johnson (1970) described "performance anxiety," the emerging field of sex therapy adopted this concept as the explanation for the enigma. This vigilant preoccupation with the state of erection keeps the

Sphere of causality	Phase of time
1. Performance anxiety	Here-and-now of lovemaking
2. Antecedent life events	Months to years ("recent" history)
3. Developmental vulnerabilities	Childhood/adolescence (remote history)

FIGURE 8.1. General model for pathogenesis of psychogenic impotence: Three spheres of causality.

typical impotent man from sensually experiencing lovemaking. Rather than giving himself over to the pleasures of touching and being touched, he thinks about whether his erection is or will be adequate. The anticipation or dread of the loss of erection is highly destructive; it precludes arousal by substituting anxiety and inattention for sensation. The man with performance anxiety goes through the motions of lovemaking, instead of participating in a relaxed, sensual manner.

Performance anxiety is a description of the here-and-now lovemaking experience of men with erectile dysfunction. It is widely agreed upon as an etiological factor, because almost no patient with any cause of impotence escapes its destructive powers. Once established, it has great power to maintain the erectile dysfunction. Although performance anxiety is the final common psychological pathway to erectile impairment, it does not provide an adequate explanation of the origin of the problem.

Sphere 2: Antecedent Life Events

The second sphere of causality consists of the life events that have preceded the development of the problem. These events usually have occurred within a few months to a few years of the time the patient seeks assistance. The man does not fully appreciate his personal responses to these events (e.g., his affects, defenses, coping devices, and adaptational shifts). Neither does he fully realize that the inciting mechanism for his impotence is contained in these responses. These life events have more affect-laden meaning to him than he realizes. He focuses on his loss of sexual confidence—that is, his performance anxiety—as the obvious cause of his problem; how he originally fell into its pernicious trap remains a mystery. The clinician has ready access to the second sphere of causality through the history of the social, familial, vocational, and medical events that have preceded the symptom.

Sphere 3: Developmental Vulnerabilities

The third sphere of causality is historically remote. It involves the professional's interest in and understanding of the reasons why this man's life events were emotionally powerful enough to undermine his potency. The language that clinicians use in these explanations depends upon their ideological assumptions. Common explanations are as follows: failed tasks of psychological development, impairments in sexual identity, vulnerabilities of the self-system, various forms of abuse, social learning difficulties, and transference. All of these explanations rest upon developmental processes that are at least several decades old.

These three spheres of causality provide a comprehensive though skeletal overview of the contributants to psychogenic impotence. The clinician adds the "flesh" during the patient's evaluation and therapy; he or she notes the extent of performance anxiety, the precipitating events, and the personal meanings of these events in terms of the man's past. Therapy rarely plumbs the depth of each sphere. Neither does it yield an exact understanding of how the spheres fit together and resonate to produce the symptom.

It is fortunate for many psychogenically impotent men that a complete understanding of the causes is not necessary. Some men spontaneously get over their problem within a short period of time without any therapy. Others respond to therapeutic suggestions that decrease performance anxiety. Some seem to improve in response to conversations that help them work through their life events; others need to work through the earlier life events that set up the meanings of the recent life changes. There are also men for whom no therapy is sufficient to restore erections with a partner.

THE LIFE EVENTS PRECEDING SECONDARY PSYCHOGENIC IMPOTENCE

The most prevalent form of psychogenic impotence develops after a sustained period of secure erectile functioning. These cases of "secondary psychogenic impotence" provide a further insight into pathogenesis within the second sphere of causality—that is, within the history of the present problem.

The events that precede secondary psychogenic impotence typically fall into one of five categories: deterioration in the nonsexual relationship with a spouse or partner; divorce; death of a spouse; vocational failure; or loss of health. Although the emotional details are different in each case, all of these processes elicit feelings that interface with potency. For much of this century, these feelings have been referred to as "unconscious conflicts," because they function in opposition to the man's wish to have intercourse and he is unaware of their presence. Today these intrapsychic states may alternatively be called "affects," "conflicts," or "dilemmas"; nevertheless, the result is that the patient thinks he wants to have intercourse and something within him does not allow it. The clinician's responsibility is to define that "something."

Deterioration in the Nonsexual Relationship

The self-declaration of impotence in the face of alienation, mutual hostility, lack of psychological intimacy, and partner unreceptivity is a testimony to the man's expectation that he and his penis ought to be able to function under any conditions. Such optimism is not warranted, even though a shocked man may emphasize that in his last marriage he was able to have intercourse when divorcing. It is reasonable for the clinician to presume that such a man's impotence involves some of the following: resentment; loneliness; confusion about who is correct about the couple's unresolved differences; guilt over his role in their troubles; reaction to his partner's anger and unreceptivity; and/or fear of abandonment.

> *Case Vignette*
> A successful 37-year-old lawyer became impotent with his wife, had his first extramarital affair, and was impotent with his lover for 2 months. Once he recovered fully, he divorced his wife and married his lover. "I didn't realize how angry I was at my wife, but I did know how guilty and unsure I was with my lover at first. I was angry at my wife because nothing I did was good enough; everything was a hassle with her, including my having to beg for sex." When asked to state the single most powerful reason for his anger at her, he replied, "She stopped liking me! Without that, I could not function."

Divorce

Many divorcing and divorced men are surprised by their embarrassing sexual difficulty. Initially, they cannot relate their bitterness, guilt, or fear of future attachment to their erection problem. They, too, expect their penises to operate autonomously. It is reasonable for the clinician to presume that such a man's impotence involves some of the following: love for his wife; fear of his rage; doubt about his lovability; doubt about his ability to love; despair over his children's pain and alienation; and/or wariness that a new partner will eventually turn into an impossible person, as his wife did.

> *Case Vignette*
> A gentle, highly principled man who did not want a divorce slowly came to perceive that he was the victim of his cruel, materialistic wife, who by cunning and guile took his assets and turned his two young sons against him. Although he felt he knew the real reason for her requests for extra funds and frequent family crises that required her to be away, he always acceded to her requests. His lawyer felt he was crazy for not taking steps to preserve his wealth. However, he was doing what he felt

was correct to maximize his attachment to his sons and to give his wife a chance for a happier life. When he eventually began dating, he was impotent. Although he acknowledged only sadness about his wife's behavior, he had nightmares about violence and terror. He eventually learned that he was enraged; expressing that rage frightened him and threatened his basic concept of himself as a kind, gentle, peace-loving person.

Death of Spouse

Most widowers are at least in their 50s. A widower's feelings about resuming a sexual life with a new partner are influenced by many factors, such as the duration and quality of the marriage, and the cause of the wife's death. Many of these men have been through slow deaths from cancer, and began mourning well before the actual event. Because there are many partners available to physically healthy widowers, many men use dating as a distraction from being home alone and other inevitably difficult aspects of grief. It is reasonable for the clinician to presume that the impotence of a recent widower involves some of the following: unresolved grief; guilt about impulses to have multiple partners; a sense that he belongs only to his wife; confusion about his new freedom; and/or discomfort about his children's and friends' reactions to his dating and the specific women he dates.

Case Vignette

In the case of one widower, his wife's breast cancer began when she was 47, and took her life 7 years, four surgeries, and two chemotherapy courses later. Their sexual life persisted for 6 years after the first mastectomy, but ended eventually because of her weakness. Three months after her death, the widower had his first date with a woman he quickly recognized was not going to be a candidate for his second wife. Sex was aproblematic. Three months later, he had one date with a nice woman who had had a mastectomy; he felt he could not "go through it again" and never called her back. When he found a woman he thought he might eventually be able to marry, he was impotent for the first time in his life.

Vocational Failure

Vocational adequacy is central to most men's identity and self-esteem. Vocational failure or threatened vocational failure creates feelings of despair, uncertainty, anxiety, unworthiness, and guilt, which may be most apparent when a man attempts to make love. "I don't feel worthy of her any longer" may lurk behind the recent impotence of men with employment problems.

Case Vignette

One year prior to retirement, a usually prudent businessman made a bad investment and lost 25% of the money he and his wife were intending to live on during retirement. The remaining funds were adequate for their lifestyle, but the "added luxuries" were probably not going to be possible. His wife was not nearly as disturbed by this loss as he was. Neither partner recognized that his new impotence was related to this business problem, because he had weathered financial difficulties in the past without sexual symptoms. This man blamed himself for foolishly trusting another man who promised him too much. He felt that he was not worthy of his loving wife, who was loyal, proud, and ever respectful of him.

Loss of Health

Psychogenic potency problems are common after major health events, such as myocardial infarction, open heart surgery, stroke, or cancer. Fear of death during sexual activity or a heightened awareness of the recent close call may be most apparent to the man during lovemaking. The partner's reactions to the man's illness and new health status may not be completely worked through, and can create a subtle sexual unreceptivity that triggers erectile failure and performance anxiety. Since sexual life within couples takes place within a delicately balanced equilibrium (Levine, 1989), the deterioration of the partner's health may also lead to erectile impairment because of his new perceptions of his partner.

Case Vignette

A retired man whose major occupation had become caring for his wife, who had Alzheimer's disease, became impotent during the second year of her care. Their sexual life had continued despite her increasing difficulties fueled by their new closeness, the loss of her previous pattern of delaying responding to his request for sex, and the fact that she seemed to enjoy their physical interaction. As she developed incontinence and began aimless nocturnal wanderings, he began having erectile failures. He simultaneously understood and was mystified by his impotence: "It just was not right any more; she was too sick."

A Summary of the Pathogenesis of Secondary Psychogenic Impotence

Secondary psychogenic impotence occurs under diverse social and psychological circumstances. It is triggered by the destructive impact of dimly perceived feelings that successfully compete for arousal during sex play. These feelings initially stem from the life event itself (e.g., job failure or loss of health). The man typically does not recognize the emotional significance of this event or its relationship to his potency. The affects that distract him during lovemaking represent the contribution from the second sphere of causality. Soon, however, the significance of the affect-laden trigger event is amplified by its association with similar past developmental experiences. In this way, the third sphere of causality becomes interactive with the affects from the second (Figure 8.2).

What makes secondary impotence so mysterious to the patient is that he usually is only aware of his performance anxiety during the here-and-now of lovemaking. This first-sphere contribution to the pathogenesis usually occurs after the first or second episode of erectile failure. The patient remains relatively unaware of the feelings that originally competed with arousal and their immediate and historical sources.

Performance anxiety is labeled the first sphere of causality because the patient becomes aware first of its contribution to his problem. The antecedent life events are labeled the second sphere because the patient usually becomes aware of them next when his history is skillfully elicited. The developmental vulnerabilities are labeled the third sphere because they are the most subtle background factors for the problem and are usually the last contributions to be appreciated by the patient.

This interactive model of pathogenesis requires two fundamental assumptions: (1) The man possesses the expectation that he ought to be able to perform sexually, regardless of social circumstances; (2) The man is unable to experience his affects quickly and to understand what he feels. Both of these assumptions seem to apply to a great many adult men.

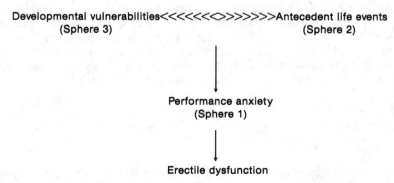

Developmental vulnerabilities<<<<<<<<>>>>>>>>Antecedent life events
(Sphere 3)   (Sphere 2)

Performance anxiety
(Sphere 1)

Erectile dysfunction

FIGURE 8.2.   Pathogenesis of secondary psychogenic erectile dysfunction.

A REVIEW OF THE CONCEPT
OF THE SEXUAL EQUILIBRIUM

Discerning the pathogenesis of secondary psychogenic impotence is difficult in some cases because of a rarely discussed complexity: the sexual equilibrium. Each person brings six sexual components or characteristics to lovemaking. Three of these—gender identity, orientation, and intention—involve sexual identity. These are generally stable characteristics that, unless they are mismatched with the partner in some way, do not feel relevant to the person as he or she behaves sexually. The other three components are sexual function characteristics: intensity of desire, ease of arousal, and ease and means of orgasmic attainment. These three characteristics are not usually stable; desire, arousal, and ease of orgasm fluctuate from sexual experience to experience.

The sexual equilibrium is the delicate balance between two partners' sexual characteristics. When a sexual partnership is formed, each person's sexual characteristics accommodate, influence, and interact with those of the partner. The product of this interaction is the sexual equilibrium (Figure 8.3).

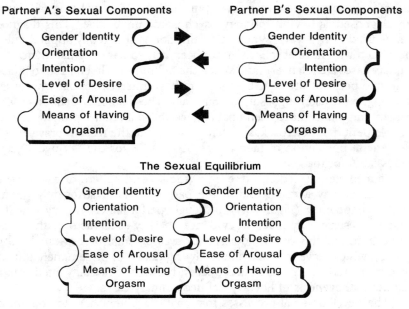

FIGURE 8.3.   The origins of the sexual equilibrium.

For fortunate couples, a good fit exists between each person's comparable components. They react to each other's characteristics with a comfortable acceptance and are able to make love in a sensuous, joyful manner. In other couples, however, the partners react negatively to each other's components. One partner's disappointment over the other's desire, arousal, or orgasm leads to tension, which limits sexual pleasure. Over time, this poor fit can change the sexual characteristics of the partner. Thus, a man may become impotent after he loses his motivation to make love to a woman who is rarely aroused. Potency may become unreliable in response to a man's demoralization over his rapid ejaculation, which he and his wife use as an explanation for her anorgasmia.

Clinicians use the concept of the sexual equilibrium to explain the fact that both partners contribute to the pleasure or tension in their sexual lives. The clarity of the three-sphere model for the pathogenesis of secondary impotence is superimposed on this basic fact of sexual life within a couple.

THE CAUSAL SPHERES
OF PRIMARY PSYCHOGENIC IMPOTENCE

The experience of heterosexual potency is a rite of passage that enhances a man's masculine identity and sense of personal adequacy. Those who consistently fail to negotiate this developmental step for psychological reasons are diagnosed as having "primary psychogenic impotence." This diagnosis can be used in two ways. When this definition is stringently applied only to those men who have absolutely never been able to have vaginal intercourse, primary cases are relatively rare. When the definition is liberalized to include men who occasionally have been able to have intercourse, but who usually cannot, the prevalence goes up dramatically. These liberally defined cases of primary impotence have been unable to establish a secure, prolonged, comfortable period of heterosexual potency. A guess at the relative prevalence in the general population of men at age 30 is 0.5% for the "stringent" cases versus 5.0% for the "liberal" ones.

Immediate antecedent life events (the second sphere of causality) do not seem to play a major role in the pathogenesis of stringently defined primary impotence (Figure 8.4). Although performance anxiety (the first sphere) is usually very much in evidence, the key elements of pathogenesis derive from childhood and adolescent developmental processes (the third sphere), which leave the male unusually frightened of or genuinely uninterested in intercourse. Issues from the second sphere of causality often complicate the pathogenesis of liberally defined primary cases.

The developmental processes that enable a potent man to contain his fear while aroused with a woman have not been positively identified. Some

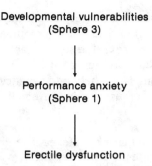

FIGURE 8.4.   Pathogenesis of primary psychogenic erectile dysfunction.

clues are available from the patterns recurrently noted among men with primary impotence.

Gender Identity Problems

Gender identity problems are the least common of the sexual identity difficulties that lurk behind a complaint of primary impotence. Most men with this type of difficulty are considered transvestites. Such a man may acknowledge having recurrent fantasies of being a woman, cross-dressing in private, discovering that their potency is assured by wearing a female garment during lovemaking, or thinking that their partner's breasts and vagina are their own.

> *Case Vignette*
> An impotent man who had been married for 3 months confessed to his sturdy, alcohol-dependent, "let's get to the bottom of this" wife that he had been cross-dressing since age 14. Much to his surprise, she asked to see him dressed. They talked a great deal and became closer than ever. When he asked whether he could make love wearing "his" slip, they were able to consummate their relationship. Her tolerance for his cross-dressing waxed and waned; when he could not wear "something," his potency was impaired or marginal, as was his desire for lovemaking.

Homoeroticism

Many men who have responded with arousal to male bodies and repeatedly masturbated to male images cannot calmly make the transition from their homoeroticism to a homosexual identity and lifestyle. Some of them attempt a heterosexual relationship and fail at intercourse, seemingly because the motivational aspects of their sexual desire are lacking. They may never have revealed their homoeroticism to their partners and often will not spontaneously reveal it to the clinician. Their performance anxiety seems to grow when they cannot sustain arousal during lovemaking.

Case Vignette
   A highly successful corporate executive, active in Alcoholic Anonymous for 15 years since attaining sobriety, masturbated to homoerotic images when he was away on his frequent business trips, but had never had sexual contact with a man. Although he had intercourse with his wife of 18 years, the frequency had been once or twice a year during the past decade. In the early years of marriage, the highest frequency of attempts had been monthly, and he had been impotent about half the time. When potent, he felt he needed to "get it over with" as quickly as possible. He typically responded with silence to his wife's entreaties for an explanation, or simply said, "I don't know why, but I can't." He resisted her requests for professional help until he thought she was going to abandon him. The first therapist failed to ask about his eroticism, and the patient never volunteered the information.

Paraphilia

Men with long-standing, highly arousing, unusual erotic fantasies that are associated with a compulsion to masturbate or act out with a partner usually have some impairment of conventional heterosexual function as well (Levine, Risen, & Althof, 1990). This impairment is most often manifested as an avoidance of lovemaking, but it also commonly involves impotence or inability to ejaculate in the vagina. Many paraphilic men have difficulty in immediately revealing their unusual eroticism to a professional. Thus, as with other sexual identity problems, the presence of the paraphilia usually must be directly elicited from the patient by careful questioning.

Case Vignette
   Before the acquired immune deficiency syndrome (AIDS) epidemic, a sheepish high school teacher in his late 50s asked to be put in contact with a sex surrogate because he wanted to be able to have intercourse once before he died. Although he dated occasionally for social reasons, he had never had any physical intimacy with anyone but a prostitute. His eroticism was dominated by the image of being spanked. He masturbated several times a day to variations on this theme, and had arranged elaborate means of hurting himself during masturbation. All attempts at

intercourse with prostitutes had failed; during the last decade, he had only requested to be yelled at and spanked for his naughtiness.

Abuse History

Heterosexual potency requires two capacities: to be aroused by a woman, and to be able to neutralize the ordinary fear and nervousness about entering her body. The three types of sexual identity problems outlined above limit the capacity to respond to women with arousal; when those who have such problems are excluded, there remains a group of masculine, heterosexual males without perversion who cannot neutralize their anxiety about lovemaking. Such a man transfers feelings about his parents or other earlier significant attachments to his partner because of the unconscious assumption that she will hurt him just as "they" did. The hurt may have been the result of egregious psychological abandonment, beatings, or sexual abuse. The patient's problem indicates that he is pessimistic about finding anyone who is trustworthy enough to share his bodily experience with him.

Case Vignette

A 48-year-old, never-married, never-potent, heterosexual public relations specialist was raised by his enema-fixated grandmother while his busy parents ran their business. Now a knowledgeable man about legal issues involving mental health, he looked back on his upbringing and felt certain that his mother's periodic nervous breakdowns and hushed-up disappearances were due to manic episodes. Until his teenage years, he was given frequent enemas by both his mother and grandmother. He remembered moments during adolescence when his generally seductive mother insisted that he wash her back while she was in the bathtub. Before his grandmother died, her enema preoccupation intensified, and she was placed in a psychiatric hospital. "I know why I have troubles, Doctor. My family was nuts. The question is, is it too late to help me?"

Diagnosable Mental Illness

Unlike secondary impotence, in which there is no necessary relationship between a *Diagnostic and Statistical Manual of Mental Disorders*, third edition, revised (DSM-III-R) diagnosis and the sexual dysfunction, primary impotence is often (though not invariably) associated with a diagnosable major condition. Most of these conditions are Axis II diagnoses, such as obsessive-compulsive disorder, schizoid personality disorder, or borderline personality disorder; some, however, have a significant Axis I problem, such as depression, psychosis, or anxiety disorder.

A Summary of the Causes of Primary Psychogenic Impotence

The causes of primary psychogenic impotence are related to those factors that explain the man's private sense of himself as an inadequate person and his strong, inarticulate fears of closeness to a woman. These powerful yet hard-to-define developmental vulnerabilities (the third sphere of causality) generate an emotional state that either precludes arousal entirely or overwhelms the physiological impact of arousal. It is intriguing that arousal does not reliably occur with a consenting female partner, but does when the man is alone, is cross-dressed, is with a male, or is with a victim.

A clinician should always carefully consider each of the three components of sexual identity when a man presents with primary impotence. The clinician should not be surprised when, after an initial denial of unconventional sexual identity, the patient reveals his unconventional eroticism involving gender identity, orientation, or intention. Similarly, primary impotence presents the clinical challenge of evaluating deficiencies in sexual desire (Levine, 1987). Although some of these problems seem to involve both drive and motivational aspects of sexual desire, most of these men will prove to have adequate sexual drive manifestations. Their clinical situation is usually brought about by their strong motivation to avoid sexual behavior with a partner unless a special condition is met, such as wearing or caressing a female garment, conjuring a fantasy of a man, or having a fantasy of hurting a woman.

TWO OTHER FORMS OF IMPOTENCE

At the end of a comprehensive medical and psychological evaluation of an impotent man and his partner, a professional is usually able to classify the case into one of four generic categories: "psychogenic," "organic," "mixed," and "idiopathic." Organic cases are relevant to a consideration of psychogenic impotence, because potency always involves people's feelings and the meanings that they subtly give to their sexual behavior.

Mixed Impotence

The diagnosis of mixed impotence is used when a man with an organic cause, such as diabetes or antihypertensive medication, has an additional significant contribution from antecedent life events (the second sphere of causality). A medicated, hypertensive diabetic with peripheral neuropathy, for instance, may be rendered impotent as a result of four factors: marital problems, depression, diabetic neuropathy, and a calcium channel blocker. A man with supraventricular tachycardia who is treated with 120 mg of Inderal may also be dealing with the implications of a myocardial infarction, an insecure job, and a child who has just been asked not to return to college.

The diagnosis of mixed impotence is not made when a man with a clear-cut organic factor develops performance anxiety. Performance anxiety is such a universal psychological response to impotence of any origin that organic impotence is almost always influenced by it. In contrast to cases of organic impotence, mixed impotence has a significant organic factor plus a contribution from the second sphere of causality. Performance anxiety is evident in cases of both organic and mixed impotence.

Idiopathic Impotence

When the professional cannot identify the cause of a patient's erectile problem with a reasonable sense of certainty, the case is classified as idiopathic. Time often reveals the true diagnosis as organic or psychogenic (e.g., a pelvic malignancy or marital deterioration is subsequently discovered). Some idiopathic impotence is an artifact of not including the partner in the evaluation process. Even after thorough physical, laboratory, and psychological evaluations, however, there are cases in which the clinician does not know whether the problem is psychogenic, mixed, or organic.

Recently, some progress has been made in conceptualizing some of these situations. Their pathogenesis begins with changes in erectile capacity that occur during the late 50s and early 60s. Masters and Johnson's (1966) original observations—namely, that aging men normally find that their erections are slower to form, do not attain the same degree of rigidity, and do not last as long as they did a decade or less before—have recently been given rigorous scientific confirmation. Using sleep laboratory evaluation of tumescence and rigidity with happily married, physically healthy men, Schiavi, Schreiner-Engel, Mandeli, Schanzer, and Cohen (1990) documented a gradual decline in physiological capacities between 55 and 74 years of age. Two crucial ideas have become apparent as a result of their work. First, the physiological mechanisms for the decline in erectile capacity with age are unknown; second, men with the same physiological decrements can be found among the impotent and the potent.

These observations direct a clinician to the couple's sexual equilibrium. It is possible that an idiopathically impotent man may develop sufficient performance anxiety to undermine his potency in response to his own perception of erectile decline or his partner's comments about his erections. The partner may respond to the man's worries by avoiding lovemaking and quietly retiring from sex. She may do this because she wishes to prevent his humiliation or because she is happy to stop having sex with him.

Idiopathic impotence is further complicated by the decline in sexual drive that usually is apparent by the time a man is in his late 50s. Because he is not as often and as intensely aroused spontaneously or in response to lovemaking, he can comfortably not make love for longer periods of time than earlier in his life. The decline in drive and the erectile decrements summate.

Such nuances within a couple's sexual equilibrium may not be apparent during the initial evaluation. Even when a clinician sees the partners over an extended period of time, the subtle psychodynamics of their situation may be missed. Clinicians need to guard against the assumption that a pattern is organic when it is in fact idiopathic.

Nowhere in the adult life cycle is the term "impotence" more destructive to the man and his partner than among healthy men about 60 years of age. Many of these so-called "impotent" men are able to have intercourse. Their problem, however, is that their ability to have intercourse is no longer predictable or reliable. Their problem is erectile *unreliability*, not impotence. This simple shift in terminology means a great deal to these men and their partners. The term "impotence" generally implies that the capacity is lost forever; "erectile unreliability" implies that tomorrow may be a better day.

When idiopathic impotence occurs in a man younger than the early 50s, the clinician needs to worry about hidden organic and psychogenic factors. When it occurs during the late 50s, it is of great value to study the sexual equilibrium closely over time. There is likely to be a shifting balance of male and female arousability that sometimes makes intercourse possible and sometimes prevents it. Idiopathic impotence in the late 50s and early 60s may turn out to be a special variation of mixed impotence. That is, it may combine a definite (though inconstant) physiological decline with a subtly fluctuating psychological factor, which at times derives from performance anxiety and at times from emotions about the social changes in the man's life.

AGE AND EASE OF DIAGNOSIS

The presence of a stand-up, rigid, lasting erection when intercourse is not being attempted usually alerts the clinician to psychogenic impotence. These adequate erections occur during the night or early morning, during kissing or petting behaviors, during masturbation, with certain partners, in response to magazines or videos, or spontaneously. When the history clearly indicates the presence of periodic normal erections, the clinician looks for an organic factor that might explain the inconstant pattern. Such factors include periodic substance abuse, medication use, or exacerbations of chronic diseases (e.g., the "pelvic steal syndrome," congestive heart failure, or multiple sclerosis). Of course, the clinician also needs to identify any psychological factors that might explain the problem.

Age has a dramatic influence on the psychogenically impotent man's ability to demonstrate normal erections. The diagnosis is easiest to make in young men, because their drive, ease of arousal, and degree of responsiveness to erotic stimuli are great; rigid, lasting, stand-up erections are frequently present. As some men become middle-aged, their sexual neurophysiology slows in responsivity. Marital problems, vocational disappointments, and concerns over children compete more powerfully with the slower, less intense arousal, and the typical psychogenic pattern of erections is more difficult to discern. Clinical judgment weighs the infrequently present adequate erection against the man's emotional situation. This is particularly striking in some men over 55 who have psychogenic impotence, yet have a history of no adequate erections under any circumstances for many months. In these common situations, the clinician should be most influenced by what can be seen in a patient's antecedent life events. If little has changed in the man's life and adequate erections are rarely in evidence, the presence of organic impotence may be suspected. If, however, much has changed in the man's life before the onset of the erectile problem and there are no adequate erections for months at a time, the clinician should not rule out psychogenic impotence.

Youth and young adulthood make the diagnosis of psychogenic impotence easy. Between 35 and 55, the diagnosis is not usually difficult to perceive, even though the man's life is complex and his sexual physiology may have become less insistent. Beginning in the middle to late 50s, however, misdiagnoses are common because the normal, weakened sexual physiology is confused with organic impotence. Some of those who are misadiagnosed have mixed impotence, in which the psychological contribution is the significant and treatable factor. Others, however, have pure psychogenic impotence in the face of a normal (but slower and less intense) physiological expression.

The effects of age on potency and the ease of diagnosis underscore the difference between what is practical in busy clinical settings and the actual pathogenesis of any form of erectile function. The schema of four generic types of impotence—organic, psychogenic, mixed, and idiopathic—is useful, but not entirely accurate. Psychogenic factors are always subtly involved in erectile dysfunction. This may explain why the presence of the same organic factor (to the same extent) ends the sexual life of some men and only modifies that of others.

Busy clinicians often oversimplify the issue of causality by declaring impotence to be *either* organic *or* psychogenic. The need to keep medical reports from being too complicated helps to perpetuate this overly simple notion. To be most accurate, clinicians should be able to specify all the organic and psychogenic contributants to any older man's erectile problem.

BEYOND IMPOTENCE: FREUD ON MALE SEXUALITY

A mental health professional who sees patients in psychotherapy has many opportunities to consider patterns of male and female sexuality. Psychogenic impotence is just one of many problems that affect men. As such, it is always embedded in the larger psychological contexts of male sexuality, female sexuality, and the way in which society construes relationships. Freud was concerned about the developmental processes that shaped men's lives and the resulting patterns of their sexuality. Three of his observations follow.

Degradation Enhances Potency

Freud (1912/1957) pointed out that the potency of many men is enhanced by their perception of their sexual partners as not being their equals. When a woman is perceived as being in a lower social class, less intelligent, of lesser status or power, or otherwise degraded, this perception enhances a man's ability to abandon himself to sensuality and maximizes his potency. This pattern is privately noticed by many men during their development. A clinician does not have to be in practice very long before running into a man who loses his potency shortly after becoming engaged or married. This situation, in which the partner is perceived as "too good" to have sex with, is sometimes referred to as the "madonna–whore" complex. Typically, the man presents with impotence but actually has a more dramatic motivation to avoid all sexual contact with his beloved partner; this is currently diagnosed in DSM-III-R as "inhibited sexual desire."

Maturity Requires Uniting Affection and Excitement

Freud (1905/1953) conceived of the Oedipal phase as the time of a boy's life when he is able to have deep affection for, and physical excitement over, his mother. His growing awareness that this ideal situation is untenable because of his powerful father leads to the splitting apart of the affection and sexual excitement. The affection stays with his mother, while his sexual excitement is displaced outside the family. Much of adolescent sexual experimentation involves attempts to bring the two currents together in one person. Sexual maturity is attained when this was accomplished. "Sowing of wild oats" is an exploration of sex without affection, or sex with the deception of affection; this phase continues until the person can "get it all together" (i.e., in Freud's terms, unite the two currents of his libido as they once existed during his Oedipal phase). Clinicians encounter many men

symptom resolution. When treatment has not been efficient and effective, the patient or couple need the therapist's sustaining optimism even more. This time, however, it must be tempered with the understanding of the nature of the psychological obstacles. It is one matter to grasp the nature of a man's intraspychic problem; it is entirely another matter to work it through. Therapists often lose hope faster than patients when they merge these two concepts. Discouraged patients often respond with hope when a therapist summarizes the forces that have converged to produce the problem.

Sometimes, a man's potency does not improve in therapy or with his current partner. The therapist does not know how to catalyze the symptom's resolution. From the beginning of therapy, the clinician should be aware that psychogenic impotence is not one disorder with a uniform pathogenesis. Statements about prognosis should be couched in terms reflecting awareness that the cause of the problem, rather than the diagnosis per se, will influence the outcome. Some degree of therapeutic optimism is usually in order at all stages of the relationship.

Sensate Focus Exercises

The essence of the sensate focus technique is the prohibition of intercourse. The man can then relax and concentrate on sensation because his mind can be free of images of failure. Sensate focus instructions are a powerful tool for the elimination of performance anxiety. They can be simply given as a suggestion to make love for several weeks without intercourse, as the 18th-century physician John Hunter (1788) suggested, or they can be more elaborately structured, in the way made famous by Masters and Johnson (1970). Masters and Johnson reported taking each couple through stages of physical intimacy that always included body touching: no access to breasts and genitals; breast stimulation; genital stimulation; quiet containment of penis in vagina; intercourse.

There are several problems with these exercises. Inexperienced therapists tend to think that these exercises *are* the treatment. Experienced therapists sometimes forget that their dutiful patients are still following the last set of instructions. Patients can be demoralized if they fail to get consistent erections during their "homework assignments."

Therapist's Knowledge

The therapist needs to know that even though the patient has psychogenic impotence, his problem can also be conceptualized as an unrecognized motive to avoid intercourse. The therapist must be able to use the concepts of sexual drive, motivation, and wish, and to understand that they blend together in various combinations to produce sexual desire.

Erectile dysfunction brings the patient for help. However, other sexual dysfunctions, such as limited motivation to make love, premature ejaculation, or retarded ejaculation, may have been present or may appear during the recovery process. The therapist need not entirely reconceptualize the problem; these difficulties are usually produced by the same psychodynamic forces that have generated the erectile dysfunction.

Although sensate focus techniques are a useful tool, the therapist needs to know that their power lies in the judgment about when to use them and skill in handling the resistances to them. Whether treatment is conducted with the man alone or with the couple, its success depends upon the clinician's fundamental therapeutic skills and his or her comfort and willingness to discuss sexual matters openly and factually. Many people who seek help for psychogenic impotence have been in psychotherapy for the problem with therapists who are generally competent but lack the comfort to deal with sexual matters directly.

Men with this problem often want its cause to be organic and treatable with a pill. Therefore, therapists need to know about penile anatomy, physiology, pharmacology, and the organic conditions that produce impotence, as well as the medical and surgical treatments that are available to patients regardless of their diagnoses. Often a man has to be reassured several times during therapy that his problem is psychogenic.

Ten Powerful Ideas

Therapy is a process that occurs between the therapist and the patient, as well as within the mind of the patient. What the therapist says, how it is said, what it means to the patient, and how it affects his psychic life are all related but distinct phenomena. The mechanisms of therapeutic success are never quite understood; the therapist is never certain what is heard and when, if ever, it will have an impact upon the patient. I have found, however, that a few ideas have been helpful to numerous men with this problem:

1. The penis is attached to the heart.
2. Trying to be a rooster in a hen house, eh?
3. In some Polynesian languages, there is no word for impotence. When a man cannot get an erection, he concludes that he must not have felt like it after all.
4. I think your penis knows something that you don't know.
5. This limp penis of yours if your friend; let's try to find out how it is protecting you.

6. More than 200 years ago, the medical recommendation to cure impotence was to go home and have six "amatory experiences" without coital connection. Although the language has changed a bit in two centuries, the idea of making love for a while without attempting intercourse has not. I'd like you to try this time-honored tradition.

7. The penis is the organ of attachment.

8. Almost everyone finds that making love for the first time with a partner is like a two-horse race: Fear runs against Excitement.

9. I know you want to get better yesterday, but I worry when a man is too quickly cured. I'd much rather help you stay potent than help you to have intercourse a few times.

10. I think you will eventually be fine!

Results

The most important skeptics about the value of psychotherapy for this problem are those who work with these patients and their partners. They recognize that psychogenic impotence is not one problem. They have had numerous experiences of watching potency return, disappear, and return. They have had couples drop out of therapy. They have occasionally recognized that they have made mistakes in diagnostic assessments. These therapists have seen divorces among those who were temporarily better and those who did not improve. Recently, they have begun to suggest using a vacuum pump or injections in occasional cases of persistent performance anxiety (Turner & Althof, in press). They have seen some couples return to lovemaking with therapy, but not to secure potency or to potency with ejaculation. And they have seen complete successes that have lasted at least as long as the final follow-up visit.

Such experienced but skeptical therapists have a difficult time translating the diversity of clinical problems into the narrow parameters of results: "unchanged," "improved," or "excellent." However, such studies show other skeptics that talking with people in psychotherapy has value.

Clinical experiences have led to a few generalizations about success rates that ring true. Secondary psychogenic impotence is generally much easier to help than primary psychogenic impotence. Recent-onset impotence is easier to help than chronic impotence. When impotence is related to interpersonal problems, men who have been faithful are easier to help than those who have been unfaithful. A partner's unreceptivity is a poor prognostic indicator, particularly when it is reflected in her refusal to participate in the evaluation. Men who do not recognize their feelings or continue talking about their lives only with great unease often drop out of therapy prematurely.

Masters and Johnson (1970) reported that about two-thirds of men were helped with the innovative treatment format they used in the 1960s. When I studied the results of my treatment style with 16 couples in the 1970s (Levine & Agle, 1978), only one man remained securely potent without temporary relapse during the ensuing year—even though the majority of men were "improved." The understanding of psychogenic impotence has evolved considerably during the last several years. Today, I am more interested in questions such as "What is the natural duration of widowers' or divorced men's impotence?" and "What impact does therapy have on the time course?" I am less interested in such questions as "How effective is one brand of psychotherapy or another for psychogenic impotence?", because it now seems clear to me that mental health professionals of various ideological preferences have success with some cases of psychogenic impotence. I suspect that the pathogenesis of the man's impotence is more important than the language the therapist uses to conceptualize the problem and its management.

PSYCHOGENIC IMPOTENCE: A SUMMARY

The Deeper Dilemma

To the patient, psychogenic impotence means that he cannot have intercourse. To the professional, however, it usually means that it is not safe for this man to emotionally attach himself to another person through this means. The symptom is his mind's way of resolving a hidden drama. Since potency is vital to the man's experience of himself as competently masculine, the presence of the symptom assaults his innermost conscious system of self-esteem. It reverberates to his gender identity. Its pathogenesis probably always involves emotional resonance among contributions from each of the three spheres of causality. Although performance anxiety and the assault on gender identity are the most obvious consequences that maintain the symptom, issues specific to the man are typically involved in the origin of the problem.

Frequency of Incomplete Resolution

Therapists often prefer to work with recently impotent men who can be quickly helped, but these are not the most common types of cases encountered. In many more chronic cases of secondary psychogenic impotence, the patients do not attain fast or complete symptomatic relief. This experience has led to the impression that impotence can be a very difficult symptom to resolve completely and lastingly. It is likely that many men never entirely get over their psychogenic impotence; that is, the previous resolution of their drama is permanent. A therapist always has to be concerned whether a treatment plan gives the patient enough opportunity to understand and resolve the problem. Many factors, such as a patient's fear of talking, poor insurance coverage, a therapist's inability to conceptualize the cause, or a spouse's lack of cooperation, can interfere with resolution. Even when conditions are ideal, the results may not be attained efficiently.

CASE EXAMPLE: TED

The following case of secondary psychogenic impotence illustrates contributions from each of the three spheres of causality. It briefly describes the therapeutic process and the time and focus required to give this very able man an opportunity to understand, feel, and deal with the interplay among the emotional forces stimulated by the precipitating life events, his childhood experiences, and his characteristic manner of dealing with any affects that threatened his rationality.

Ted became impotent when he became a cuckold. He was 50, robustly healthy, rich, handsome, athletic, a successful chief executive officer, kind, intelligent, generous, a good father, a devout Christian—a star at almost everything he had ever attempted. He and his wife were building their dream home. During his preoccupation with a business crisis and the back-to-back deaths of his father and uncle, she and the architect of the house began an affair. Brief marital therapy ensued; she was unwilling to give up the relationship, and within several months this ended Ted's willingness to stay married. He sought psychotherapy first to help his wife come to her senses, then to process his devastation, and soon to deal with his many children. Therapy was helpful; eventually he became engaged to another woman, and discovered that in the 3 years since his last intercourse, he had become impotent. He could not work out the problem with his own psychotherapist or in brief conjoint therapy with another one during the first 2 years of the second marriage. His only erections were transient, were less than rigid, and occurred in the morning once every several months.

At our 2-hour psychiatric evaluation, I told him that it seemed that he, an angerless man, worshipped at the altar of reason, and that his penis knew something about his feelings that he did not. After three emotionally powerful psychotherapy sessions—during which he elaborated upon his struggle to be fair with the divorce settlement (so as not to limit his children's opportunities further), his father's infidelity when he was 12, the extreme goodness of fit with his new wife, and his extended family's dependence upon him—he reported the presence of good, though transient, erections with his wife. I encouraged him to compose a "letter" to his ex-wife to express what he thought about her behavior, and to do it in a style that reflected his earthy humanity rather than his cultured, analytic rationality. One paragraph from his eight pages of compelling prose follows:

> I despise you for desecrating me as a person and everything I worked for and stood for all of my life. In the vernacular, you are a BITCH, a JERK, an ASSHOLE. My vocabulary of profane and vulgar descriptors is somewhat limited, so let's just leave it that you are a TURKEY TURD! But don't be so naive as to believe that my anger goes only as deep as a few expletives. No, my rage goes to the depths of my intellect and to the heights of my emotion. You are too shallow to comprehend the full extent of the fury your cruelty has ignited, but some day you will come to understand your own petty insignificance when you see yourself as a groveling turkey turd looking up at soaring eagles gliding in noble and loving skies of peace and joy.

After several weeks of better intercourse and occasional failures, his erectile capacity disappeared. I suggested that his anger at his first wife continued to be a part of the problem. He replied, "I understand, but I don't feel it!" Months later, while Ted was plowing snow, his jeep landed in a ditch and he responded with uncharacteristic rage. "Where did it come from?" he wondered. Later in the session, he spoke of his frustration about his new wife's refusal to stick to the budget they had agreed upon. He was devoted to building up his estate for her, while she preferred to live to the hilt now. This focus did not help his erections, which were occasionally present. Secure potency followed 3 months later, after we had discussed his morality, his father's "ladies' man" behavior, and his adolescent determination to disgrace his father by being the finest human being possible.

Although Ted's performance anxiety was strong, his gender identity was relatively intact because the rest of his life was so successful. The precipitant, his first wife's infidelity, not only created an array of feelings that he suppressed; it stirred up his feelings about his inept, morally reprehensible father. Ted's ability to think his way through life contributed to the mystery of his impotence. The ability of the therapy to have him feel the impact of his being a cuckold, a divorced father, an irritated new husband, and an enraged, morally superior son enabled his potency to return.

This formulation, based on 15 hours of therapy (sometimes spaced 3 weeks apart), is not necessarily complete or correct. I expect that some experienced therapists would phrase Ted's psychodynamics differently. It is possible that the key elements that maintained the problem were never identified. The problem with psychological pathogenesis is that one is never certain one has the full story.

CONCLUSION

This chapter has provided one clinician's views on a common male sexual dysfunction. It has posited a skeletal model for understanding the pathogenesis of secondary and primary impotence. Since every patient's life is unique in numerous ways, it is up to the clinician to put the "flesh" on the model in a manner that provides the patient with dignity, understanding, and feeling. Understanding the deeper meanings of psychogenic impotence gives the patient an opportunity to find a less burdensome manner of expressing his private feelings about himself and his dilemmas. Such an approach provides clinicians with the opportunity to help some men to secure potency, to help others to psychological improvements short of lasting potency, and to help themselves to continuing fascination about the mental processes of still others.

REFERENCES

Freud, S. (1953). Three essays on the theory of sexuality. In J. Strachey (Ed. and Trans.), *The standard edition of the complete psychological works of Sigmund Freud* (Vol. 7, pp. 135–243). London: Hogarth Press. (Original work published 1905)

Freud, S. (1957). On the universal tendency to debasement in the sphere of love (Contributions to the psychology of love II). In J. Strachey (Ed. and Trans.), *The standard edition of the complete psychological works of Sigmund Freud* (Vol. 11, pp. 179–190). London: Hogarth Press. (Original work published 1912)

Hunter, J. (1788). *Treatise on venereal disease.* London: Nicol & Johnson.

Levine, S. B. (1987). More on the nature of sexual desire. *Journal of Sex and Marital Therapy, 13*(1), 35–44.

Levine, S. B. (1989). *Sex is not simple.* Columbus, OH: Psychology Publishing.

Levine, S. B., & Agle, D. P. (1978). Effectiveness of therapy for chronic secondary psychogenic impotence. *Journal of Sex and Marital Therapy, 4,* 235–258.

Levine, S. B., Risen, C. B., & Althof, S. E. (1990). The diagnosis and nature of paraphilia. *Journal of Sex and Marital Therapy, 16*(2), 89–102.

Masters, W., & Johnson, V. (1966). *Human sexual response.* Boston: Little, Brown.

Masters, W., & Johnson, V. (1970). *Human sexual inadequacy.* Boston: Little, Brown.

Schiavi, R. C., Schreiner-Engel, P., Mandeli, J., Schanzer, H., & Cohen, E. (1990). Healthy aging and male sexual function. *American Journal of Psychiatry, 147*(6), 766–771.

Turner, L. A., & Althof, S. E. (in press). A 12-month comparison of the effectiveness of two treatments for erectile dysfunction: Self-injection versus external vacuum devices. *Urology.*

9

Couples Therapy for Erectile Disorders: Observations, Obstacles, and Outcomes

Sandra R. Leiblum and Raymond C. Rosen

> A basic premise of the therapeutic approach . . . is the concept that there is no such thing as an uninvolved partner in any marriage in which there is some form of sexual inadequacy.
> —Masters and Johnson (1970, p. 2)

While most of the chapters in this book explore the medical, hormonal, and physical factors involved in erectile difficulties, this chapter highlights the critical importance of relationship issues. It was Masters and Johnson who emphasized the fact that there is rarely an uninvolved partner in a situation where erectile failure occurs. Yet the recent tendency among the medical community is to minimize or ignore the dyadic nature of these problems. Nevertheless, couples issues are clearly pivotal in the genesis and maintenance of erectile problems. Power struggles, betrayal of trust, waning sexual chemistry, role conflicts, and other couples issues are often implicated. It is our experience that firmer erections are rarely, if ever, the solution to a deteriorating relationship and usually the presence of erectile problems signals the fact that something is awry within the couple.

In this chapter, we suggest that four domains are particularly important to explore when treating erectile complaints, namely, status and dominance issues, struggles with intimacy and trust, feelings of waning sexual chemistry and desire, and sexual script incompatibilities. Although problems within these domains are not unique to the development of erectile failure, one or several of them are usually implicated. For example, clinicians often observe that erectile problems are an effective distance regulator in a relationship. Failure to achieve or keep an erection can maintain a tolerable level of closeness in a relationship where one or both partners would be overwhelmed by greater intimacy. Similarly, where there are

unwelcome shifts in the power balance between partners, a not uncommon conse-
quence is difficulty with sexual performance, or even a loss of sexual desire.

Assessing the sexual script is important whenever sexual dissatisfaction exists,
but it can be particularly helpful when dealing with couples with erectile difficulties.
Often the sexual script becomes attenuated or rigidified in these cases as both
partners focus on the presence and strength of the male's erection rather than on
the sensuality of their sexual interaction. Talking about and modifying the sexual
script usually can help rekindle intimacy even if it does not directly alter erectile
response.

Finally, we address the perplexing question of when and if marital therapy
should supersede sexual therapy. Such considerations as commitment to the rela-
tionship, degree of marital conflict, existence of extramarital affairs and other
secrets, and the presence of concurrent medical or psychiatric illness are relevant
issues when making the decision to begin either sexual or marital therapy.

Sandra R. Leiblum, Ph.D., is Professor of Clinical Psychiatry and Co-Director
of the Sexual Counseling Service at Robert Wood Johnson Medical School. She is
widely known for research and writing in the field of sexuality and is coeditor of
Principles and Practice of Sex Therapy *(1980, with L. Pervin),* Sexual Desire
Disorders *(1988, with R. C. Rosen), and* Principles and Practice of Sex Therapy
(2nd edition): Update for the 1990s *(1989, with R. C. Rosen).*

Raymond C. Rosen, Ph.D., is Professor of Psychiatry and Medicine and Co-
Director of the Sexual Counseling Service at Robert Wood Johnson Medical School.
He has written extensively on human sexuality and sex therapy and is coauthor of
Patterns of Sexual Arousal: Psychophysiological Processes and Clinical Appli-
cations *(1988, with J. G. Beck) and coeditor of* Sexual Desire Disorders *(1988,*
with S. R. Leiblum) and Principles and Practice of Sex Therapy (2nd edition):
Update for the 1990s *(1989, with S. R. Leiblum). He is the Past President of the*
International Academy of Sex Research.

The role of relationship issues in the evaluation and treatment of erectile
failure cannot be overstated. Couples issues are clearly pivotal in the genesis
of many sexual difficulties, as power struggles, betrayal of trust, waning sexual
chemistry, role conflicts, and a wide spectrum of related problems often
contribute to the development or maintenance of sexual disorders. Similarly,
couple distress is among the most frequent sequelae of sexual dysfunction,
because the strain of coping with sexual incompatibility often leads to a
breakdown of trust and intimacy in the relationship, and may motivate one
partner or the other to seek sexual gratification outside of the relationship.
Sexual difficulties remain a leading cause of separation and divorce, even in
our "postmodern" sexual era of the 1990s. In fact, couple dynamics are

perhaps the single most important determinant of therapy prognosis. In our experience, couples with strong, committed, and supportive relationships typically develop effective coping strategies in the face of even the most severe sexual dysfunctions. By contrast, uncommitted couples with major relationship conflicts seem to derive little or no benefit, even from the most advanced medical, surgical, or psychological interventions. It is a basic truism of sex therapy that firmer erections are rarely, if ever, the sole solution to a deteriorating relationship.

Despite the obvious importance of these factors, couples issues have been surprisingly underemphasized in much of the contemporary literature on erectile failure (e.g., Segraves & Schoenberg, 1988; Montague, 1988; Tanagho, Lue, & McClure, 1988). Several reasons might account for this omission. First, major innovations in the medical and surgical approaches to erectile failure in the past decade (see Chapters 10 and 11, this volume) have clearly directed attention away from both intrapsychic and interpersonal determinants. Unfortunately, organic and psychogenic factors are all too often perceived as mutually exclusive foci of therapeutic intervention. It has been our experience, however, that even in the most obvious cases of organic erectile failure, relationship issues must be addressed.

Second, there is an unfortunate lack of consensus in the field regarding the choice of theoretical models or intervention strategies for dealing with couples conflicts, and this lack of consensus has undermined more widespread acceptance of these approaches. Thus, some sex therapists have formulated couples issues from a psychodynamic perspective (e.g., Kaplan, 1974; Scharff, 1988; Levine, 1988); others have preferred a cognitive–behavioral perspective (e.g., LoPiccolo & Friedman, 1988; McCarthy, 1989); and still others have argued for a family systems approach (Verhulst & Heiman, 1979; Hof, 1987). This lack of agreement concerning both the theory and practice of couples therapy has impeded efforts to develop more standardized approaches for dealing with couples issues in erectile dysfunction. Finally, male patients seeking help for erectile failure typically minimize or deny the role of relationship issues as a cause of their sexual difficulty. It appears more comfortable for a man to attribute erectile problems to a medical or stress-related condition than to a basic failure in the marital relationship. Many therapists unwittingly "buy into" this attributional framework, thereby neglecting to address critical relationship issues.

After briefly reviewing the origins of couples therapy approaches in contemporary sex therapy, the present chapter examines in depth the role of relationship factors in the development and maintenance of erectile failure. In addition to presenting concepts and interventions from several theoretical perspectives, our goal is to highlight specific clinical issues and dilemmas that confront the practicing clinician. Several case studies are presented to illustrate these issues. In general, it is our firm belief that adequate and comprehensive treatment of erectile failure *demands* a close attention to the role of couples dynamics throughout.

SYSTEMS APPROACHES TO ERECTILE FAILURE

In the past, many so-called experts attributed the causes of erectile failure to excessive masturbation (e.g., Ryan, 1835; Bloch, 1908), neural degeneration (Krafft-Ebing, 1893), constitutional factors (Gross, 1887; Allen, 1949), or castration anxiety (Freud, 1910/1957; Ferenczi, 1913). It remained for Masters and Johnson (1970) to place couples issues squarely in the forefront of our current understanding of erectile failure. From the beginning of *Human Sexual Inadequacy*, couples dynamics are emphasized. In addition to the importance of relationship factors in the development of erectile failure, the response of the partner is seen as crucial in determining treatment outcome. In particular, Masters and Johnson observe that wives of men with erectile failure are severely affected by the "crippling tensions in the marital relationship" that inevitably accompany the onset of the problem:

> Her constant concern is that when her husband is given adequate opportunity for sexual expression, he will be unable to achieve and/or maintain an erection. She has grave fears for his ability to perform. . . . Additionally, wives of impotent men are terrified that something they do will create anxiety [in], or embarrass, or anger their husbands. (1970, p. 12)

From their observations of the importance of couples dynamics, Masters and Johnson formulated their well-known "conjoint therapy" approach, in which a dual-sex therapy team is assigned to work with every couple, regardless of the nature of the presenting problem. In dealing with cases of erectile failure, Masters and Johnson encouraged the female clinician in the conjoint therapy team to align herself with the wife in an empathic and reassuring manner. Once the wife is reassured that she has the full understanding and support of the female therapist, according to Masters and Johnson, the path is generally cleared for effective sex therapy to begin. Additional couples interventions introduced by Masters and Johnson include the well-known "sensate focus" exercises, with the emphasis on nondemanding, sensual interaction between the partners, and the use of "guided" stimulation techniques, in which partners are instructed to communicate sexual needs and desires through verbal and nonverbal means.

Building upon the basic Masters and Johnson framework, Kaplan (1974) has offered a more in-depth account of couples issues, or "dyadic causes" for sexual dysfunction. Several key areas of dyadic conflict are identified, such as lack of trust, power struggles, partner rejection, contractual disappointments, and sexual sabotage. In each of these areas, conflicts are seen primarily as transferential extensions of unresolved familial issues:

> Much of the anger and fear of loss characterizing marital relationships is not so much the product of "here and now" reality, but rather stems from recreating old family relationships. . . . Parental transferences towards the spouse result in abandonment fears and excessive dependencies and demands. (1974, p. 158)

Transferential issues such as these are typically outside of the conscious awareness of the individual, and will need to be addressed in couples or individual therapy. Psychodynamic therapy, transactional analysis, or conjoint marital therapy approaches are all recommended by Kaplan for this purpose.

Can couples issues be ignored or "bypassed" in treating some cases of sexual dysfunction? In contrast to the position taken by Masters and Johnson that couples conflicts must be addressed in *all* cases, Kaplan considers a number of situations in which couples conflicts can be bypassed, and therapy can be focused directly on the sexual dysfunction: "Often it is possible to 'bypass' marital problems. Nodal points of trouble are identified and the couple is charged with the responsibility of 'keeping them out of the bedroom' prior to final resolution" (p. 168). Specific instructions are given to couples, such as these: "You can have your choice—fight or make love tonight. But don't try to do both. It probably won't work." On the other hand, Kaplan also recognizes that such "bypassing" strategies are doomed to failure in certain instances, where underlying couples conflicts are so severe that no movement on the sexual problem is possible. Unfortunately, she fails to provide more specific guidelines for determining when "bypassing" strategies can be employed.

Another of Kaplan's key contributions is the observation that not all couples issues are necessarily resolvable. In particular, she notes that lack of attraction can be an insurmountable problem in some couples, as can deeply ingrained patterns of hostility:

> Many persons seem to feel that they should be able to function sexually with anyone or under any circumstances. . . . [However,] couples who are clearly physically or mentally incompatible or are frankly hostile to each other are not good candidates for sexual therapy. One simply cannot create a functional sexual system under such circumstances. (pp. 156–157)

Lack of sexual attraction is indeed a critical factor in many cases, and we return to this important issue in a later section.

Several authors have incorporated a systems–interactional perspective in dealing with couples issues in sex therapy. For example, Verhulst and Heiman (1979) have presented a systemic model of sexual dysfunction, based upon concepts from social ethology and general systems theory (Riggs, 1978; von Bertalanffy, 1968). According to Verhulst and Heiman, four specific categories of dyadic interaction need to be evaluated in each case of sexual dysfunction:

1. *Territorial interactions* refer to rights of ownership or access to each other's body or body space. In a typical sexual interaction, each partner is expected to grant access or control of his or her body to the other, which may be associated with a variety of emotional reactions. For example, "giving one's body out of a sense of duty, fear, guilt or the grim determination of martyrdom is not giving from a sense of ownership and is likely to lead to resentment" (Verhulst & Heiman, 1979, p. 26).

2. *Ranking-order interactions* are interactions centered around the establishment of status and control in the relationship. Verhulst and Heiman note that difficulties in this area are frequently manifested as power struggles in the relationship, because "the issue in ranking order interactions is the control over the relationship and over the communication itself" (1979, p. 26). Thus, men with erectile failure frequently complain that their partners are critical or domineering, or that they feel undermined in key areas in the relationship (e.g., child rearing, household finances, or choice of social and recreational activities). Feelings of inferiority or submissiveness may also be experienced in the sexual situation itself. Ranking-order interactions are not always overtly addressed, but are present to varying degrees in most cases of sexual dysfunction.

3. *Attachment interactions* center around the affiliative bonds between the partners. Included in this category are interactions dealing with love, commitment, and intimacy in the relationship. Attachment or intimacy may be lacking in either the sexual or nonsexual aspects of the relationship for a variety of reasons (e.g., distrust, jealousy, anger), and can seriously impair the quality of the sexual interaction. Lack of commitment in the relationship is another issue frequently associated with erectile failure in men.

4. *Exploratory and sensual interactions* are those patterns in the relationship "having to do with sensate experiences and with the teaching and guiding of the partner" (1979, p. 24). Because of difficulties in communication or touch aversion, partners may be severely restricted in their ability to give and receive sensual pleasure to each other. Noting that this presents a major obstacle to effective sexual stimulation, Verhulst and Heiman recommend techniques such as sensate focus for building and strengthening a couple's repertoire of exploratory sensual interactions.

According to other systems theorists (e.g., Fish, Fish, & Sprenkle, 1984), a sexual dysfunction such as erectile failure can serve a positive function as a "distance regulator" in a relationship. Drawing upon the family therapy concepts of Bowen (1978), these authors observe:

> All couples find ways to create intimacy and distance in their relationships that is syntonic with their joint level of emotional maturity. If the couple is fearful that too much intimacy will produce fusion and lack of differentiation as individuals, one or both partners will need to create distance. (Fish et al., 1984, p. 5)

In such cases, the sexual dysfunction provides a rationale for the couple's lack of sexual or emotional intimacy, and may even be used as a justification for terminating the relationship. In a similar vein, other authors have emphasized the potential secondary benefits of erectile failure in protecting the female partner from her own difficulties with sexual intimacy. Althof (1989), for example, has discussed the concept of a "sexual equilibrium," which functions to maintain critical levels of distance or intimacy in the relationship:

> The power of the sexual equilibrium surprises many therapists. Often couples seem to take one step back for each step forward. For example, as a man begins to get firmer erections, his partner suddenly loses her sexual desire. This trading of symptoms between partners occurs with such frequency that we refer to it as the "hot potato syndrome." (Althof, 1979, p. 254)

The notion of a "sexual equilibrium," or the interaction between sexual dysfunction in one partner and feelings of ambivalence or sexual anxiety in the other, is a critical aspect of the couples approach to erectile failure. Whereas medical and physiological treatment approaches to erectile failure frequently neglect such reactions in the partner, couples therapists attend closely to partner responses, both during initial evaluation and throughout the course of subsequent therapy. In fact, the focus of therapy must be shifted at times to dealing directly with the negative reactions (e.g., inhibited desire) of the partner. This issue is explored more fully by LoPiccolo (Chapter 7) and Levine (Chapter 8) in the present volume.

Case Vignette

Alex B. was a 62-year-old accountant, remarried for the past 7 years to a wife 17 years his junior. Prior to getting married, the couple's sexual life was limited by Alex's protracted divorce settlement. Although they enjoyed a brief period of sexual contentment after marriage, Alex soon began to experience erectile difficulties of increasing frequency and severity. He responded with embarrassment and avoidance, leading to increasing anger and resentment on the part of his wife, Sharon. "If not for his problem, we would be having sex every chance we could," she complained bitterly during the first evaluation session. Several months later Alex was instructed in the use of a vacuum pump device, and reported his complete readiness to resume sexual intercourse. Sharon responded with uncharacteristic hesitancy and reluctance, leading to several individual sessions to explore her growing anxieties about resuming sexual intercourse at this time. During these sessions it emerged that Sharon had begun to develop feelings of sexual attraction to a coworker, and was seriously reconsidering her commitment to the marriage.

Many couples are lacking in basic communication and conflict resolution skills, and this also can contribute in various ways to the development and maintenance of sexual dysfunction. This point was first emphasized by Masters and Johnson (1970), who noted: "Usually the failure of communication in the bedroom extends rapidly to every other phase of the marriage. When there is no security or mutual representation in sexual exchange, there rarely is freedom of other forms of marital communication" (1970, p. 15). Among the various approaches to building communication skills, Masters and Johnson particularly emphasized the use of modeling techniques by the cotherapy team. The goal is for therapy to serve as a "catalyst" to more effective communication between the couple, which in turn facilitates direct treatment of the sexual dysfunction.

Kaplan (1974) views communication difficulties as either superficial in nature, or more deeply rooted in underlying couples dynamics. In either event, the therapist needs to work directly with the couple to help establish a direct and empathic style of communication:

> Sometimes it is possible to accomplish this by simple methods, confronting the spouses with their inadequate communications and by setting an example of openness and lack of defensiveness about sexual matters. . . . At times, however, more basic dyadic problems must be dealt with before open trusting communications can be established. (p. 167)

In the latter case, Kaplan recommends analytic or transactional therapy for resolving the underlying "dyadic conflict" before communication problems or sexual dysfunctions are addressed directly.

Conflict management skills are often lacking in sexually dysfunctional couples, and specific interventions may be required. Communication deficits set the stage for a "snowballing" effect: Conflicts in one area of the relationship, such as control of family finances, may escalate into major power struggles in which sexual approach or initiation becomes impossible. As noted by Hof (1987), "Without the ability to manage conflict effectively, angry and resentful feelings have a way of remaining unresolved and ever-present, serving as an effective means for undermining sex therapy" (p. 14). Hof recommends the incorporation of problem-solving techniques such as emotional awareness exercises, empathy training, and behavioral contracting for resolving couple conflicts.

Finally, the potential effect of extended-family or multigenerational influences on sexual dysfunction have been described by Regas and Sprenkle (1984), Berman and Hof (1987), and others. Family messages and values regarding sexuality, the presence of sexual "secrets" in the family, expectations regarding masculinity and femininity, and the potential occurrence of incest or other forms of sexual abuse have all been emphasized. In order to assess the possible role of family-of-origin factors in determining sexual dysfunction, Hof and Berman (1986) have recommended the use of a "sexual genogram." This can be briefly defined as a diagrammatic representation of the family tree of each member of the couple, in which sexual relationships, tensions, or issues are especially highlighted. According to this approach, couples are encouraged to make a "family journey" and to carefully reassess their relationships with all relevant family members, prior to addressing the sexual complaint directly. Although such family-of-origin interventions may not be indicated in *all* cases of erectile failure, there are some instances in which little therapeutic progress can be made until such issues are addressed.

Case Vignette

Roberto B., a 60-year-old lawyer of Puerto Rican descent, contacted the Sexual Counseling Service after several years of unsuccessful psychoanalytic therapy for his erectile difficulties. He complained of inability to achieve or sustain erections with his second wife since their marriage 6 years earlier. Although sex had been lusty and problem-free during their courtship, the couple had begun to experience sexual difficulties soon after marriage. At about the same time, Roberto developed symptoms of severe prostatitis, which necessitated two separate surgical interventions. Following each operation, he experienced intermittent episodes of bleeding during urination, which frightened and distressed him. Although fully recovered from surgery, he continued to feel hesitant about resuming sexual activity, and noted that ejaculation was accomplished with difficulty because of his tendency to "hold back."

A sexual genogram was taken during the initial evaluation, which revealed a major concern about privacy during his childhood and adolescence. Roberto had been raised in a small, two-family house with his parents, his mother's sister, and two brothers. In fact, his sleeping alcove was between that of his parents and his aunt, so that he regularly overheard the bedroom activities of both. His father, whom he admired as a successful enterpreneur and "ladies' man," frequently boasted of his sexual exploits with other women. Roberto was well aware that his father enjoyed sex with a mistress throughout most of his marriage, whereas his mother was a devout Catholic and a sexually puritanical woman. Her younger sister, who lived with them, was quite different from his mother. She was described as sexually liberated and uninhibited—a woman who loved to laugh, flirt, and play.

In talking about his earliest childhood memories, Roberto recalled his father's ongoing bouts of prostatitis and concomitant complaints about urination. He remembered his father occasionally passing blood during urination, which he witnessed at times, since his father kept a bucket for this purpose in his bedroom. Roberto recalled feeling sexually conflicted and uncomfortable during most of his adolescence. He was sexually stimulated by thoughts and fantasies of his aunt and her various boyfriends, as well as his father's extramarital exploits. At the same time, he felt sympathetic and loyal to his mother, who was always affectionate and loving toward him and kept the household running.

During his first marriage, Roberto had remained sexually faithful to his wife, despite her lack of warmth and sexual receptivity, until after his children were grown and had left the house. At this point, he had begun a series of extramarital affairs, including sexual liaisons with several women at a time, much like his father. Several months following his divorce, however, he became involved with the woman who was to become his second wife. She was married at the time, but agreed to a weekly sexual rendezvous. With her, Roberto enjoyed intense sexual and emotional gratification. However, after she decided to leave her husband and children to be with him permanently, Roberto began to experience episodes of erectile failure.

The couple's sexual difficulties rapidly escalated following their marriage, and the development soon thereafter of Roberto's prostate symptoms (at about the same age at which his father's prostatitis emerged). His emotional reaction to erectile failure was profound, although his wife continually reassured him of her sexual satisfaction in the marriage. She was orgasmic with oral sex and manual stimulation, and considered him an attentive and caring lover. Nevertheless, Roberto felt inadequate and depressed, and was not reassured by her protestations of love and support.

During the course of therapy, it became clear that Roberto's response to his intermittent erectile difficulties was determined in large part by his belief that sexual competence implied performing like his father (i.e., being sexually active and interested under any and all circumstances). At the same time, he felt conflicted by the two very different models of female sexuality he had been exposed to—his sexually permissive and uninhibited aunt, and his puritannical, straight-laced mother. It was difficult for Roberto to feel sexual abandonment with his former lover, although their sexual relationship had been trouble-free prior to marriage. Finally, the coincidence of his developing severe prostatitis at the same time in life as his father, and the implications of this condition for his concerns about aging and loss of masculinity, became key issues for exploration in individual therapy.

CORE ISSUES IN COUPLES THERAPY

In our therapy program for couples with erectile difficulties, we have observed four major facets of a couple's relationship that are typically implicated in the development or maintenance of erectile failure. Any of these four areas may be involved in a given case, regardless of the presence of other psychogenic or organic factors. Furthermore, couples therapy focuses on these areas in conjunction with more direct medical, surgical, or sex therapy approaches for control of erection. The specific topics to be addressed are (1) status and dominance issues, (2) intimacy and trust, (3) sexual attraction and desire, and (4) sexual scripts. Although we acknowledge the different theoretical contributions of other authors (e.g., Kaplan, 1974; Verhulst & Heiman, 1979; Hof, 1987) to our understanding of the first two areas, there has been relatively little attention in the literature to the role of sexual attraction or sexual script factors in the development and maintenance of erectile failure.

Status and Dominance Issues

Case Vignette

Arthur M., a 53-year-old tax attorney with a 6-year history of intermittent erectile failure, described his marital relationship as follows: "Since this problem developed, I can no longer stand up to my wife in an argument. She has the edge on me every time, all the time!" For Arthur, the loss of his erectile ability was associated with a drastic change in status in the relationship, leading to a growing sense of his being "one-down" in nonsexual as well as sexual situations. His loss of status was similarly associated with a progressive decline in sexual desire for his wife, in addition to a growing sense of despair regarding the future of his marriage. Conflicts in the area of status and dominance may be viewed as either a cause or an effect of erectile failure.

Social status and dominance may be linked to sexual expression in males in a number of ways. At a biological level, for example, there is growing evidence that social status directly influences circulating testosterone levels in both nonhuman (Eberhart, Keverne, & Meller, 1980; McGuire, Brammer, & Raleigh, 1986) and human (Mazur & Lamb, 1980; Gladue, Boechler, & McCaul, 1989) males. In one recent study, Gladue et al. (1989) manipulated the success rates of college males in a competitive laboratory task, and found that winners had consistently higher testosterone levels than losers. On the basis of their findings from this and other similar studies, Gladue et al. (1989) conclude: "A male's testosterone and cortisol levels change when his status changes, rising when he achieves or defends a dominant position, and falling when he is dominated" (p. 410). Changes in mood state were also found by these authors to vary significantly with social status. Although the specific links to erectile failure remain to be demonstrated, changes in status or dominance clearly have significant effects on circulating androgen levels, mood state, and other psychoendocrine responses in the male.

At a sociocultural level, males are socialized from an early age to be competitive and status-oriented in a wide variety of interpersonal situations. Studies of play activity patterns in boys and girls, for example, reveal striking differences in the interpersonal styles of each gender, as described by sociolinguist Deborah Tannen (1990):

> These worlds of play shed light on the world views of men and women in relationships. . . . The chief commodity that is bartered in the boys' hierarchical world is status, and the way to achieve and maintain status is to give orders and get others to follow them. A boy in a low-status position finds himself being pushed around. So boys monitor their relations for subtle shifts in status by keeping track of who's giving orders and who's taking them. (p. 47)

As adults, most men experience a sense of dominance or superiority in at least one aspect of their primary relationship. For example, a man may be older, of higher professional status or income, better educated, or even physically stronger or larger than his partner. Such differences reinforce his sense of dominance—an attribute that most women have been socialized to believe is more characteristic of men than of themselves. At a psychodynamic level, Levine (Chapter 8, this volume) suggests that the "potency" of many men is enhanced by their perception that their sexual partners are not their equals, but are inferior to them in some way. Levine argues that "this perception enhances a man's ability to abandon himself to sensuality and maximizes his potency."

When the power balance shifts—either because of external factors such as the loss of a job and unemployment, or because of internal factors such as depression or loss of self-esteem—sexual difficulties are often the result. In many couples presenting with complaints of erectile failure, the problem can be traced to the male's perception of himself as "one-down" in his primary relationship. Of course, we should bear in mind that status in a relationship is a relative issue, and has little to do with the absolute level of power or dominance. Rather, it relates to the male's perception of his status relative to his mate's, as well as the woman's perception of her status relative to his. To the extent that both partners are satisfied with the balance of power between them, or experience the relationship as symmetrical, relative harmony (sexual and otherwise) exists. If one or the other becomes dissatisfied, emotional conflict and sexual dysfunction may ensue.

Just as shifts in the power balance of a relationship can trigger emotional conflict and sexual dysfunction, we have frequently observed that erectile failure itself is a major source of demoralization and loss of status for the male. As time goes by, his partner may become increasingly frustrated and openly critical of him, thus compounding his sense of sexual inadequacy further. This can set off a vicious cycle of erectile failure leading to feelings of inadequacy and sexual incompetence, which in turn increase his sense of being "one-down" in the relationship. Not surprisingly, the first task of treatment in these situations is to restore the male's sense of confidence and self-respect.

Case Vignette

Joan and Philip enjoyed a mutually satisfying sexual relationship for the first 15 years of their marriage. Philip was a nonpracticing attorney who worked primarily as a free-lance business consultant. When business was brisk, he made a good living. During slow periods, however, the partners modified their expenditures and got by with less. Sexually, they described their relationship as friendly and compatible, with weekly intercourse throughout most of their marriage.

Troubles began when Joan returned to graduate school for her M.B.A. degree. She had always been an excellent scholar (Philip suspected that she was more intelligent than he), but she had chosen to forgo her professional career to raise their two children. Now, at age 43, she embarked on her delayed quest for professional recognition and success. Within 4 years, she had received an M.B.A. from a leading business school and was earning almost twice the income of her husband. Joan now felt somewhat superior to Philip, and was more openly critical and dismissive when she felt he had failed to perform—either in bed or out of it. His behavior became increasingly submissive and tentative with his wife, which only fueled her sense of indignation. Sexually, he began to experience erectile difficulties on occasion. Although Joan was initially tolerant and supportive of her husband, she became increasingly abusive about his sexual "inadequacy," which further compounded Philip's feelings of failure and humiliation. Finally, after a year of intense sexual frustration, the couple sought sex therapy.

In cases such as this, status and dominance issues are a major source of relationship conflict, and a clear contributing factor to the presenting complaint of erectile failure. At times, conflicts in these areas can become so intense that therapeutic progress becomes impossible. Kaplan (1974), for example, observes: "Incredible anger and rage may be mobilized by power struggles in the relationship. When such a struggle is a dominant theme in a couple's relationship, all other life goals become secondary" (p. 160). In other instances, conflicts over status and control operate at a more covert level, subtlely undermining the couple's ability to work together toward overcoming the sexual complaint. Furthermore, given the overall male sensitivity to issues of status or dominance in a relationship (Tannen, 1990), it is not surprising that problems in this area remain a central focus in current sex therapy approaches for erectile failure.

Intimacy and Trust

For most individuals, sexual intimacy involves exposure of one's most private self. The feeling of vulnerability that this entails can be a major source of sexual insecurity or inhibition, particularly in the presence of distrust, anger, or resentment toward one's partner. There is "nowhere to hide" in the bedroom, and most individuals have difficulty in maintaining sexual interest or receptivity when experiencing feelings of anger or distrust. Particularly for a man who is sexually tentative or insecure to begin with, feelings of distrust or lack of intimacy with a partner may be sufficient to tip the balance into sexual dysfunction and erectile failure.

In our culture, it is not uncommon for males to experience difficulty in maintaining relationships involving emotional intimacy and open expression of feelings (Tannen, 1990; Zilbergeld, 1992). Many reasons for this have been noted, including cultural prescriptions for appropriate "masculine" behavior, the lack of effective male role models in the society, and the potential adverse effects of early deprivation and developmental traumas. During adolescence, males frequently experience difficulty in negotiating the emotional aspects of their relationships. All too often, they lack both tools and training. Feelings of love and tenderness are expressed physically through touch, rather than verbally. When sexual difficulties arise or when relationship conflicts thwart physical intimacy, many men are unable to verbalize their difficulties. They lack the words to describe feelings, and many men feel too embarrassed, ashamed, or humiliated to offer a verbal articulation of their concerns. At other times, failure to achieve or maintain an erection may be a symbolic declaration of ambivalence, resentment, or internal conflict in the relationship.

Women, on the other hand, are raised in our culture to crave intimacy—verbal, physical, and emotional—from early childhood on. When faced with partners who are emotionally constricted or withholding, many women become frustrated, angry, and even verbally abusive. Others withdraw and become emotionally distant and unavailable themselves. Paradoxically, the more female partners in a relationship complain about the lack of intimacy, the more difficult it usually is to achieve it. Studies of marital communication styles, for example, have shown that whereas men are reactive and responsive to positive messages from their partners, they become unresponsive and increasingly avoidant with critical feedback (Gottman, Markman, & Notarius, 1977). Sadly, the strategy many women employ in attempting to secure their partners' confidences usually backfires, and they often feel themselves to be living in a hostile enemy camp. Erectile failure in these instances is a potent signal of marital discord. Often, the more basic issue is an erosion of intimacy and trust between partners.

Erectile difficulties can also serve to protect the female partner from her own feelings of vulnerability or distrust. In such instances, the male may unwittingly participate in an elaborate "intimacy dance," as described by Treat (1987):

> The intimacy dance is a metaphor for the means by which each member or a couple maintains a safe distance from the other, protecting his own and often his partner's vulnerabilities. Often, as one partner steps toward the other partner, the other partner collusively steps back. . . . The intimacy dance is designed to avoid greater intimacy. Fear of intimacy can include fear of hurt, abandonment, rejection, intrusion, and loss of self. (p. 62)

As the man begins to show progress in treatment, it is not uncommon for the woman to become increasingly critical or hostile in other aspects of the relationship. From a couples therapy perspective, the underlying issue is the need for maintenance of a critical level of intimacy in the relationship.

Case Vignette

Henry and Susan had been married for 11 years. They began dating in high school, and both were virgins at the time of marriage. According to Susan, she was attracted by Henry's "good looks and easygoing personality." During the early years of the marriage, the central foci of the relationship were the birth of their two children and the development of Henry's career as a dentist. As time went by, however, Susan began to complain about Henry's lack of verbal responsivity and interest in her emotional needs. The couple's sexual relationship also showed signs of strain at this time, as Henry began to experience premature ejaculation and intermittent erectile failure.

The growing emotional and sexual distance in the relationship culminated in Susan's entering into a protracted extramarital affair with Jack, a neighbor and friend of her husband's. This relationship lasted for 2 years, and was experienced by Susan as intensely gratifying at both a physical and an emotional level. For his part, Henry became increasingly suspicious of the inexplicable changes in his wife's behavior, and eventually engaged the services of a private detective. Once the details of her affair were revealed, Susan broke down and promised never to see Jack again. However, she made it clear that Henry's "coldness" and sexual ineptitude were what had "pushed" her outside the marriage, and insisted that they seek counseling for the problem.

During initial assessment, it became obvious that major trust and intimacy issues needed to be addressed. Although Henry accepted his wife's invitation to enter therapy together, he remained distrustful of her affection and was frequently suspicious of her behavior. For her part, Susan could not forgive her husband for having her followed, and secretly yearned for the emotional connection and sexual gratification she had found with Jack. Not surprisingly, Henry's erectile difficulties were greatly exacerbated during this time, and sexual interaction between the couple ground to a complete halt.

In such cases, the first priority for treatment is to rebuild a sense of trust and intimacy in the relationship. A new "marriage contract" may need to be negotiated (Sager, 1976), and specific commitments offered by each partner. For instance, it was imperative for Susan to promise her husband that she would not return to seeing Jack under any circumstances. Henry, in turn, undertook to deal directly with intimacy problems in their relationship, and to remain in sex therapy until their sexual relationship was significantly improved. In addition, specific tasks were assigned for enhancement of emotional communication in the marriage. Like most couples with intimacy problems, Susan and Henry tended to avoid the use of present-tense, first-person communications, and relied heavily on intellectual discussions of past events. Techniques such as role playing, communication training, and guided touch exercises (Treat, 1987) are useful interventions for dealing with such "roadblocks to intimacy."

Sexual Chemistry and Desire

Time and again, clinicians are told: "I love him [her] deeply, but he [she] just doesn't turn me on!" For such individuals, a lack of "sexual chemistry" may present a major obstacle to sexual expression. As noted by Levine (1984), there may be a wish or "cognitive aspiration" for sexual desire, but little or no arousal occurs with the anticipation of sexual contact. A lack of physical attraction or sexual chemistry typically leads to low desire, which in turn may greatly reduce or inhibit sexual arousal in such individuals (Rosen & Leiblum, 1987).

Sexual chemistry is an elusive entity. Why one person is perceived as sexually exciting or attractive, while another elicits little or no sexual interest, can be difficult if not impossible to explain. The topic has been relatively neglected in scientific research on sexuality (Rosen & Hall, 1984; Kachadurian, 1989), and little is known about the nature and origins of sexual attraction. Clinically, we frequently observe men who are strongly attracted to female partners with whom they have little in common, and whom they would never dream of marrying. The "madonna–whore" or "good woman–bad woman" dichotomy is sometimes implicated in these cases, but more often the source of attraction to one woman rather than another is more subtle and difficult to articulate. Unfortunately, with the exception of recent research on paraphilic attractions, more is known at present about the nature of love and romance than about the wellsprings of sexual attraction (Walster & Walster, 1978; Money, 1986).

Men who complain that they rarely or never experience sexual attraction to their mates present a special challenge for sex therapy. Many such men report "loving" their wives, but note a distinct absence of sexual attraction. At times, the excitement of meeting and the thrill of a new relationship may be sufficient to override a lack of sexual chemistry. At other times, the wish to be married or to share a stable, coupled lifestyle leads to a minimization of the importance of sexual attraction. Over time, however, as the novelty of the new relationship inevitably wanes, the lack of basic attraction can play a major role in the development of erectile difficulties.

Case Vignette

John R. was a hard-working, serious-minded 33-year-old stockbroker, married to his college sweetheart, Amy. When they first met, both partners were sexually inexperienced but receptive. She had grown up in a traditional Protestant family with conservative sexual values, including a strong endorsement of premarital virginity. John, too, had been raised in a Midwestern community that valued chastity and monogamy. When they met, he found Amy appealing—like a chum. He felt comfortable and safe with her, although not passionate. She felt similarly about him: He was a "good guy, a guy you could count on." Although he was sexually awkward, she knew he was "someone you could rely on for the long haul." They married and experienced several years of satisfactory if dispassionate sex. Over time, however, his interest in sex waned, and with it his erections. He blamed his sexual difficulties on his 3-hour daily commute to the city and on severe allergies, which he found increasingly debilitating. It was only when couple sessions hit an impasse, and Amy expressed reluctance to continue treatment, that John finally admitted (with considerable chagrin and embarrassment) that he was not, and in fact never had been, sexually attracted to Amy.

John explained that as a teenager, he had "devoured" *Playboy* magazines. He had enjoyed an active fantasy life centered around "bunnies with huge breasts and large asses," whom he imagined as sexually assertive and voluptuous. His favorite repetitive fantasy involved having a tall, mysterious, full-bosomed woman tantalizingly coax him into her bed and caress him erotically, while he lay passively in her arms. With Amy, in contrast, he found himself in the dominant and sexually aggressive role. Furthermore, he found Amy's "choirgirl" appearance, petite body, and small breasts to be a sexual turnoff. He could not imagine her in a sexually seductive or alluring role. In fact, he said, he would collapse into helpless laughter if she appeared in sexy lingerie or struck an erotic pose. Jeans and princess collars, rather than sexy negligées and plunging necklines, were her fashion trademarks.

Therapeutic progress was made as John articulated his sexual wishes to Amy and agreed, in turn, to experiment with increased flexibility in his erotic repertoire. In particular, John was pleasantly surprised by his ability to achieve erections by touch stimulation alone, rather than his past reliance on visual or fantasy means of stimulating arousal. Sex was infrequent, but took place often enough to satisfy Amy and to insure the possibility of pregnancy (something that Amy very much desired). Privately, John continued to enjoy an active fantasy (and masturbatory) life, full of voluptuous "bunnies" cavorting in disreputable dens of sexual iniquity!

Couples may be sexually mismatched not only in terms of physical attraction, but also in terms of sexual desire. We have devoted a separate volume to the assessment and treatment of sexual desire disorders (Leiblum & Rosen, 1988). Among the various factors to be considered in this regard are the effects of physical or mental illness, hormonal deficiency, a history of sexual abuse or other developmental traumas, and a variety of intrapsychic and interpersonal issues. However, desire discrepancy issues are also important to consider when treating cases of erectile failure. In some instances, the problem can be traced to a chronic or global lack of desire in the male partner. In other situations, the problem is partner-specific: The man may desire sex with someone other than his present partner. Even in those instances where the erectile failure occurs consistently across situations and partners, the problem may be traced to an underlying lack of desire.

Case Vignette

George H. was a happily married 50-year-old construction worker. Although he and his wife had been together for more than 20 years, he had lacked sexual interest throughout their relationship. He masturbated infrequently, had few sexual thoughts and fantasies, and rarely initiated sex with his wife. In other respects, George presented as a rather anhedonic personality, who was stoical, self-contained, and dispassionate about most things in life. During his infrequent sexual interactions with his wife, George had generally been able to function adequately, but with little or no sensual pleasure. Recently, with the onset of recurrent prostatitis, he reported diminished erectile functioning. Although he was not overtly concerned with this difficulty, it bothered his wife greatly, especially since George appeared to be using his erectile "unreliability" as an excuse to avoid all forms of sexual contact and physical intimacy between them.

In such cases, erectile failure should be viewed as secondary, or symptomatic of a more fundamental problem of low desire. Rather than focusing on George's erectile difficulty per se, we would recommend careful assessment of the possible intrapsychic and relationship factors that might be contributing to his underlying lack of desire. Various treatment approaches have been advocated for problems of desire, ranging from individual psychodynamic therapy to couples therapy. For a complete review of current treatment approaches, the reader is referred to Leiblum and Rosen (1988).

Sexual Scripts

The "sexual script" is a concept drawn from contemporary sociology (Gagnon & Simon, 1973); it refers to both the organization of sexual activity and the circumstances under which such activity occurs. Sexual scripts define the range of sexual behaviors that are acceptable, with whom, under what circumstances, and with what motives. The sexual scripts of partners in a relationship may vary considerably, and this lack of congruence frequently paves the way for the development of a sexual dysfunction or desire disorder. Couples facing erectile difficulties, in our experience, are often unable to negotiate a sexual script that is compatible and satisfying to both partners. Elsewhere, we have written about the "scripting" approach to problems of sexual desire and ejaculation (Gagnon, Rosen, & Leiblum, 1982; Rosen & Leiblum, 1988), and script incompatibilities are frequently seen in cases of erectile dysfunction as well.

When applied clinically, script analysis begins with an assessment and comparison of both the "performative" and "cognitive" dimensions of the script (Rosen & Leiblum, 1988). The "performative" script refers to the overt or actual sequence of behaviors typically characterizing a sexual encounter, whereas the "cognitive" script comprises the covert or imaginal aspects, including sexual thoughts, fantasies, beliefs, and attitudes. The cognitive script may be synonymous with an ideal or fantasy script, and can include persons, situations, or behaviors not deemed acceptable or desirable in real life. In fact, to the extent that there is a large discrepancy between fantasy and performative scripts, performance difficulties are likely to ensue. For example, men with recurrent homosexual or sadomasochistic fantasies may have difficulty in achieving erections in conventional heterosexual situations.

The performative script includes all those activities that take place during a typical sexual encounter. We have previously suggested that performative scripts should be analyzed in terms of four major script dimensions: complexity, rigidity, conventionality, and satisfaction (Gagnon et al., 1982). In couples with chronic sexual dysfunctions, performative scripts are likely to become increasingly restricted, repetitive, and inflexible, with little satisfaction for either partner. This narrowing and restrictiveness of the performative script can pose a major problem for the older male, who may require an increased range and intensity of stimulation in order to achieve adequate erections. For example, if the man or his partner believes that erections should be spontaneous and should not require any "laying on of hands," they are likely to encounter difficulties when visual stimulation or the proximity of a partner alone is not sufficient to elicit prompt erectile responses. Older men who reject oral sex as an acceptable form of stimulation may need to encourage their partners to provide more manual stimulation as a means of generating sufficient arousal for an erection to occur.

When assessing the sexual scripts of couples presenting with erectile failure, clinicians often discover significant conflicts between the partners in terms of their ideal and actual sexual scripts. Although the dissatisfaction each mate feels with the way in which sex occurs may not be the immediate cause of the erectile problem, it usually plays a salient role in sexual avoidance, lack of interest, and lack of arousal. For this reason, it is important to assess and compare the partners' perceptions of their current and ideal scripts early in treatment, so that therapy sessions can focus directly on the process of script renegotiation and modification.

CASE EXAMPLE

The following case study illustrates several key issues regarding couples conflicts in sex therapy. The couple, Arnold and Phyllis C., reported significant marital discord as well as script incompatibility. In private sessions, Arnold complained about what he perceived as his wife's critical and domineering behavior, whereas Phyllis worried about her lack of physical attraction toward her husband. The dissatisfaction that each partner experienced with the sexual script functioned as a "final nail in the coffin" for this couple, causing them to avoid all forms of sexual exchange. Script incompatibility also contributed directly to Arnold's erectile failure, since he was generally unaroused by the couple's performative script or by fantasies of lovemaking with his wife.

Arnold C. was a successful accountant, who had met his current wife following his divorce from a woman he described as tyrannical, unfaithful, and cold. According to Arnold, he had remained married to his former wife for 14 years because of inertia and a wish to keep his family together. However, his wife eventually left him for another man, and divorce became inevitable. Although lacking in self-confidence generally, and with a limited repertoire of sexual skills, Arnold was gratified to discover that he had no difficulty in developing new relationships. Before long, he became seriously involved with a divorcée, Phyllis, whom he described as attractive, out-spoken, and intelligent. Although Phyllis was the mother of three children, she supported her family by working full-time as an executive secretary.

The excitement of being with an attractive and seemingly accepting woman permitted Arnold to enjoy a reasonably active, albeit unimaginative, sexual relationship. He felt prepared to commit himself to matrimony, as long as he would not be "taken advantage of" in the relationship: He wished to avoid assuming financial responsibility for his new wife, but was willing to encourage her own career development. He saw Phyllis as inferior to him educationally and economically, a perception that enhanced his feelings of sexual self-confidence. The fact that she was unable to achieve orgasm during intercourse did not trouble him, since he tended to be quite self-centered regarding sexual satisfaction.

Over the years of their marriage, Phyllis eventually left her job as a secretary to set up her own business. Arnold was reluctant to support this decision, however, fearing a loss of income as a result of her career switch. She resented his lack of emotional and financial support, but nevertheless decided to go ahead. In a few years, Phyllis had succeeded beyond her wildest dreams and soon found that her income far exceeded her husband's. She felt less dependent on him, and increasingly dissatisfied with his lack of emotional support. At this point Phyllis entered into an extramarital affair, which she found highly gratifying. For the first time, she became optimistic about experiencing orgasm during intercourse. Feeling intensely conflicted, she decided to enter individual therapy to evaluate the sources of her sexual and marital dissatisfaction with her husband, and to overcome the pyscho-logical inhibitions preventing orgasm with her lover.

During the course of individual therapy, Phyllis made rapid progress in overcoming her orgasmic inhibitions. Initially, she was successful in achiev-ing orgasm with vibrator stimulation, and then during oral sex with her lover. This ability transferred to oral sex with her husband, although she com-plained repeatedly about her lack of attraction to Arnold. In fact, the more she contrasted the passionate and lengthy sexual encounters she enjoyed with her lover, and the lackluster and routinized sex she experienced with her husband, the more critical of Arnold she become. She complained also about his early ejaculations, his lack of foreplay, and his "selfishness" in bed and out. Not surprisingly, Arnold began to develop intermittent erectile difficulties and to avoid sex. For her part, Phyllis gradually came to recognize the potentially destructive effects of her affair. During therapy, she decided to terminate her extramarital affair and to devote serious efforts to enhancing her marital and sexual life with her husband.

Several sessions were devoted to helping Arnold and Phyllis to articulate their marital resentments, and to tracing the antecedents of these resentments in earlier family-of-origin relationships. Arnold had been raised in a family in which his mother was dominant and critical, and his father felt continually henpecked. Arnold's feelings of sexual and physical inadequacy could be traced back to his teenage years, during which he was teased about his skinny physique and shy personality. He had always felt insecure about dating and developing relationships with women.

Several parallels emerged in Phyllis's family background. Her mother was also critical and domineering, and was physically abusive on occasion. Phyllis harbored feelings of rage toward her mother, but simultaneously craved her mother's love and approval. She described her father as "a real shit," who was strong-willed and verbally abusive, and who had deserted her mother when Phyllis was 14. Moreover, Phyllis's first husband had been similar in many ways to her father—arrogant, strong-willed, and insensitive. She had married Arnold in the hope that he would provide the nurturance and support she had never received from either her parents or her first husband.

During the conjoint sessions, Phyllis and Arnold developed a greater understanding and appreciation of each other's family backgrounds. This new level of understanding increased their tolerance and sensitivity to the frustrations, insults, and disappointments they each had sustained. When the level of marital conflict subsided as a result, they indicated a willingness to address their sexual difficulties directly.

The first step was to conduct an extensive script analysis, during which the partners were invited to write out their perceptions of both the current performative script and their ideal or fantasy sexual scripts. Although somewhat embarrassed and uncomfortable with the assignment, they both complied fully. When the resulting scripts were compared during the next therapy session, a marked discrepancy was noted between their ideal scripts and what was actually taking place. Arnold, for example, fantasized about being made love to by a sexually dominant partner who would lovingly perform oral sex on him for long periods of time, leaving him totally free to enjoy his erotic pleasure without any need to reciprocate. In his fantasies, he longed for a situation of total sexual passivity. In turn, Phyllis fantasized about having a spontaneous and dominant lover who would make passionate love to her for extended periods, while she too lay passively, abandoning herself completely to erotic sensations. They each desired all-giving lovers who would selflessly and endlessly provide stimulation. Needless to say, their ideal scripts bore little relationship to their current reality. Arnold was "expected" to orchestrate and please Phyllis orally and vaginally, so that she could achieve her newly won orgasms. Phyllis would reciprocate out of a sense of obligation and with little emotion or desire; furthermore, she would not permit him to touch her head or face while performing oral sex with him, so that he felt emotionally isolated and cut off.

They both acknowledged that drastic changes were needed if their sexual relationship was to become satisfying. Each agreed to devote more time and effort to foreplay activities, and to approach lovemaking in a more active and involved fashion. Phyllis consented to being touched and stroked while performing oral sex, and they both elected to experiment with new intercourse positions so that they could feel more "connected" in bed. Phyllis was counseled about the importance of "building up" her husband, rather than being critical or blaming, so that he could develop greater feelings of self-confidence. Although she found it hard to praise Arnold, she did become less demeaning and occasionally provided a genuine compliment. Arnold, in turn, eventually recognized that his sexual insecurities predated his current relationship and could be traced back to developmental experiences with his mother; feeling humiliated about his body as a teenager; and feeling resentful toward his first wife. He acknowledged that his wife's newly achieved orgasmic ability was somewhat threatening, since he now felt responsible for providing her with sufficient stimulation to achieve orgasm.

Together, Arnold and Phyllis continued to work on family-of-origin issues with their respective parents, and became more tolerant and sympathetic of each other's vulnerabilities. They were able to "take turns" sexually, so that each received increasing amounts of stimulation during lovemaking. Slowly, over a period of months, Arnold developed more satisfying erections, although he continued to experience intermittent periods of erectile failure. Nevertheless, they reported satisfaction with the progress they had made. Phyllis was less enthusiastic about the therapy outcome than Arnold, but acknowledged that their relationship had improved, and that Arnold was sincerely making efforts to change. Although she toyed with the idea of having another extramarital affair, she recognized that it could signal the end of her marriage, and she therefore resisted the temptation to act on her fantasy.

CASE COMMENTARY

Some cases have less than perfect endings. The lack of sexual chemistry that Phyllis felt for her husband showed little alteration over the course of therapy, although she became more accepting of his efforts to please her. She reasoned that no marriage was perfect, and that she was fortunate to have a loyal, faithful, and committed mate. Arnold remained sexually vulnerable; occasional business or marital stresses were enough to trigger erectile insufficiency. However, he was reassured that he could function adequately on most occasions. He became somewhat more willing to use oral or manual stimulation techniques when his penis was "out of commission," and he was always successful in ejaculation. He acknowledged being threatened by the shift in power between him and his wife, but he also expressed relief that she was financially self-sufficient. He decided that freedom from financial concern was a fair trade for the power shift in his relationship. Finally, he was more satisfied than he had expected to be with the couples therapy, although he felt they had "had enough for the time being." The therapist concurred that this couple had made considerable gains, considering their initial stance.

SEXUAL SEDUCTION

One aspect of the sexual script that is frequently overlooked by therapists is the issue of sexual initiation or seduction. Couples who enjoy compatible and mutually satisfying sexual relationships generally report little or no difficulty with sexual initiation. Initiation is often equally shared by both partners, either through direct verbal invitation or by means of body language signals. In couples where sexual difficulties exist, however, sexual initiation can be a major problem. The wife of a man experiencing erectile failure, for example, is often reluctant to initiate sexual activity, because she wishes to protect either herself or her partner from the anxiety and humiliation of erectile failure. The male often feels so anxious and insecure that he avoids sexual initiation altogether. Over time, sexual frequency declines, and over-coming the mutual reluctance to initiate sex becomes a major roadblock in overcoming erectile difficulties.

Apfelbaum (1988) has highlighted the importance of sexual seduction skills for both functional and dysfunctional couples. According to Apfelbaum, most individuals are relatively unskilled in techniques of seduction, and are moreover generally unaware of their deficits in this regard. This leads to a situation, he suggests, in which one partner becomes frustrated and angry when the other is not promptly and automatically aroused. Some individuals respond to this dilemma by resorting to increasingly coercive or abusive forms of sexual initiation. Others become depressed and withdrawn. Men with erectile failure are particularly vulnerable to such feelings of personal inadequacy. Initiation can become a major ordeal; they may become incapable of making a sexual overture, even when experiencing a high level of sexual desire.

Case Vignette

Joseph Y., a sexually anxious man of 25, married a woman who was clearly more experienced and sexually comfortable than he was. Although he was capable of successful (and frequent) masturbation without erectile difficulties, he felt unable to initiate sexual encounters with his wife. He anticipated rejection and humiliation. Even when she acted seductively by walking around naked after showering and lying in provocative poses on the bed, he found himself avoiding her. When actively caressed by her, he frequently experienced erectile failure.

In individual therapy sessions, it became apparent that Joseph had a lifelong history of guilt about sexual activity. He was the youngest child and had five older female siblings. He grew up in a family of women, surrounded by female "artifacts" (sanitary pads and makeup, lingerie and clothing), and he had trained himself to avoid being sexually aroused by not looking and not touching. Now that he was in a situation where sexual interest and curiosity were appropriate, he was unable to overcome his earlier inhibitions. He was totally incapable of being sexually "seductive" himself, or even of responding to the sexual overtures of his wife.

COUPLES VERSUS SEX THERAPY:
TO TREAT OR NOT TO TREAT?

A basic dilemma in many cases of erectile failure is the question of whether couples conflicts and tensions need to be fully resolved prior to the initiation of sex therapy, or whether such problems can be "bypassed" and sexual therapy interventions introduced directly, as suggested by Kaplan (1974). This can be an extremely challenging issue at times, and we have found assessment of the following dimensions to be useful in providing clinical guidelines for making this decision.

1. *Relationship commitment.* Partners who are able to express clear and unequivocal commitment to each other, and to their relationship, are generally more amenable to sex therapy than partners who feel disillusioned and uncertain about their future. When a couple has actively contemplated separation and divorce, or where a lack of commitment exists in an unmarried couple, relationship issues need to be addressed prior to active sex therapy.

2. *Degree of marital conflict.* In a similar vein, when the level of marital conflict and disagreement is high, little progress is usually made. In particular, specific sex therapy assignments are likely to be sabotaged unless major sources of conflict are identified and resolved. When tensions run high outside the bedroom, it is unlikely that much progress can be made inside it. In some instances, long-standing frustrations and resentment toward the partner is suppressed, especially when a patient fears a loss of control. Nevertheless, overt expressions of disappointment and anger may help to "clear the air" and pave the way for greater intimacy.

3. *Extramarital affairs and other secrets.* Survey data from several sources indicate that approximately 30–40% of men and women engage in sexual

liaisons outside of marriage (Blumstein & Schwartz, 1983; Reinisch, 1990). Certainly, in many of the couples presenting for sex therapy, one or both partners have been or are currently involved in extramarital affairs. These and other secrets in the marriage are poor prognostic indications for successful sex therapy. Careful attention to the impact of such secrets on the relationship is necessary before sex therapy can be undertaken.

Secrets come in various shapes and sizes. Addictions (e.g., gambling or alcoholism), paraphilias or fetishistic preferences, financial liabilities, and similar problems all place limits on intimate exchange in a relationship. The more energy devoted to keeping the secret, the less available mates are to each other, and the greater the feeling that something is "not quite right." Even when a mate is not certain or consciously aware that a secret exists, it can have a palpable impact on the quality of the relationship. Although we do not routinely or universally recommend the sharing of secrets, we have found that ignoring certain secrets can severely handicap treatment.

Case Vignette
Following the untimely and sudden death of his wife, Bob P. felt lonely and bereft. He urgently desired companionship and sexual intimacy, but was only attracted to women significantly younger than himself. Although 62 years old, he had always been told that he looked and acted "younger than his age." When he was introduced to an attractive 41-year-old divorcee, Nancy, Bob decided to "take 10 years off" his age, and told her that he was 52.

Throughout the courtship, Bob lived in constant fear that Nancy would discover his true age and terminate the relationship. Not surprisingly, he began to experience performance anxiety and intermittent erectile failure. Although a number of factors contributed to his concerns about sexual performance (including unresolved feelings of grief for his deceased wife), his fear of discovery about his age clearly exacerbated this anxiety and reinforced his feelings of sexual inadequacy. Naturally, his true age was eventually revealed when Nancy (now his fiancée) accidentally came across his driver's license and confronted him with his deception. Although humiliated, Bob was nonetheless relieved by the disclosure, and was able to make a real commitment to therapy.

4. *External pressures on the sexual relationship.* At times, couples may experience a sense of desperation about achieving successful sexual intercourse. For instance, partners who are trying to conceive a child can become performance-oriented to a degree that drastically undermines sexual spontaneity and ease. In such instances, erectile failure is not uncommon. At other times, the pressure to be sexually functional is more subtle, but nonetheless operative. Women who feel that "penis-in-vagina sex" is the only type that matters, for example, frequently place inordinate demands on their sexually

insecure male partners. Similarly, men who feel that their manhood rests on the strength of their erections are seldom comfortable in bed. The intense pressures that such gender-related beliefs exert on sexual performance need to be addressed at the outset of therapy.

5. *Concurrent medical or psychiatric illness.* In some cases, serious medical illness or psychiatric disorders can limit both couples therapy and sex therapy interventions. In such cases, sex therapy may need to be postponed until the more immediate medical or psychiatric difficulties are resolved. Some couples appear to use sexual dysfunctions as the "ticket of admission" to treatment, but in-depth clinical evaluation may indicate more fundamental emotional problems.

In general, there are few immutable rules for determining when couples therapy is needed instead of, or as an adjunct to, sex therapy. In fact, it is seldom entirely clear when sex therapy alone will suffice or when couples work must take precedence. At times, sex therapy is undertaken despite our awareness of significant relationship conflicts, and it quickly becomes obvious that progress cannot be achieved without "time out" for additional couples work. At other times, progress in the sexual realm alleviates pre-existing relationship problems. Time and again, we have found that the best treatment approach is a flexible one, with a willingness to shift back and forward from couples work to sexual exploration and back again, as needed.

REFERENCES

Allen, C. (1949). *The sexual perversions and abnormalities.* London: Oxford University Press.

Althof, S. E. (1989). Psychogenic impotence: Treatment of men and couples. In S. R. Leiblum & R. C. Rosen (Eds.), *Principles and practice of sex therapy* (2nd ed.): *Update for the 1990s* (pp. 237–268). New York: Guilford Press.

Apfelbaum, B. (1988). Sexuality: Intimacy or illusion. In W. Eicher & G. Kockott (Eds.), *Sexology* (pp. 229–233). Berlin/Heidelberg: Springer-Verlag.

Berman, E. M., & Hof, L. (1987). The sexual genogram: Assessing family-of-origin factors in the treatment of sexual dysfunction. In G. R. Weeks & L. Hof (Eds.), *Integrating sex and marital therapy: A clinical guide* (pp. 37–56). New York: Brunner/Mazel.

Bloch, I. (1908). *Sexual life in our times.* London: Rebman.

Blumstein, P., & Schwartz, P. (1983). *American couples: Money, work, and sex.* New York: Morrow.

Bowen, M. (1978). *Family therapy in clinical practice.* New York: Jason Aronson.

Eberhart, J. A., Keverne, E. B., & Meller, R. E. (1980). Social influences on plasma testosterone levels in male talapoin monkeys. *Hormones and Behavior, 14,* 247–266.

Ferenczi, S. (1913). *Sex in psychoanalysis*. Boston: Richard C. Badger.

Fish, L. S., Fish, R. C., & Sprenkle, D. H. (1984). Treating inhibited sexual desire: A marital therapy approach. *American Journal of Family Therapy, 12*, 3–12.

Freud, S. (1957). Leonardo da Vinci and a memory of his childhood. In J. Strachey (Ed. and Trans.), *The standard edition of the complete psychological works of Sigmund Freud* (Vol. 11, pp. 59–137). London: Hogarth Press. (Original work published 1910)

Gagnon, J. H., Rosen, R. C., & Leiblum, S. R. (1982). Cognitive and social aspects of sexual dysfunction: Sexual scripts in sex therapy. *Journal of Sex and Marital Therapy, 8*, 44–56.

Gagnon, J. H., & Simon, W. (1973). *Sexual conduct: The social sources of human sexuality*. Chicago: Aldine.

Gladue, B. A., Boechler, M., & McCaul, K. D. (1989). Hormonal response to competition in human males. *Aggressive Behavior, 15*, 409–422.

Gottman, J., Markman, H., & Notarius, C. (1977). The topography of marital conflict: A sequential analysis of verbal and nonverbal behavior. *Journal of Marriage and the Family, 39*, 461–477.

Gross, S. (1887). *A practical treatise on impotence and sterility*. Edinburgh: Y. J. Pentland.

Hof, L. (1987). Evaluating the marital relationship of clients with sexual complaints. In G. R. Weeks & L. Hof (Eds.), *Integrating sex and marital therapy: A clinical guide* (pp. 5–22). New York: Brunner/Mazel.

Hof, L., & Berman, E. M. (1986). The sexual genogram. *Journal of Marital and Family Therapy, 12*, 39–47.

Kachadurian, H. (1989). *Human sexuality*. New York: Holt, Rinehart & Winston.

Kaplan, H. S. (1974). *The new sex therapy*. New York: Brunner/Mazel.

Krafft-Ebing, R. von. (1893). *Psychopathia sexualis*. London: Rebman.

Leiblum, S. R., & Rosen, R. C. (Eds.). (1988). *Sexual desire disorders*. New York: Guilford Press.

Levine, S. B. (1984). An essay on the nature of sexual desire. *Journal of Sex and Marital Therapy, 10*, 83–96.

Levine, S. B. (1988). Intrapsychic and individual aspects of sexual desire. In S. R. Leiblum & R. C. Rosen (Eds.), *Sexual desire disorders* (pp. 21–44). New York: Guilford Press.

LoPiccolo, J., & Friedman, J. M. (1988). Broad spectrum treatment of low sexual desire: Integration of cognitive, behavioral, and systemic therapy. In S. R. Leiblum & R. C. Rosen (Eds.), *Sexual desire disorders* (pp. 107–144). New York: Guilford Press.

Masters, W. H., & Johnson, V. E. (1970). *Human sexual inadequacy*. Boston: Little, Brown.

Mazur, A., & Lamb, T. A. (1980). Testosterone, status and mood in human males. *Hormones and Behavior, 14*, 236–246.

McCarthy, B. W. (1989). Cognitive-behavioral strategies and techniques in the treatment of early ejaculation. In S. R. Leiblum & R. C. Rosen (Eds.), *Principles and practice of sex therapy* (2nd ed.): *Update for the 1990s* (pp. 141–167). New York: Guilford Press.

McGuire, M. T., Brammer, G. L., & Raleigh, M. J. (1986). Resting cortisol levels and the emergence of dominant status among vervet monkeys. *Hormones and Behavior*, *20*, 106–117.

Money, J. (1986). *Lovemaps: Clinical concepts of sexual/erotic health and pathology, paraphilia, and gender transposition in childhood, adolescence, and maturity*. New York: Irvington.

Montague, D. K. (Ed.). (1988). *Disorders of male sexual function*. Chicago: Year Book Medical.

Regas, S. J., & Sprenkle, D. B. (1984). Functional family therapy and the treatment of inhibited sexual desire. *Journal of Marital and Family Therapy*, *10*, 63–72.

Reinisch, J. M. (1990). *The Kinsey Institute new report on sex*. New York: St. Martin's Press.

Riggs, B. (1978). System C: An essay in human relatedness. *American Journal of Psychotherapy*, *32*, 379–392.

Rosen, R. C., & Hall, E. (1984). *Sexuality*. New York: Random House.

Rosen, R. C., & Leiblum, S. R. (1987). Current approaches to the evaluation of sexual desire disorders. *Journal of Sex Research*, *23*, 141–162.

Rosen, R. C., & Leiblum, S. R. (1988). A sexual scripting approach to problems of desire. In S. R. Leiblum & R. C. Rosen (Eds.), *Sexual desire disorders* (pp. 168–191). New York: Guilford Press.

Ryan, M. (1835). *Lectures on impotence and sterility*. London: W. R. Lucas.

Sager, C. J. (1976). *Marriage contracts and couple therapy*. New York: Brunner/Mazel.

Scharff, D. E. (1988). An object relations approach to inhibited sexual desire. In S. R. Leiblum & R. C. Rosen (Eds.), *Sexual desire disorders* (pp. 45–74). New York: Guilford Press.

Segraves, R. T., & Schoenberg, H. W. (Eds.). (1988). *Diagnosis and treatment of erectile disturbances: A guide for clinicians*. New York: Plenum.

Tanagho, E. A., Lue, T. F., & McClure, R. D. (Eds.). (1988). *Contemporary management of impotence and infertility*. Baltimore: Williams & Wilkins.

Tannen, D. (1990). *You just don't understand: Women and men in conversation*. New York: Morrow.

Treat, S. R. (1987). Enhancing a couple's relationship. In G. R. Weeks & L. Hof (Eds.), *Integrating sex and marital therapy: A clinical guide* (pp. 57–81). New York: Brunner/Mazel.

Verhulst, J., & Heiman, J. (1979). An interactional approach to sexual dysfunction. *American Journal of Family Therapy*, *7*, 19–36.

von Bertalanffy, L. (1968). *General systems theory*. New York: Brazilier.

Walster, E., & Walster, G. W. (1978). *A new look at love*. Reading, MA: Addison-Wesley.

Zilbergeld, B. (1992). *The new male sexuality*. New York: Bantam.

10

Surgery for Erectile Disorders: Operative Procedures and Psychological Issues

ARNOLD MELMAN AND LEONORE TIEFER

Surgical treatment approaches for erectile dysfunction have proliferated in recent years. In addition to the growing number and variety of penile prostheses currently available for implant surgery, new procedures have been developed for surgical correction of arterial insufficiency or venous leakage disorders. Although still imperfect, these new surgical procedures are being performed in ever-increasing numbers. From the patient's perspective, surgical treatment is frequently perceived as offering a relatively immediate and permanent solution for the problem. As one patient commented, "Who has time for months or years of therapy?"

In this chapter, Melman and Tiefer succinctly review the current range of surgical treatments for erectile disorders. These can be divided into two general categories: (1) surgical correction of reversible conditions (e.g., Peyronie's disease), and (2) implantation of a surgical prosthesis for irreversible dysfunctions. In the first category, the authors describe various procedures for surgical correction of penile chordee, or abnormal curvature of the penis during erection. These procedures are generally associated with a high success rate. Also in this category, however, are the recent surgical techniques for correction of arterial insufficiency or venous leakage problems. These techniques are highly controversial at present, and may only be applicable to a limited number of patients. Considering the lack of adequate follow-up data, it is difficult to estimate the overall success rate of vascular bypass or venous ligation surgery for erectile dysfunction.

Penile prosthesis surgery is ideally reserved for treatment of irreversible conditions. Since the early 1950s, when the first synthetic implants were developed, penile prosthesis surgery has assumed an increasingly important role in the clinical management of erectile dysfunction. Major technological innovations in the past two decades have led to a wide variety of implant devices, including several types of semirigid and inflatable models. Major advantages and disadvantages of each type of implant are briefly considered in this chapter. Among the factors to be considered in selecting an implant are the risks of mechanical failure, the possibility of postsurgical infection, changes in the size of the patient's penis, and likely response of the partner to the type of implant selected. Clearly, the ultimate success of penile prosthesis surgery depends upon careful selection of both the patient and the type of implant procedure to be used.

From their extensive clinical and research experience, Melman and Tiefer also provide guidelines for presurgical preparation and counseling of surgical patients. Patients need to be fully informed about the procedure, and unrealistic expectations ought to be addressed. For couples who have a long-standing pattern of sexual avoidance, the authors recommend presurgical counseling aimed at restoring sexual intimacy. In some instances, this counseling may even eliminate the need for surgery! Throughout the chapter, the authors argue persuasively for the integration of psychological and surgical approaches for erectile dysfunction.

Arnold Melman, M.D., is Professor and Chairman of the Department of Urology and Director of the Center for Male Sexuality, Montefiore Medical Center and Albert Einstein College of Medicine, Bronx, New York. He has conducted extensive research on the physiology and pharmacology of male erection, and has more than 20 years of clinical experience in the treatment of erectile dysfunction.

Leonore Tiefer, Ph.D., is Clinical Associate Professor of Urology and Psychiatry at Montefiore Medical Center and Albert Einstein College of Medicine. She has published widely in the field of sexuality and sex therapy for over 20 years.

The goals of surgery for erectile dysfunction are to reconstruct or repair the penis so that coitus can be resumed. The type of repair is directed by whether or not the defect is reversible, so that, once repaired, the erectile mechanism can function normally. If the dysfunction is not reversible, then the surgical treatment of choice is a penile prosthetic implant. Erectile dysfunctions that are potentially reversible through surgery include (1) chordee, (2) arterial fistulae or insufficiency, and (3) venous corporal incompetence.

In all spheres of medicine, appropriate treatment resulting in maximum patient satisfaction requires more than just correct diagnosis and appropriately chosen and properly delivered treatment. The health care provider must take into account those aspects of psychological functioning relevant to the presenting complaint and its resolution. Taylor (1983) discusses some of the complex psychological events set into motion by a personal threat (e.g., illness or sexual dysfunction), and alerts us to the ways in which individual patients and couples search for meaning, mastery, and repaired self-esteem (i.e., how they "cope" with their situation and choices). To maximize patient satisfaction with sexual surgeries such as those discussed in this chapter, we need to attend to the many and complex psychological sequelae and accompaniments of sexual dysfunction and sexual medical treatment as we deliver appropriate diagnostic and operative services.

SURGERY FOR CHORDEE

"Chordee" is defined as a curve of the penis during erection. The two common diseases of adults that cause such curvature are hemihypertrophy and Peyronie's disease.

Hemihypertrophy is a rare congenital enlargement of one of the two corpora cavernosa. It results in a deformed erection, in which one side of the penis lengthens more than the other, causing the penis to bend. In this condition, there is no actual physical abnormality of the erectile tissue, so that the erectile mechanism functions normally. The surgical repair is necessary in order to achieve cosmetic straightening of the penis, because some patients with this condition are embarrassed by the curve and avoid attempts at coitus.

Peyronie's disease, a far more common condition, is an inflammatory process of the tunica albuginea (dense tissue covering the erectile bodies of the penis) and underlying erectile tissue (Metz, Ebbehoj, Uhrenholdt, & Wagner, 1983). The inflammation causes fibrosis (scarring) of the erectile tissue. Because fibrotic erectile tissue is not elastic, the tumescent penis bends around the region of the scar, with a resultant chordee in the majority of patients. Peyronie's disease is thought to be initiated by trauma or urethral infection, but in many patients there is no identifiable predisposing event. There may be an association with other fibrosis-creating diseases, such as Dupytren's contracture of the palms or soles or carcinoid, and some have suggested that fibrotic conditions may result from use of the popular beta-blocking antihypertensive agents.

Peyronie's disease may manifest itself as an asymptomatic mass in the penile shaft. This diagnosis can be made by palpation, ultrasound, computed axial tomography scan, magnetic resonance imaging, or cavernosography. However, a mass that involves the corpus spongiosum may signify carcinoma of the urethra, and this diagnosis should be ruled out. In addition, Peyronie's disease may be manifested as a mass in the penis, causing pain during erection; as curvature of the penis during erection, with or without pain; as total erectile dysfunction or soft phallus distal to the plaque; or as subclinical fibrosis.

Clinically, it is most important to reassure the patient that he does not have cancer and that the disease is self-limiting. There is no specific proven effective medical treatment for Peyronie's disease. High-dose vitamin E therapy (2,000 units/day) has been recommended in some cases (Scardino & Scott, 1949).

Plication Repair for Chordee

Patients who have a painless mass or minimal curvature need no treatment. Patients who have plaque that causes severe penile curvature, but who can still have a rigid erection, can be most easily treated with a Nesbit plication (Nesbit, 1965; see Figure 10.1). More extensive disease with penile rigidity may require plaque excision and grafting. The disease should be present for

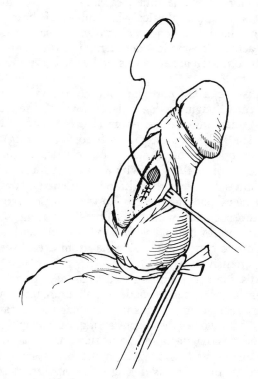

FIGURE 10.1.   Illustration of the Nesbit plication technique for correction of severe penile chordee. The tunica of the penis is excised and shortened, so that the longer, nonaffected side of the penis is drawn in during erection. A high success rate is associated with this technique.

at least 12 months before surgical therapy is initiated. Persistent severe pain has also been successfully treated with low doses (1,000 rads) of radiation (Landthaler, Kodalle, & Braun-Falco, 1983). Patients with penile flaccidity distal to the plaque require treatment with a penile prosthetic implant (see below).

The Nesbit plication is the treatment of choice for either the chordee of hemihypertrophy or Peyronie's disease. A Nesbit plication is an operative procedure in which either one or more small (about 1-cm) segments of tunica albuginea are removed from one side of the penis, or a tuck (invagination) is made on the side opposite the penile curve. The results are shortening of the longer side and subsequent straightening of the penis. The procedure can be done as ambulatory surgery with local anesthesia. Unless there is progressive or new disease, the procedure is almost uniformly successful.

Grafts and Inlays for Chordee

When the fibrosis of the penis is so severe that a Nesbit plication is not practical because significant penile shortening would result, a dermal graft procedure may be an option (Coughlin, Carson, & Paulson, 1984; Devine & Horton, 1983). In this operation, fibrotic tissue is excised and replaced with a segment of dermis harvested from the nearby inguinal area. This procedure should be performed only in patients with documented penile rigidity. Unfortunately, it runs the risk of converting a patient capable of obtaining a rigid but bent erection into one with erectile dysfunction. The success rate of removing the fibrotic plaque and creating a soft, pliable, pain-free penis is quite high. However, the reported success rates of the surgery are extremely variable, with reports of postoperative potency ranging from 0% (Melman & Holland, 1978) to 80% (Devine & Horton, 1983).

SURGERY ON PENILE ARTERIES: REVASCULARIZATION PROCEDURES

The concept of arterial bypass surgery, in cases where arterial insufficiency is the cause of erectile failure, was first proposed by Michal, Kramer, Popsichal, and Hejhal (1973). There have been many variations in surgical technique and much elaboration of the diagnostic methods to detect arterial defects since that time. The surgery that Michal et al. originally proposed was to join an artery not normally affected by atherosclerotic plaquing—the epigastric artery—directly into the side of one corpus cavernosum. Problems with priapism (permanent erectile rigidity) or scarring and closure of the anastomosis have caused that particular procedure to be abandoned.

In a recent paper, Sohn, Sikora, Bohndorf, and Deutz (1990) summarized the results of the largest operative series reported by vascular surgeons and urologists performing the 15 variations on Michal et al.'s original theme. The surgeons report a "success" rate varying from 50% to 80%. However, "success" in most of the reports is neither long-term nor objectively measured. There is little standardization in the analysis of diagnostic or surgical techniques, or in the evaluation of results from center to center. For example, not all of the centers use nocturnal penile tumescence (NPT) testing to document organic dysfunction.

The lack of standardized diagnostic methodology and the lack of normal baseline measures are causes for concern about overdiagnosis of arterial abnormalities. Decreased arterial blood flow as measured by duplex sonography, for example, or abnormal penile plethysmography in conjunction with an abnormal pudendal angiogram, should not necessarily be considered diagnostic of arterial abnormalities as the cause of erectile dysfunction. Abnormal pudendal angiograms and abnormalities in other indirect measures of penile blood flow are not *absolute* measures of erectile dysfunction. The reason is that anatomic abnormalities do not necessarily translate into functional erectile abnormalities. Therefore, the diagnosis of arterial insufficiency may be oversubscribed.

One particular pattern of diagnostic test results that clinicians should watch for is that in which the patient has normal NPT and yet shows an arterial deficiency known as the "pelvic steal syndrome." This is a syndrome in which blood flow normally destined for the penis during coitus is shunted to the thighs and pelvic muscles because of arterial narrowing (the latter muscles "steal" the blood). It can be simulated in the flaccid penis by testing the patient's penile blood flow before and after pelvic exercise (see Schiavi, Chapter 6, this volume).

Since Michal et al.'s (1973) original surgical suggestions, other techniques have been developed for penile revascularization. These include anastomosis of the epigastric artery to the cavernous artery (abandoned because of the problem of corporal fibrosis) and anastomosis to the dorsal artery and/or to the deep dorsal vein. The latest variation, as suggested by Hauri (1986), is to connect the epigastric artery to the dorsal artery and vein as a tripartite union (see Figure 10.2). The rationale is that the tripartite joining allows a continuous high-flow state. Presumably, this would eliminate one of the major causes of surgical failure, thrombosis of the anastomosis because of a low flow rate (the dorsal penile artery is less than 1 mm in diameter).

The best results of arterial bypass surgery are obtained when the surgery (epigastric artery to dorsal penile artery) is performed in young men who have obstruction of the pudendal arteries after pelvic trauma. Patient selection for the arterial bypass surgery should utilize the following selection criteria:

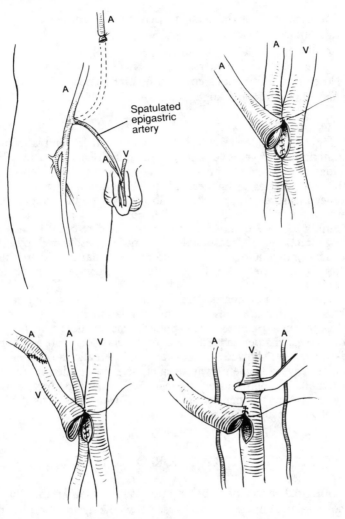

FIGURE 10.2. Illustration of the Hauri procedure for arterial bypass surgery of the penile vessels. The top left panel shows the epigastric artery brought down to the penis and joined to an artery and vein. The top right panel is a close-up view of the site of anastomosis. The lower left panel shows a vein graft interposed between the artery and the anastomosis. The lower right panel shows the end of the epigastric artery being sutured to the side of the deep dorsal vein. It can also be sutured to the adjacent dorsal artery.

1. Abnormal NPT or diagnosis of pelvic steal syndrome.
2. Age under 60 years.
3. No diabetes mellitus.
4. No neurological disorders.
5. No evidence of venous corporal incompetence.
6. Abnormal pudendal angiogram.

Case Vignette

Mr. A. T., a 60-year-old obese teacher with a complaint of erectile dysfunction for 7 years, underwent an initial evaluation in 1985. This included a physical examination, a hormone profile, glucose tolerance testing, NPT testing using mercury-in-rubber strain gauges, and a simple Doppler measure of penile blood flow with a penile-artery-to-brachial-artery index. This index was 0.78, considered a normal ratio. The remaining tests were either normal or, in the case of NPT, showed long-lasting erections of "reasonable rigidity" (as estimated by the sleep technician). Psychological evaluation revealed marital discord and severe performance anxiety. Mr. T. and his wife were sent for conjoint sex therapy.

They were not heard from for the next 5 years; they returned in 1990, stating that they now had a better relationship but that the erectile complaints had persisted. The patient was restudied with the newer technologies. His penile plethysmography was considered abnormal; his Rigiscan testing showed inadequately rigid erections of brief duration. Dynamic cavernosometry was normal. Selective pudendal angiography showed bilateral penile artery stenosis. He underwent anastomosis of the epigastric artery to deep dorsal vein, and the couple has subsequently been able to resume successful coitus.

SURGERY FOR VENOUS CORPORAL INCOMPETENCE

Since the original report of Ebbehoj and Wagner (1979), the diagnosis of venous corporal incompetence as a cause of erectile dysfunction has received increasing attention. The diagnosis is established by first confirming that the patient has erectile dysfunction and then performing cavernosometry and cavernosography to identify the site of the leaking vein. However, despite the ability of many investigators to identify the presence and even the location of apparent venous leakage from the corpora cavernosa, surgical repair has not achieved uniformly successful results. Although some authors do report improvement with venous ligation surgery in as many as 80% of patients (Wespes & Schulman, 1985), other investigators report success in only 20% (Rossman, Mieza, & Melman, 1990).

It should be noted that the concept of venous insufficiency as a cause of erectile dysfunction actually dates back to the turn of the century, when it was first suggested that ligation of the dorsal veins of the penis might be an effective treatment for erectile dysfunction (Lydston, 1908). However, it is only with the advent of dynamic cavernosometry and cavernosography that our ability to accurately diagnose and treat these patients has developed (see Figures 10.3 and 10.4). By monitoring intracavernosal pressure during the pharmacological induction of an erection and rapid fluid flow, the presence of venous corporal incompetence can be demonstrated. Dynamic cavernosography enables the surgeon to pinpoint the actual site of venous leakage. It can be manifested as shunts from the corpora cavernosa to the corpus spongiosum or glans, or alternatively as leakage directly into the dorsal, crural, or pudendal veins (Melman, 1988).

The pathophysiology of venous incompetence is incompletely understood at present. Presumably the problem lies in improper closing of the subtunical venous plexus by the corporal smooth muscle. As a result, blood is not trapped in the plexus, and the penis loses rigidity. The surgical approach

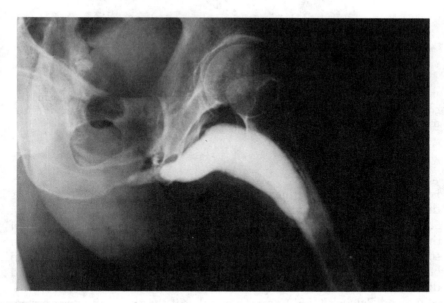

FIGURE 10.3. A normal corporal cavernosogram, showing the corpora filled with contrast material. The contrast medium is contained entirely in the sinusoidal spaces and does not drain into the glans or veins of the penis.

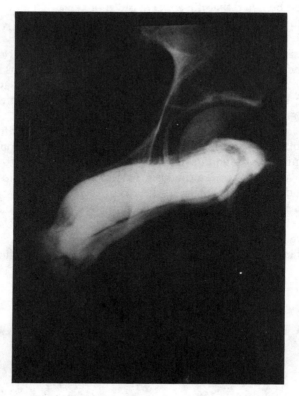

FIGURE 10.4. An abnormal cavernosogram showing contrast in the glans penis and corpora spongiosa (the tissue surrounding the urethra). This shows a site of exit of the contrast medium, which may represent an abnormal venous shunt.

is thus far limited to either ligating or cauterizing the abnormal veins draining the corpora, as diagnosed by cavernosometry and cavernosography. Some surgeons have recommended enhancing defective venous drainage of the penis by injecting a sclerosing agent into the superficial penile veins in some patients. Alternatively, several radiological groups have attempted to block the penile venous outflow with occlusive balloons or coils placed directly into the veins draining into the pelvis. However, Puech-Leao, Reis, Glina, and Reichelt (1987) have shown that if the dorsal drainage system alone is ligated, a shift to the perineal crural veins occurs. This suggests that both veins must be ligated for a successful surgical outcome. The perineal veins are not approachable with either of the nonoperative approaches.

Lewis (1991) has reviewed several reasons for the limited success in the surgical treatment of venous incompetence to date:

1. Inability to diagnose concomitant arterial disease.
2. Inability to ligate or fulgurate the veins draining the defective area of the corpora.
3. The development of collateral circulation.
4. The possibility that venous corporal dysfunction is not the true abnormality in the particular patient; rather, the abnormality may lie in the corporal smooth muscle.

Case Vignette

A 58-year-old dentist complained of a 10-year history of gradually increasing inability to maintain erection. There was no history of marital discord, diabetes, hypertension, smoking, alcoholism, or past pelvic surgery. His penile plethysmography was normal. The patient had been treated unsuccessfully with intracorporal injection of papaverine by another physician. During the course of two nights of Rigiscan testing, he did not demonstrate rigid erection on either night of study. Psychological evaluation failed to demonstrate any evidence of potential psychological factors.

The patient then underwent dynamic cavernosometry and cavernosography. A rigid erection was not obtained during cavernosometry. Cavernosography revealed multiple veins draining from the corpora 5 minutes after intracorporal injection of 60 mg papaverine. On the basis of these findings, the patient underwent penile vein ligation. He was capable of sustained, rigid erections for a period of 6 months. However, he returned to the office 9 months after surgery with complaints similar to those he had had prior to the operation. He did not achieve an erection after intracorporal injection of a mixture of papaverine–phentolamine or prostaglandin E_1. Repeat cavernosography showed evidence of new venous corporal incompetence. The patient subsequently received an inflatable penile prosthesis.

PENILE PROSTHESES

Types of Prostheses

When treatment (including surgery) cannot correct the organic defect that is causing erectile dysfunction, penile rigidity sufficient for intercourse can be restored through the use of a penile implant. The first successful penile prosthetic implant was developed by Goodwin and Scott (1952). The device was a flat acrylic rod that did not have long-term usefulness because it was so rigid as to be uncomfortable (see Figure 10.5). However, the facts that the implant was not rejected by the patient's body, and that it did allow satisfactory coitus, were extremely important.

The development of silicone rubber implants was the next major advance in penile prosthetic surgery. Pearman (1967) described the insertion of a new prosthesis, which was flexible but sufficiently rigid to allow coitus, and which was safe and practical to install surgically (see Figure 10.6). The Pearman device consisted of a single rod, placed in the midline of the corpora, that extended from the glans to the pubic symphysis.

The Small–Carrion implant was the next significant improvement in prosthetic design (Small, Carrion, & Gordon, 1975). That device consisted of two rods, one implanted in each corpus cavernosum (see Figure 10.7). It was available in several lengths and diameters. The Small–Carrion implant had the disadvantage of keeping the patient's penis in a constant erect state, and was of limited rigidity. The implant represented a major improvement, however, and was widely used.

At about the same time, Scott, Bradley, and Timm (1973) reported the development of an inflatable silicone-based, hydraulic implant, which provided improvement in both rigidity and girth (see Figure 10.8). The inflatable cylinders, although of constant length, allowed the patient a soft penis until

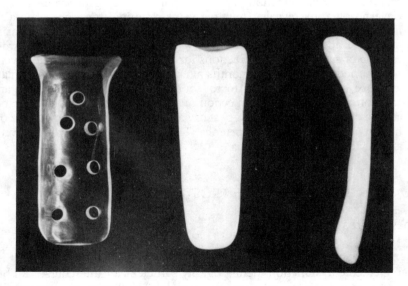

FIGURE 10.5.   A photograph of the first synthetic penile prosthesis, invented by Dr. Willard E. Goodwin. The right panel shows a side view of the device. (Photo courtesy of Dr. Goodwin.)

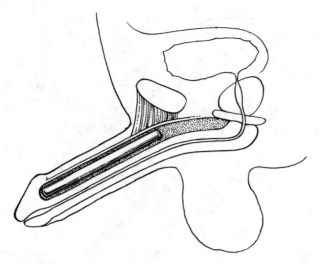

FIGURE 10.6.   A sketch of the Pearman prosthesis in the penis. A single rod was placed in the center of each corpus from glans to pubic symphysis.

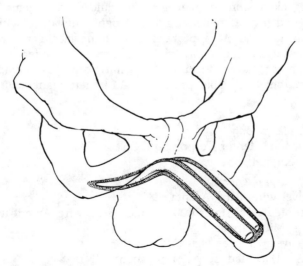

FIGURE 10.7.   A sketch showing the Small–Carrion implant, a set of two semirigid prostheses filling the entire corpora.

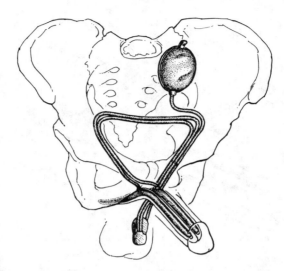

FIGURE 10.8. A sketch showing placement of the three-component inflatable prosthesis in the body. The pump was located in the scrotum; the reservoir was placed in the space in front of the bladder and behind the abdominal muscles.

the pump mechanism was activated. The cylinders then became filled with fluid, allowing expansion in diameter. The fluid-filled systems were not compressible and thus extremely rigid. The penis implanted with the hydraulic systems had a normal appearance in both the flaccid and erect states.

Today the surgeon has a wide variety of implants to offer the prospective patient. The prostheses include both semirigid and hydraulic devices. The list of currently available prostheses and their manufacturers is as follows:

Semirigid, silicone only
Small–Carrion (Mentor Corporation, Goleta, CA)
Flexirod (Surgitek, Racine, WI)

Semirigid, metal interior
Jonas (silver wire; Bard, Atlanta, GA)
American Medical Systems 600 (stainless steel wire; American Medical
    Systems, Minneapolis, MN)
Mentor (silver wire; see Figure 10.9)
Duraphase (Dacomed Corp., Minneapolis, MN)
Omniphase (Dacomed)

Inflatable
Two-piece (combined pump–reservoir and cylinders)
    Uniflate 1000 (Surgitek)
    GFS Mark II (Mentor)
Three-piece (pump, reservoir, and cylinders)
    American Medical Systems 700
    American Medical Systems Ultrex
    Mentor
Self-contained (cylinders, pump, and reservoir as one piece)
    Flexi-flate (Surgitek)
    Dynaflex (American Medical Systems; see Figure 10.10)

Choice of a Prosthesis

Surgeon's, Patient's, and Partner's Preferences

Once the decision is made to proceed with a penile prosthetic implant as the method of treatment for erectile dysfunction, the type of implant to be used must be decided upon. In this era of informed consent, the patient must be

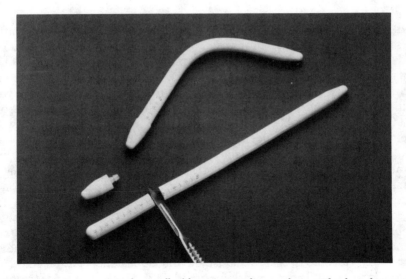

FIGURE 10.9. A present-day malleable (semirigid) prosthesis. The length is trim-mable, so that the device can be customized to size in the operating room. (Photo courtesy of Mentor Corporation, Goleta, CA.)

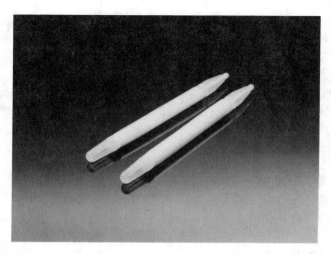

FIGURE 10.10. A self-contained inflatable prosthesis. The expandable cylinders contain fluid in an inner chamber that is pumped into a space beneath the surface, and causes increased rigidity. (Photo courtesy of American Medical Systems, Minneapolis, MN.)

told in detail about the availability and characteristics of each of the prostheses. Frequently, patients have written to one or more of the manufacturers and have based their choice upon the manufacturers' information. Other considerations include personal preference of the surgeon, the surgeon's technical ability, and limitations imposed by the hospitals. The average cost of the inflatable devices is about $3,000; that of the semirigid devices is about $1,000. It is not possible for hospitals to have a full range of sizes (with backup) for each type of device. Most operating rooms stock one type of semirigid device and the inflatable prosthesis used most often by the implanting surgeons. If the patient desires an unstocked device, usually a company representative will bring several sizes to the operating room on a per-case basis.

It is frequently helpful to provide the patient or couple with literature prepared for the lay public, with sketches of the different devices (see "Guidelines for Preoperative Preparation," below). Also, postoperative photographs or videotapes that demonstrate the appearance and method of manipulation or inflation are helpful in aiding the patient's choice, since it may be difficult to imagine squeezing either the penis or scrotum to generate an erection. Some patients are repulsed by the idea of going about in a constant state of erection.

In a follow-up study in which patients and their partners were interviewed after prosthetic surgery (Tiefer, Pedersen, & Melman, 1988), no difference was found in satisfaction ratings of men with semirigid or inflatable models. However, their female partners' satisfaction ratings were significantly lower when the patients had semirigid devices. We have also found that most men believe there is some change in penile size after the insertion of implants (Pedersen, Tiefer, Ruiz, & Melman, 1988). When queried, 50% of men thought that their penises were smaller and 19% believed that their penises were larger after surgery. Those men with the perception of smaller penile size were less satisfied with their devices. Thus, the patient's penile size has some bearing on his (and his partner's) ultimate satisfaction with surgery. It has been our recommendation to men on the low and high side of the bell-shaped curve of penile size to use the three-component inflatable device. The majority of men should be equally satisfied with either type.

In terms of ultimate penile rigidity, the three-component inflatable devices (American Medical Systems, Mentor) provide the greatest range of flaccidity and rigidity, as well as ease of inflation. The two-component devices (Mentor, Surgitek) offer about 85–90% of the rigidity of the three-component prostheses (see Figure 10.11). The self-contained inflatable cylinders offer both limited inflation and deflation. Their foremost advantage is ease of insertion. The Omniphase and Duraphase mechanical rods offer both good rigidity and flaccidity.

Other Considerations in Prosthesis Choice

Age of the Patient. Age is not a significant factor for choice of type of device. The patient must have sufficient intelligence, hand strength, and dexterity to use the inflatable variety successfully. Therefore, men with arthritis, stroke victims, and men with Parkinson's disease may be more satisfied with a semirigid, nonhydraulic, system. Also, men with large abdominal bulk may not be able to see or reach over their abdomens to inflate the cylinders.

Other Disease. Prior abdominal surgery (e.g., colectomy, cystectomy) or radiation should influence whether a retropubic reservoir is placed, as is needed with the three-component inflatable devices. Severe hypertension or other limitations for general or regional anesthesia may require that the procedure be performed with local anesthesia. Although local anesthesia can be employed for the placement of any of the prostheses, the penis-only cylinders are most easily inserted in that circumstance.

Risk of Complications. The complication rates of the different types of prostheses should also be considered in the choice of an implant (Fallon,

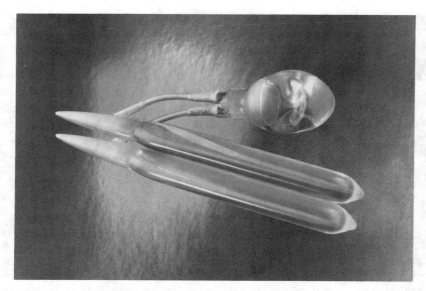

FIGURE 10.11.   A two-component inflatable prosthesis. The pump and reservoir are combined into a single structure and placed into either side of the scrotum. (Photo courtesy of Mentor Corporation, Goleta, CA.)

Rosenberg, & Culp, 1984). The patient at greatest medical risk for surgery should choose a device with the least risk of failure in order to minimize the risk of repeat operation(s). The devices with the smallest risk of failure are the pure-silicone models; there is no risk of mechanical failure with these implants. There are no published data on the long-term success of the mechanical implants. Because of their complicated internal linkages, there is a greater probability of stress wear of their metal components with time. We (Pedersen et al., 1988) noted a 28% failure rate with the unmodified Jonas (an early malleable) prosthesis (including wire breakage or unwanted rotation of the device). Long-term evaluations of the newer Jonas implant or of the American Medical Systems and Mentor semirigid devices are lacking.

In the past, the inflatable implants were susceptible to long-term rates of failure as high as 50% (McLaren & Lewis, 1990). Newer-generation implants have reduced many of the causes of failure by eliminating tubing connectors (Mentor) and by adding stronger triple-ply expansive cylinders (American Medical Systems). Although the failure rates seem much lower with the newer devices, they have not yet been objectively evaluated over the long term (at least 5 years).

Perioperative infections are a minor risk of surgery. In one large series, Montague (1987) reported a rate of infections of approximately 2.7%, whether or not the patients were diabetic. The infections occurred despite meticulous preoperative preparation and use of prophylactic antibiotics. *Staphylococcus epidermidis*, a ubiquitous skin contaminant, is the most frequent cause of infections.

Although the goal of the penile implant—to recreate a rigid phallus—is met to varying degrees with each of the prostheses now available, this is not the only or even the primary benefit of the penile implant. We found that the majority of men with successful implants, whatever their frequency of use, benefited most from the sense of restored manhood (Pedersen et al., 1988). The correction of their impotence (in the broad sense) returned their sense of masculine pride and was of greater importance than the device itself. The feeling of being *capable* of coitus, whether or not the device was used to accomplish successful intercourse, was reported by many of the men in the study as a prime benefit of surgery.

POSTSURGICAL FOLLOW-UP STUDIES

Postsurgical follow-up studies constitute a major source of information on psychological issues related to sexual surgeries. Careful research can identify problems that need to be addressed before surgery. Unfortunately, most published follow-up studies of sexual surgery have focused narrowly on the issue of surgical outcomes, with scant attention to patients' or partners' subjective experiences and evaluations. We and others who have reviewed the follow-up literature have deplored the dearth of well-designed and detailed interview studies of patients and partners who have experienced penile prosthesis implantation (Tiefer et al., 1988; Mallon & Williams, 1987; Schover, 1989). Most postoperative studies on penile prostheses include only superficial and global satisfaction information, which is subject to numerous psychological distortions (e.g., the need to justify past decisions to maintain self-esteem) (Tiefer et al., 1988; Schover, 1989; Teger, 1980).

Moreover, most follow-up studies have neglected to obtain information independently (if at all) from partners. This is especially important, since partners' reports indicate that they often have relevant information to provide about patients' experiences, as well as about their own reactions (Tiefer & Melman, 1983; Kramarsky-Binkhorst, 1978; Beutler et al., 1984). For example, in our current study of men with repaired prostheses, the typical couple has not usually communicated anxieties about having a "foreign object" in the male's body, or about the dangers of further surgery. Yet both partners' privately held feelings affect their enjoyment, as well as their performance of sexual activity (Tiefer, Moss, & Melman, 1991).

To date, there are no psychological studies focusing on effects of surgical treatments other than penile implants. A recent review of the various new surgeries for erectile dysfunction presents the results of seven papers on arterial surgeries and nine papers on venous surgeries; however, none of these provides any but the most superficial psychological information (Lue, 1990). It appears that we are in a phase of rapid technical expansion, but collection of psychological information on the experience of these treatments must become a priority in years to come. The best we can do at present is to generalize from studies of sexual and psychological coping with the penile implant and with other, nonsexual surgical procedures (Schover & Jensen, 1988).

CLINICAL EXPERIENCES

Tiefer (1990) has recently noted that interactions between patient and provider regarding erectile problems and available treatments are complex negotiations involving different symbolic universes, different interaction goals, and different discourse strategies. A rational, problem-solving approach typically dominates the provider's script: Identify the problem(s), find the cause(s), choose appropriate remedies based on etiology, and apply the remedy. In the provider's universe, erections are measurable realities; penises are standardized machines with parts that may or may not work properly; and sexuality can be reduced to a universe of acts and attitudes (Tiefer, in press).

To the extent that the patient shares the clinician's class and educational background, a similar outlook will generally prevail. However, patients with different backgrounds may approach erectile dysfunction consultations with different cultural beliefs and values from those of the clinician. They may also be preoccupied by self-esteem or security needs, and may accept or reject diagnoses or treatment suggestions on the basis of psychological defenses rather than rational problem-solving approaches.

Schover (1989) has recently stated the problem many of us have faced in this regard:

> As a clinician who has spent much of the past 10 years evaluating men with erectile dysfunction, I have noticed a recurrent paradox: the man who wants a penile prosthesis the most is usually the one who will benefit from it the least. . . . The typical man who wants a prosthesis has a very performance-oriented view of sex. He feels his erection is a gauge of his manhood. Foreplay is merely an inconvenient prelude to intercourse and the less needed, the better. He assumes that women share his opinion and are searching for the man with the biggest, hardest, and longest-lasting erection. (p. 93)

These "beliefs" are deeply held convictions, and Schover (1989) has identified postsurgical problems that may result for the man with such convictions (e.g., disappointment with penile size or rigidity). These same
problems have been reported in a number of follow-up studies (Tiefer et al.,
1988; McCarthy & McMillan, 1990; Gerstenberger, Osborne, & Furlow,
1979; Steege, Stout, & Carlson, 1986; Kaufman, Boxer, & Quinn, 1981;
Hollander & Diokno, 1984). We have recently found that the specific belief
that women are most interested in men with "superior" erections is a
significant motivation for reoperations in some men whose penile prostheses have malfunctioned (Tiefer et al., 1991). These men (often divorced
or widowed) feel vulnerable to rejection because of their diminished erectile
performance, and turn to medical technology to provide security. Even with
new or repaired prostheses, some of these men continue to feel insecure
over their partners' sexual satisfaction—a finding also reported by
McCarthy and McMillan (1990).

SELECTION OF PATIENTS FOR SEXUAL SURGERY

Controversies in the Field

There is significant disagreement in the literature over criteria for selecting
patients for penile prostheses. Very little has been written about selection
criteria for other surgical procedures, but it seems likely that the same
differences of opinion will prevail. The two extremes of opinion are represented by the following quotations. The first one is from a urological follow-
up study of 24 patients with semirigid implants:

> Our study suggests that the patient or partner who would make a poor
> psychologic adaptation is either effectively screened out by the careful but
> unaided urologist, or, as the lack of case material suggests, such maladapta-
> tion is a rare event in the larger patient population, or both. . . . Many
> clinics *grossly overevaluate men psychologically* by requiring extensive inter-
> views, psychologic testing, and overnight tumescence studies. . . . Penile
> implantation is not especially dangerous, among elective surgical proce-
> dures, from a psychologic point of view. (Blake, McCartney, Fried, &
> Fehrenbaker, 1983, pp. 255–256; emphasis added)

The opinion at the other end of the continuum is represented by
Schover (1989), a psychologist and sex therapist who recommends screening
for the "risk factors" presented in Table 10.1, and who then recommends "a
preventive course of brief sex counseling" for men and couples who evidence
these risk factors. She reports that men with erectile problems frequently

TABLE 10.1. Common Risk Factors for Postimplantation Sexual Dissatisfaction

Risk factor	Impact after surgery
Belief that size of penis is crucial in sex	Disappointment with penile length, girth, or rigidity
Belief that foreplay is a nuisance	Inability of either partner to reach orgasm because intercourse is begun without high sexual arousal
Poor sexual communication	Inability to modify sexual caressing or intercourse techniques to compensate for differences between penile prosthesis and a natural erection
Premature ejaculation	Intercourse still is too brief for satisfaction or man feels compelled to continue thrusting without arousal
Decreased orgasmic intensity	Orgasms remain disappointing to the man
Male low sexual desire	Frequency of sex remains very low
Female low sexual desire	Bickering about the frequency of sex increases, and the husband may initiate an affair
Untreated postmenopausal vaginal atrophy	The woman has severe dyspareunia
Erectile dysfunction was psychogenic	Because psychogenic problems often serve a function, a technical "cure" destabilizes the relationship or leads to a new sexual problem, such as psychogenic pain or inability to reach orgasm

Note. From "Sex Therapy for the Penile Prosthesis Recipient" by L. R. Schover, 1989, Urologic Clinics of North America, 16, 91–98. Copyright 1989 by W. B. Saunders Co. Reprinted by permission.

have concurrent psychological, interpersonal, or additional sexual difficulties, which will interfere with their successful utilization of penile prostheses.

It is probable that these differences reflect the differing perspectives of surgeons and mental health care providers. If the goal is merely to restore rigid erections, then very little screening seems necessary—perhaps just enough to eliminate patients who are grossly psychotic or litigious. However, if the goal is to restore satisfactory sexual functioning, then many more issues need to be taken into consideration.

Only further follow-up research will clarify the extent to which different types of patient screening and preoperative preparation lead to different sexual surgery outcomes. In such screening research, both patients who have received careful screening and preparation and those who have not should be included for proper interpretation of follow-up results. It is inappropriate to conclude from follow-up research that does not compare screened and unscreened patients that no screening is necessary *if* the patients who are being followed are carefully chosen in the first place. For example, one cannot conclude from our own postoperative research that high postoperative satisfaction rates indicate that the penile prosthesis is a good treatment for many or most patients. Our rates of satisfaction are only generalizable to patients who are carefully screened and prepared by a urologist–psychologist team. Many of our patients requesting surgery have been steered toward other options.

Guidelines for Selecting Patients

In general, the more criteria listed in Table 10.2 that a couple meets, the better the chances are for good results. These criteria are best assessed in separate interviews of the patient and the partner, since we have shown that information important for a proper diagnosis and choice of treatment emerges only when the sexual partner is interviewed separately (Tiefer & Melman, 1983).

The criteria are based on follow-up study results and clinical experience. The most controversial is probably the final criterion listed, "Identifiable organic cause for the erectile dysfunction." This derives from a few worrisome studies that show poor results with patients whose dysfunction is either wholly or primarily psychogenic (see Collins & Kinder, 1984, for a review of this issue). On the other hand, there are several studies clearly showing no difference in outcome relating to dysfunction etiology. Again, the differences reported may have more to do with the screening process and criteria for evaluation than with the etiologies themselves.

Another criterion requiring some discussion is "History of continued sexual activity despite erectile difficulty." Many couples cease all lovemaking activity when intercourse is not possible, and often come for evaluation and treatment after they have had no sexual activity for months or years. The

TABLE 10.2.   Criteria for Selecting Patients (and Their Partners) for Sexual Surgeries

1. Good general psychological coping and flexibility.
2. Basic knowledge about sexuality and capacity to understand the nature of both problem and treatment.
3. Cooperative and communicative lovemaking style.
4. Relationship satisfaction.
5. History of continued sexual activity despite erectile difficulty.
6. Realistic goals for postoperative sexual capacity.
7. Mutual decision for surgery.
8. Identifiable organic cause for the erectile dysfunction.

history in such cases may be of little clinical use. Details about lovemaking technique that could alert the clinician to contributory factors are unavailable. Moreover, these couples' heavy reliance on intercourse for sexual satisfaction is worrisome, given the prevalence of mixed postoperative reports about prostheses. Thus, part of good preoperative preparation includes encouraging such couples to resume nonintercourse sexual activities, as we discuss below. Not surprisingly, some couples find that their dysfunction is no longer present, and are able to proceed without further treatment.

It would be most helpful to be able to identify how these criteria should be modified in accordance with the ethnic, religious, and cultural backgrounds of patients and couples, since we know that sexual and relationship values vary enormously among different cultural and subcultural groups (McGoldrick, Pearce, & Giordano, 1982). Unfortunately, sexual medicine that takes cultural differences into account is all but nonexistent. We were able to show in our prosthesis follow-up study that ethnicity made a difference in choice of prosthesis model and in whether the partner participated in the follow-up interviews, but small numbers precluded more detailed analyses of the results (Tiefer et al., 1988).

In addition, since all studies show a wide age range in patients seeking these sexual surgeries, it would be helpful to have some idea of differential criteria based on age. Beaser, Van der Hoek, Jacobson, Flood, and DeSautels (1982), using questionnaire data from diabetic patients, suggested that men in midlife are more satisfied with penile prostheses than are younger or older men. However, there is almost no research at all in this important area of age differences in treatment choice and satisfaction.

GUIDELINES FOR PREOPERATIVE PREPARATION

Obviously, preoperative preparation must include complete information about the planned procedures, their possible risks, and their potential benefits, as well as sufficient information about relevant anatomy and physiology. Choice of vocabulary is especially important here, since misunderstandings frequently occur when a common sexual and medical vocabulary is assumed. The use of visual materials is an asset where possible, and commercial booklets, although not perfect in terms of content, do have excellent diagrams (e.g., *Understanding Impotence: A Common and Treatable Problem*, available from Krames Communications, 312 90th St., Daly City, CA 94015).

In addition to providing information, adequate preparation should include combating unrealistic expectations—a process that requires more time and effort than merely offering facts. Barrett and Furlow (1985) and Tiefer (1986) have both emphasized the misinformation available in the popular media. Men desperate for help are vulnerable to misreading even accurate information; overestimating success rates; or underestimating complications, cost, pain, or extent of physical intervention. Men with sexual problems tend to blame all of the difficulties in their lives (especially relationship difficulties) on their sexual "failure," and to hope inappropriately for magical effects even from successful treatments (Rieker, Edbril, & Garnick, 1985).

We have already mentioned the importance of resuming sexual activity if there has been a long-term cessation. This allows for some of the risk factors mentioned in Table 10.1 (e.g., poor communication, low sexual desire on the part of either partner) to be assessed and addressed, if necessary, before surgery.

CONCLUSION

Selection and preparation of patients are extremely important; they should be based more on the results of appropriate research than on clinical impressions and anecdotes. With our field in the midst of a technological explosion, however, new diagnostic and treatment modalities are emerging without concomitant information about psychological experiences. At the moment, awareness of the complex psychological and interpersonal impact of these procedures, and awareness as well of the differing and sometimes conflicting disciplinary emphases, at least provide a beginning.

REFERENCES

Barrett, D. M., & Furlow, W. L. (1985). Penile prosthesis implantation. In R. T. Segraves & H. W. Schoenberg (Eds.), *Diagnosis and treatment of erectile disturbances* (pp. 219–240). New York: Plenum.

Beaser, R. S., Van der Hoek, C., Jacobson, A. M., Flood, T. M., & DeSautels, R. E.

(1982). Experience with penile prostheses in the treatment of impotence in diabetic men. *Journal of the American Medical Association, 248*, 943–948.

Beutler, L. E., Scott, F. B., Karacan, I., Baer, P. E., Rogers, R. R., & Morris, J. (1984). Women's satisfaction with partner's penile implant. *Urology, 24*, 552–558.

Blake, D. J., McCartney, C., Fried, F. A., & Fehrenbacker, L. G. (1983). Psychiatric assessment of penile implant recipient: Preliminary study. *Urology, 21*, 252–256.

Collins, G. F., & Kinder, B. N. (1984). Adjustment following surgical implantation of a penile prosthesis: A critical overview. *Journal of Sex and Marital Therapy, 10*, 255–271.

Coughlin, P. W. F., Carson, C. C. C., & Paulson, D. F. (1984). Surgical correction of Peyronie's disease. *Journal of Urology, 131*, 282–285.

Devine, C. J., Jr., & Horton, C. E. (1983). Surgical treatment of Peyronie's disease with a dermal graft. *Journal of Urology, 111*, 44–49.

Ebbehoj, J., & Wagner, G. (1979). Insufficient penile erection due to abnormal drainage of cavernous bodies. *Urology, 13*, 507–510.

Fallon, B., Rosenberg, S., & Culp, D. A. (1984). Long-term followup in patients with an inflatable penile prosthesis. *Journal of Urology, 132*, 270–271.

Gerstenberger, D. L., Osborne, D., & Furlow, W. L. (1979). Inflatable penile prosthesis: Followup study of patient-partner satisfaction. *Urology, 14*, 583–587.

Goodwin, W. E., & Scott, W. W. (1952). Phalloplasty. *Journal of Urology, 68*, 903–908.

Hauri, D. (1986). A new operative technique in vasculogenic erectile impotence. *World Journal of Urology, 4*, 237–249.

Hollander, J. B., & Diokno, A. C. (1984). Success with penile prosthesis from patient's viewpoint. *Urology, 23*, 141–143.

Kaufman, J. J., Boxer, B., & Quinn, M. C. (1981). Physical and psychological results of penile prostheses: A statistical survey. *Journal of Urology, 126*, 173–175.

Kramarsky-Binkhorst, S. (1978). Female partner perception of Small-Carrion implant. *Urology, 12*, 545–548.

Landthaler, M., Kodalle, W., & Braun-Falco, O. (1983). Radiotherapy of induratio penis plastica. In P. O. Hubinont (Ed.), *Progress in reproductive biology and medicine* (Vol. 9, pp. 73–77). Basel: Karger.

Lewis, R. (1991). Results of surgery for veno-occlusive disease. *Journal of Sex and Marital Therapy, 17*, 129–135.

Lue, T. F. (1990). Impotence: A patient's goal-directed approach to treatment. *World Journal of Urology, 8*, 67–74.

Lydston, G. F. (1908). The surgical treatment of impotency. *American Journal of Clinical Medicine, 15*, 1571–1573.

Mallon, D. S., & Williams, C. F. (1987). A review of patient and partner perceptions of the penile prosthesis. *Journal of Urological Nursing, 6*, 17–26.

McCarthy, J., & McMillan, S. (1990). Patient/partner satisfaction with penile implant surgery. *Journal of Sex Education and Therapy, 16*, 25–37.

McGoldrick, M., Pearce, J. K., & Giordano, J. (Eds.). (1982). *Ethnicity and family therapy.* New York: Guilford Press.

McLaren, R. H., & Lewis, R. H. (1990). The reoperated penile implant. *International Journal of Impotence Research, 2*(Suppl.), 463–464.

Melman, A. (1988). The evaluation of sexual dysfunction. *Urologic Radiology, 10,* 119–128.

Melman, A., & Holland, T. F. (1978). Evaluation of the dermal graft inlay technique for the surgical treatment of Peyronie's disease. *Journal of Urology, 120,* 420–422.

Metz, P., Ebbehoj, J., Uhrenholdt, A., & Wagner, G. (1983). Peyronie's disease and erectile failure. *Journal of Urology, 130,* 1103–1104.

Michal, V., Kramer, R., Popsichal, J., & Hejhal, L. (1973). Direct arterial anastomosis to the cavernous body in treatment of erectile impotence. *Rozhledy v Chirurgii, 552,* 587–591.

Montague, D. K. (1987). Periprosthetic infections. *Journal of Urology, 138,* 68–69.

Nesbit, R. M. (1965). Congenital curvature of the phallus: Report of three cases with description of corrective procedure. *Journal of Urology, 93,* 230–232.

Pearman, R. O. (1967). Treatment of organic impotence by implantation of a penile prosthesis. *Journal of Urology, 97,* 716–719.

Pedersen, B., Tiefer, L., Ruiz, M., & Melman, A. (1988). Evaluation of patients and partners one to four years following penile prosthesis surgery. *Journal of Urology, 139,* 956–958.

Puech-Leao, P., Reis, J. M. S. M., Glina, S., & Reichelt, A. C. (1987). Leakage through the crural edge of corpus cavernosum. *European Urology, 13,* 163–165.

Rieker, P. P., Edbril, S. D., & Garnick, M. B. (1985). Curative testis cancer therapy: Psychosocial sequelae. *Journal of Clinical Oncology, 3,* 1117–1126.

Rossman, B., Mieza, M., & Melman, A. (1990). Penile vein ligation for corporal incompetence: An evaluation of short-term and long-term results. *Journal of Urology, 144,* 679–682.

Scardino, P. L., & Scott, W. W. (1949). The use of tocopherols in the treatment of Peyronie's disease. *Annals of the New York Academy of Sciences, 52,* 390–396.

Schover, L. R. (1989). Sex therapy for the penile prosthesis recipient. *Urologic Clinics of North America, 16,* 91–98.

Schover, L. R., & Jensen, S. B. (1988). *Sexuality and chronic illness.* New York: Guilford Press.

Scott, F. B., Bradley, W. E., & Timm, G. W. (1973). Management of erectile impotence: Use of implantable inflatable prosthesis. *Urology, 2,* 80–82.

Small, M. P., Carrion, H. M., & Gordon, J. A. (1975). Small–Carrion penile prosthesis: New implant for management of impotence. *Urology, 5,* 479–486.

Sohn, M., Sikora, R., Bohndorf, K., & Deutz, F.-J. (1990). Selective microsurgery in arteriogenic erectile failure. *World Journal of Urology, 8,* 104–110.

Steege, J. F., Stout, A. L., & Carlson, C. C. (1986). Patient satisfaction in Scott and Small–Carrion penile implant recipients: A study of 52 patients. *Archives of Sexual Behavior, 15,* 393–399.

Taylor, S. E. (1983). Adjustment to threatening events: A theory of cognitive adaptation. *American Psychologist, 38,* 1161–1173.

Teger, A. I. (1980). *Too much invested to quit.* Elmsford, NY: Pergamon Press.

Tiefer, L. (1986). In pursuit of the perfect penis: The medicalization of male sexuality. *American Behavioral Scientist, 29,* 579–599.

Tiefer, L. (1990, March). *Beyond diagnosis: Patient–doctor rhetoric in the evaluation of sexual dysfunction.* Paper presented at the annual meeting of the Society for Sex Research and Therapy, Baltimore.

Tiefer, L. (in press). Critique of the DSM-III-R nosology of sexual dysfunctions. *Psychiatric Medicine.*

Tiefer, L., & Melman, A. (1983). Interview of wives: A necessary adjunct in the evaluation of impotence. *Sexuality and Disability, 6,* 167–175.

Tiefer, L., & Moss, S., & Melman, A. (1991). Follow-up of patients and partners experiencing penile prosthesis repairs, removals and replacements. *Journal of Sex and Marital Therapy, 17,* 113–128.

Tiefer, L., Pedersen, B., & Melman, A. (1988). Psychosocial follow-up of penile prosthesis implant patients and partners. *Journal of Sex and Marital Therapy, 14,* 184–201.

Wespes, E., & Schulman, C. C. (1985). Venous leakage: Surgical treatment of a curable cause of impotence. *Journal of Urology, 133,* 796–798.

11

Self-Injection Therapy and External Vacuum Devices in the Treatment of Erectile Dysfunction: Methods and Outcome

STANLEY E. ALTHOF AND LOUISA A. TURNER

Physical interventions for erectile failure are widely used nowadays, both for men with organic dysfunction and for some individuals with psychogenic difficulties. In the past decade, two methods in particular have become increasingly popular: self-injection therapy and external vacuum devices. These two approaches were first made available for clinical use in the mid-1980s, and despite the absence of reliable data, it appears that self-injection therapy and vacuum pump devices are currently among the preferred first-line treatments in many centers.

In this chapter, Althof and Turner provide a comprehensive, well-balanced review of the advantages and disadvantages of these highly popular treatment methods. Injection therapy, they point out, grew out of early studies on pharmacological control of bladder function. At the present time, three drug substances are used in different combinations; papaverine hydrochloride, phentolamine mesylate, and prostaglandin E_1. Althof and Turner recommend a combination of papaverine and phentolamine to produce erections that are sufficiently rigid and long-lasting. Dosages need to be carefully regulated, however, especially for patients with neurogenic erectile dysfunction, who may display hypersensitivity to vasoactive agents. Various other side effects have been reported, ranging from fibrotic nodules, scarring, and liver problems to occasional instances of priapism. Althof and Turner report that negative subjective reactions are very common with this form of therapy, which is acceptable to only 40–50% of patients in their experience. On the other hand, self-injection therapy may be combined with more traditional forms of sex therapy, and can be highly effective for restoring erectile capacity and sexual self-confidence in certain individuals. The authors provide an informative review of common partner reactions to self-injection therapy, which are illustrated in several excellent case vignettes.

Although the first prototype for an external vacuum device was patented more than a half century ago, this approach to treatment has only become clinically available in the past 5 years. Since that time, the procedure has gained rapid acceptance, and is now viewed as an effective and less invasive alternative to self-injection therapy. Althof and Turner describe five different types of vacuum devices currently available, as well as the potential side effects associated with each. Patients may experience hematomas or ecchymosis during the initial phases of learning to operate the device, although these are not usually serious. Other complaints include pulling of scrotal tissue into the cylinder, and blocked or painful erection due to constriction of the urethra. External vaccum devices are contraindicated for men with certain hematological conditions (e.g., dyscrasia) or with poor manual dexterity as a result of Parkinson's disease or other disorders. Despite these potential difficulties, external vacuum devices are well tolerated by 80–95% of patients, according to the authors. As with self-injection therapy, they recommend combining this form of treatment with psychotherapy or sex therapy for optimal results.

In addition to a highly specific and detailed comparison of these two popular methods of treatment, Althof and Turner provide a thoughtful discussion of various clinical issues associated with their use. For example, they observe that single men typically prefer self-injection therapy as less intrusive and easier to conceal with a new partner. Patients in a committed relationship may prefer the vacuum pump device as having potentially fewer serious side effects. Overall, these two approaches have added a significant new dimension to the treatment of both organic and psychogenic erectile disorders.

Stanley E. Althof, Ph.D., is Director of the Male Sexual Health Center at University Hospitals of Cleveland and Associate Professor of Psychology at Case Western Reserve University School of Medicine. He has published widely in the field of sex therapy and has conducted several recent outcome studies of self-injection therapy and external vacuum devices.

Louisa A. Turner, Ph.D., is Assistant Clinical Professor of Psychology at Case Western Reserve University School of Medicine and in private practice in Cleveland, Ohio. She has written numerous articles that address the medical and psychological impact of self-injection and vacuum pump therapy.

NEW TREATMENTS, TOUGH QUESTIONS

The 1980s ushered in several new treatments for erectile dysfunction. Previously, three options were available: (1) psychotherapy; (2) implantation of a penile prosthesis; and (3) hormone therapy. Although these treatments have all been refined and continue to be utilized, four other alternatives have been developed: (1) yohimbine; (2) vascular surgery; (3) self-injection of vaso-active substances; and (4) external vacuum devices.

When fewer options were available, the rules regarding their use were more straightforward. Patients with psychogenic erectile difficulties were referred for psychotherapy; patients who were deficient in testosterone received hormone replacement; and patients with other organic conditions were referred for penile prostheses. There was generally no second line of treatment for psychogenic patients who did not recover their potency with psychotherapy. Similarly, if a prosthesis failed, or the patient with an organic dysfunction declined the implant, no other forms of treatment were available to restore the capacity for intercourse.

Inevitably, new options raise new questions. The rules are no longer as straightforward as they once were; now clinicians need to develop thoughtful strategies for steering their way through the array of treatment choices. Even though each decision is ultimately made by the patient and his partner, as therapists we offer suggestions and have complex questions to consider. Do we make our recommendations based on efficacy, cost, side effects, patient acceptance rates, aesthetics, or irreversibility? Do we begin with the least radical alternative and proceed stepwise to more radical alternatives? Do we consider offering men with psychogenic dysfunctions self-injection or an external vacuum device? This chapter discusses these questions for two of the newer alternatives: self-injection and external vacuum pump therapy.

SELF-INJECTION THERAPY WITH VASOACTIVE DRUGS

Development

The first paper on pharmacologically induced erections appeared in the late 1970s. Domer, Wessler, Brown, and Charles (1978) were studying the autonomic nervous system's role in bladder function and noted that erections resulted from the infusion of phentolamine, phenoxybenzamine, terbutaline, and salbutamol. Their study went unnoticed until several years later, when Brindley (1983) and Virag and his associates (Virag & Virag, 1983; Virag, Frydman, Legman, & Virag, 1984) independently published papers reporting that intracavernosal injection of phenoxybenzamine and papaverine induced erection. These findings led to the development of home self-injection programs, in which men were taught to inject themselves and given syringes and medication for home use (Althof et al., 1987; Nellans, Ellis, & Kramer-Levien, 1987; Nelson, 1989; Sidi, Cameron, Duffy, & Lange, 1986; Sidi, 1988; Trapp, 1987; Zorgniotti & Lefleur, 1985).

Clinical investigations of intracavernosal injection have focused primarily on four medications: (1) phenoxybenzamine hydrochloride, (2) papaverine hydrochloride, (3) phentolamine mesylate, and (4) prostaglandin E_1. Other agents also reported to induce erection are vasoactive intestinal peptide, theophylline, thymoxamine, imipramine, verapamil, moxisylate, and nitroglycerine (Brindley, 1983, 1986; Buvat, Lemaire, Buvat-Herbaut, & Marcolin, 1989; Lue & Tanagho, 1987; Virag, 1985; Willis, Ottesen, Wagner, Sundler, & Fahrenkrug, 1981).

Phenoxybenzamine is an alpha-adrenergic blocking agent not available in the United States. Although it was one of the first drugs discovered to induce erection, it was painful to inject, was slow to produce turgidity, and resulted in penile enlargement for up to 3 days (Brindley, 1983, 1986).

Papaverine, a smooth muscle relaxant, was less painful to inject and induced erection more rapidly and for a shorter duration than phenoxybenzamine. Zorgniotti and Lefleur (1985) later showed that a combination of papaverine and phentolamine, an alpha-adrenergic blocker, was superior to papaverine alone. Most clinicians employ a combination of 15–60 mg of papaverine with 0.5–2 mg of phentolamine. A moderate erection is usually evident within 15 minutes. Turgidity further increases with sexual stimulation, resulting in an erection that lasts for 1–4 hours (Kursh et al., 1988).

Prostaglandin E_1 is a smooth muscle relaxant. The first clinical trials in humans were performed independently by Ishii et al. (1989) and by Virag and Adaikan (1987). The accepted dose levels range between 5 μg and 20 μg.

Method of Action

Papaverine relaxes the arterial and trabecular smooth muscles by inhibiting oxidative phosphorylation, blocking cyclic adenosine monophosphate phosphodiesterase, and interfering with calcium flow during muscle contraction; this increases arterial inflow and corporal veno-occlusion (Krane, Goldstein, & Saenz de Tejada, 1989). It also has an antinicotinic effect on ganglionic transmission (Poch & Kubovetz, 1971; Bauer & Capek, 1972).

Phentolamine induces smooth muscle relaxation by blocking the alpha-adrenergic receptors on cell membranes. Sexual stimulation enhances, and anxiety interferes with, the efficacy of these medications.

The mode of action of prostaglandin E_1 is less clear. It is thought to exert an inhibitory effect on adrenergic receptors by preventing norepinephrine release, thereby relaxing the smooth musculature (Waldhauser & Schramek, 1988).

Indications for Use

Self-injection of vasoactive substances should be considered a first-line treatment for mixed, idiopathic, and organic erectile dysfunctions. It is not the treatment of choice for psychogenic impotence.

Medical–Legal Issues

Neither papaverine, phentolamine, nor prostaglandin E_1 has been approved for treating erectile dysfunction by the Food and Drug Administration (FDA). Because there is little financial incentive, it is unlikely that drug manufacturers will seek FDA approval. What this means for the clinician is not entirely clear. There is some risk involved in using a medication that goes beyond the FDA-approved indications. However, what stands in the clinician's favor is a considerable body of literature that documents the efficacy and relative safety of the drugs. To minimize risk of litigation, many clinicians have their patients sign a consent form that clearly details the risks and benefits of self-injection therapy. A patient's spouse can also sign a separate form, stating that she is aware that her partner is undergoing this treatment and that she has been apprised of the gains and limitations of self-injection.

Trial Dose Procedure

Treatment begins with the trial dose procedure. The patient comes to the doctor's office to receive physician-administered injections. At each visit, the dose of medication is increased until either the man has a satisfactory erection, or the maximum dose fails to induce an adequate result.

The first trial dose is limited to 15 mg of papaverine. If the response is poor, a second injection of 0.5 mg of phentolamine is given during this first office visit. Thereafter, the following schedule of dose increases is often used: 30 mg papaverine and 0.5 mg phentolamine; 30 mg papaverine and 1 mg phentolamine; 30 mg papaverine and 2 mg of phentolamine; 45 mg papaverine and 1.5 mg phentolamine; 45 mg papaverine and 2 mg phentolamine; 60 mg papaverine and 1 mg phentolamine; and the ceiling dose, 60 mg papaverine and 2 mg phentolamine. Although some clinicians go beyond these dosage levels, our experience suggests that other options should be considered when the patient fails to respond at 60 mg of papaverine and 2 mg of phentolamine (Kursh et al., 1988).

Patients with neurogenic erectile dysfunction have denervation hypersensitivity to these medications and are at risk for developing prolonged erection. Therefore physicians often begin the trial dose procedure with less than 7.5 mg of papaverine.

Injections are given at the base of the penis at the 3 o'clock or 9 o'clock positions (posterolateral, away from the neurovascular bundle and urethra), using a disposable 1-ml insulin syringe and a 26- or 27-gauge needle. Holding the syringe perpendicular to the penis, the patient inserts the needle through the tough tunica albuginea into the left or right corpus cavernosum (Figure 11.1). A popping is usually heard and felt as the needle passes

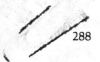

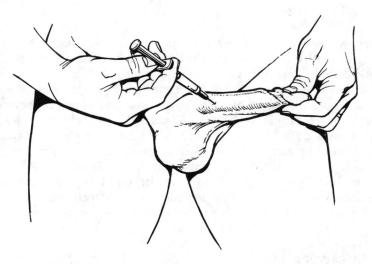

FIGURE 11.1.   Illustration of intracavernosal injection.

through the tunica into the corpora. The needle is withdrawn slightly and the medication is slowly injected. Some physicians suggest that a tourniquet be tied around the base of the penis prior to injection to reduce the venous outflow, thereby increasing the local concentration of the injected material (Sidi & Reddy, 1990).

Patients' psychological responses to the trial dose phase warrant careful attention. Because injections need to be used within 30 minutes of intercourse, and several visits to the clinic are often necessary to establish the proper dose, this may be a frustrating time for couples. Some manage these frustrations with grace, humor, and creativity; these patients joke about how they would respond to the proverbial policeman's question, "What's the hurry?", if caught speeding on the way to a motel. Others, however, are demoralized.

Case Vignette

One couple was in the midst of trial dosing at Christmas time. They planned to go from our offices in midtown Cleveland to a downtown hotel. Although the man had a good erection when the couple left the office, it unfortunately subsided on the way to the hotel. When asked at the next visit how things went, the wife vented her frustration by saying, "Let's put it this way, it was no miracle on 34th Street!"

After determining the proper dose, the patient is taught how to use sterile technique, how to draw up medication, and where and how to inject himself. This process is usually accomplished in 1 hour by a nurse educator. Should the patient be unable or unwilling to inject himself, the partner is invited to learn the technique. Once the nurse educator is satisfied that the patient and/or his partner can safely inject the drug, they are given a 1-month supply of medication and syringes.

Efficacy

Self-injection of papaverine and phentolamine has been employed as a means of temporarily reversing erectile dysfunction that is due to neurogenic, vasculogenic, hormonal, and psychological factors. This alternative is most effective for patients with neurogenic problems, such as those with spinal cord injuries (Bodner, Lindan, Leffler, Kursh, & Resnick, 1987; Sidi, Cameron, Dykstra, Reinberg, & Lange, 1987); it is least effective in men with severe corporal veno-occlusive dysfunction and/or arterial insufficiency (Krane et al., 1989).

We prospectively studied 42 patients who completed 1 year of self-injection with papaverine and phentolamine (Althof et al., 1987, 1991). Follow-up appointments with each patient and partner (when available) were scheduled for 1, 3, 6, and 12 months after beginning self-injection. The men injected themselves an average of five times per month; 83% of the injections produced satisfactory erections. It was difficult to discern all the factors that produced the 17% failure rate; the primary explanations appeared to be poor injection technique, outdated phentolamine (i.e., phentolamine that was constituted in solution more than 60 days prior to use), worsening vascular disease, and tachyphylaxis (i.e., lessening effectiveness over time of the same dose because of enhanced metabolism). When pretreatment and postinjection sexual functioning were contrasted, there were statistically significant improvements in the quality of erections, frequency of intercourse, frequency of orgasm, and sexual satisfaction. These positive gains were evident at 1 month and persisted throughout all follow-up visits.

The efficacy of intracavernosal prostaglandin E_1 was studied by Ishii et al. (1989), who reported that 62% of men achieved complete erection, 24% achieved incomplete erection, and 14% had poor responses. Waldhauser and Schramek (1988) compared erectile response to papaverine and phentolamine with the response to prostaglandin E_1 and found protaglandin E_1 to be more effective. Reiss (1989) demonstrated that prostaglandin E_1 produced erections in men who failed to achieve or maintain a good response to papaverine.

Psychosocial Impact

There are also significant psychological changes associated with self-injection therapy. In our study (Althof et al., 1991), there were significant improvements in general psychiatric symptomatology over the course of the year, as measured by the Symptom Checklist 90—Revised (SCL-90-R; Derogatis, Rickels, & Rock, 1976), and anxiety, as measured by the State–Trait Anxiety Inventory (STAI; Spielberger, Gorsuch, & Lushene, 1970). Bahren et al. (1989) reported that 78% of their sample experienced improved self-esteem as a result of self-injection therapy.

Two vignettes follow. The first describes a positive outcome with self-injection therapy; the second describes a treatment failure.

Case Vignette

A 30-year-old financial analyst hoped to save a few dollars by climbing up a 30-foot ladder to clean the gutters on his house. He fell, sustaining a spinal cord injury. Upon being told he would never walk again, he and his wife, a registered nurse, sought additional consultation. Their persistence paid off when they found a surgical team with considerable expertise. Although he never really regained control over bowel and bladder functions, he was eventually able to walk with a limp. Despite his partial response to spinal cord decompression surgery, he had unreliable, short-lived erections, decreased penile sensation, and rare ejaculations. The couple was eager to have children and was pursuing artificial insemination when first seen in our clinic.

Injections of papaverine and phentolamine induced good erections. The patient's ejaculation frequency increased to two-thirds of the time. He reported, "The injection treatment is working wonderfully. I still don't get good erections without the injections, but our reaction is different; we don't get so frustrated. What surprises us, though, is all the other effects. I feel more normal, more like there's a real place in the world for me. I am more assertive and less depressed. Our relationship is more comfortable and more loving, and the idea that we can get pregnant like everybody else and be normal parents is wonderful." His wife confirmed these changes and added, "I even feel more self-confident. It's funny; even though I knew his problems were physical, I hadn't realized how inadequate I felt and how much I thought things were my fault. You really have turned our lives around."

Case Vignette

Following radical prostatectomy, a retired accountant developed erectile difficulties. He also complained of postsurgical "hypersensitivity" of the penis and decreased sensation with orgasm. Over the 8 years following surgery, the hypersensitivity diminished; the weak orgasm remained. He chose not to be implanted with a prosthesis, fearing that surgery would reactivate the hypersensitivity. We thought that this patient was an excellent candidate for papaverine–phentolamine injections because of a good marital climate, intact sexual desire, and the spouses' admirable life coping mechanisms (they cared effectively for an adult son with Down's syndrome).

During the trial dose procedure, the patient obtained a satisfactory erection. However, he experienced a painful burning sensation on the right side of the penis, but not on the left. He fainted during the second trial dose injection; with embarrassment, he mentioned his lifelong fear of needles.

Self-injection facilitated weekly intercourse. At 1 month, the couple was pleased; the patient's only complaint was weak orgasmic sensation. By the third month, however, burning sensations had become unbearable, and the patient decided to discontinue the program. The couple felt they would learn to surmount this loss, as they had so many others in life.

Through Women's Eyes

It is essential that clinicians understand that a treatment administered to one partner affects the other. We prospectively studied the sexual and psychosocial impact on the partners of men who utilized self-injection of papaverine and phentolamine. When pretreatment status was contrasted with that at follow-up 1 year later, partners reported statistically significant positive increases in sexual satisfaction, sexual arousal, frequency of intercourse, and frequency of coital orgasm (Althof et al., 1989b).

The women also reported feeling more at ease in their marital relationships. From the women's perspective, restoration of potency led to more generalized changes in the men's self-esteem, which made it easier to be with them. Several women noted that restoration of potency made them feel closer to their husbands, and opened up new channels for communication about topics that had previously been avoided.

The women reflected upon how stressful lovemaking had been prior to their partners' initiating injection therapy. The uncertainty about erection had fostered hurried and anxious attempts at lovemaking. At the 1-year follow-up, several women spontaneously commented upon how relaxed, unhurried, assured, and even "fun" sex had become. Some characterized lovemaking as better than ever because the erection persisted after ejaculation, which allowed them time to achieve an unhurried orgasm. Said one female, "It's a real boon for women to know about. Now that I don't have to hurry up, it's like dying and going to heaven." On the other hand, one partner commented, "Two hours is a bit much."

Negative responses focused on the lack of spontaneity that accompanied injection therapy. By the 1-year follow-up, the majority of couples who continued to use papaverine had adapted to this artificial mechanism for inducing erection. Some women felt hesitant and guilty about initiating lovemaking because initiation contained a covert demand that the men inject themselves. This dilemma was solved by one woman who signaled her husband about her amorous wishes by leaving a syringe on his pillow. Some women were deeply disappointed because injection therapy did not boost their partners' sexual desire.

Side Effects

Seven potential side effects have been associated with self-injection therapy: (1) prolonged erection (priapism), (2) fibrotic nodules, (3) liver function abnormalities, (4) bruising, (5) vasovagal episodes, (6) pain, and (7) infection.

Prolonged erection from intracavernosal injection of papaverine and/or phentolamine has occurred during the trial dose phase in 2.3% to 15% of patients (Zentgraf, Ludwig, & Ziegler, 1989). "Prolonged" is defined as continuing for more than 4 hours. Priapism occurs infrequently during home self-injection, usually because a patient experiments with his medication levels. This side effect has been reported to occur less frequently with prostaglandin E_1 (Krane et al., 1989). Men with neurogenic erectile dysfunctions are most susceptible to prolonged erection. Patients are advised to return for intervention if an erection persists beyond 4 hours. Intracavernosal injection of an alpha-adrenergic receptor agonist, such as phenylephrine or epinephrine, often reverses the erectile response. If this is not effective, surgical intervention may be required.

There has been considerable variation in the reported incidence of fibrotic plaque or nodule development with papaverine and/or phentolamine. The lowest estimate is 1.5% (Padma-Nathan, Goldstein, & Krane, 1986), whereas the highest is 60% (Levine et al., 1989). Krane et al. (1989) reported a lower incidence of nodule development with prostaglandin E_1.

Although the origin of plaques is unknown, investigators speculate that they may be related to the low pH of papaverine, high frequency of injection, number of months on self-injection, and/or faulty injection technique (Levine et al., 1989). Clinicians are concerned that plaques may lead to a Peyronie-like penile curvature. When this occurs, cessation of self-injection is recommended. Also, corporal fibrosis makes later implantation of a penile prosthesis more difficult. These plaques may disappear once treatment is stopped.

The incidence of reported liver function abnormalities associated with papaverine and/or phentolamine varies from 0.4% (Zentgraf et al., 1989) to 40% (Levine et al., 1989). In Levine et al.'s (1989) study, 40% of men had at least one abnormal value in serum glutamic–oxaloacetic transaminase, bilirubin, lactate dehydrogenase, or alkaline phosphatase. None of these patients had symptoms of hepatic disease. Because papaverine is considered potentially hepatotoxic, liver function values should be monitored while patients inject themselves (Direman, 1973). No research studies have linked prostaglandin E_1 to liver function abnormalities.

From 25% to 50% of men have developed bruising, hematomas, or ecchymosis (Girdley, Bruskewitz, Feyzi, Graversen, & Gassner, 1988; Levine et al., 1989). These symptoms are usually the results of poor injection technique and do not require medical intervention.

Orthostatic hypotension has developed in 2% of patients injecting with papaverine and/or phentolamine (Sidi et al., 1986). A lower incidence of vasovagal symptoms is reported with prostaglandin E_1.

Pain is an infrequently reported occurrence with papaverine and/or phentolamine. With prostaglandin E_1, however, 75% of patients report significant pain and burning during injection and while erect (Krane et al., 1989; Waldhauser & Schramek, 1988).

Although infection is uncommon, it is most often associated with reusing needles. The only life-threatening development following intracavernosal injection of papaverine has been reported by Hashmat and Abraham (1987). One of their patients developed a pulmonary embolism following infection secondary to prolonged erection.

Patient Acceptance

Although self-injection therapy has been shown to be a safe, reliable treatment, a large percentage of patients do not accept it. Approximately 50% (Althof et al., 1989a; Sidi, Pratap, & Chem, 1988) of men who are referred for or begin treatment fail to continue. The majority of these patients drop out either after evaluation or during the trial dose phase. Once they begin home self-injection, the dropout rate significantly decreases.

In our study, the men who declined injection therapy did so because they could not accept the idea of injecting themselves and/or were concerned with the potential side effects. Those patients who dropped out after beginning trial dosing or after beginning self-injection were dissatisfied with the effectiveness of treatment. The low patient acceptance rate suggests that more time needs to be spent in assessing motivation for treatment and willingness to accept penile injection.

Psychotherapy and Self-Injection

Midway through our first efficacy study, we wondered whether injection would help patients with psychogenic erectile disorders who had not improved with psychotherapy. With some trepidation, we offered self-injection to 15 patients who had been in psychotherapy for at least 6 months without symptom remission (Turner et al., 1989). We were concerned with the potential negative effects (increased marital discord, anxiety attacks, deepening depression, and symptom substitution) of overriding an important psychological symptom, but wished to determine whether self-injection could alleviate severe performance anxiety, bypass unconscious conflict, and enhance psychological intimacy. We believed that the risks of this study were modest, because self-injection was a reversible treatment that was not likely to damage natural function.

We concluded that performance anxiety was not alleviated, because the majority of the men remained dependent upon self-injection in order to have intercourse. Most were hesitant even to try without injecting themselves. Symptom substitution did not occur. However, four men had concomitant sexual dysfunctions; three were unable to ejaculate during intercourse, and one had premature ejaculation. These men continued to manifest these dysfunctions after 6 months on self-injection. The majority of men did not demonstrate an enhanced capacity for psychological intimacy. Most of the man had voiced the hope that injection therapy would enable them to engage in a relationship or to improve their marriages; in general, restoration of potency did not effect these changes.

The following case illustrates treatment with psychotherapy and self-injection of papaverine and phentolamine.

Case Vignette

Peter, a 37-year-old divorced attorney with primary sexual dysfunction, was regularly able to achieve firm, long-lasting erections with masturbation. He had adequate sexual drive and a primarily heteroerotic fantasy life. We believed that concerns with gender identity (masculine adequacy), extreme performance anxiety, and possibly concerns with sexual orientation were at the root of his erectile dysfunction. These psychodynamic speculations were derived from the following history.

When Peter was a young boy, his father had ridiculed his body, leading him to believe that he was insufficiently manly to warrant admiration or respect. He was raised to believe that his family was superior to others, that one should be dutiful, that emotions should never be expressed, and that sex was something only for animals. The patient had vague memories of sexual abuse at the hands of his mother during early childhood, and vivid memories of repeated abuse by a female nanny at age 12. Initially, he was unclear whether these events might have had an impact on his adult development.

Rather, Peter believed his failure to maintain an erection during a college drug orgy and his subsequent humiliation by peers had laid the foundation for his current sexual problems. He subsequently joined the

Marines to "become a man." During repeated visits to the local brothel, he was unable to sustain an erection sufficient for intercourse. During this time, the patient gave in to his episodic homoerotic fantasies and once engaged in mutual masturbation with another man. Later, he married, but was unable to consummate his marriage for the 8 years of its existence. He became preoccupied with sexual failure and began to avoid any form of partner sexual interactions; eventually, he and his wife divorced.

This man was seen in weekly psychodynamically oriented psychotherapy for over a year. The patient struggled to understand his early parental relationships, recognized his split-off aggression, and began to relate deeply to his therapist. These gains generalized to relationships with others; he received feedback about being less rigid and felt more capable of intimacy. He began dating and met a vicacious 36-year-old actress named Heidi. After dating for 6 months, Peter was still unable to sustain an erection during foreplay or intercourse. He was also unable to ejaculate when manually stimulated. Peter requested to be evaluated for injection therapy.

We agreed with the therapist's belief that, in spite of the substantial gains derived from treatment, Peter's sexual problem was not likely to remit via continued psychotherapy alone. Peter had his first injection and fainted as he was starting to develop a good erection. Later he remarked, "It felt like I was losing control. I was scared. It makes me realize how much I need to stay in control." Subsequent test doses were administered without complication; however, Peter and Heidi never managed to coordinate their schedules to make use of the injection-induced erections. The patient told his therapist that he thought Heidi was purposefully planning dinner parties or buying theater tickets on the nights he received injections. It was at this point that the couple was referred for conjoint treatment.

The first few sessions addressed the couple's severe performance anxiety. Even though Peter would inject himself, he often failed to achieve an erection. It was never clear whether he employed poor injection techniques or whether his performance anxiety overrode the medication. Preoccupied with failure, Peter could not concentrate on sensation. Heidi, for her part, became obsessed with producing a good erection; the harder she tried, the more frustrated they became. In her past sexual experiences, she had considered the man's erection a sign of being pleased by her. Now she was struggling to believe that Peter enjoyed her caresses. The therapist attempted to redirect the focus of lovemaking from producing an erection to concentrating on sensation.

Peter awoke one morning with a firm erection, and Heidi was able to masturbate him to orgasm. This was the first time he was able to ejaculate in her presence. They were then able to move on to having intercourse via injection-induced erections, but Peter still could not ejaculate in the vagina. At about this time, Peter terminated individual psychotherapy.

When Heidi accepted Peter's marriage proposal, Peter disclosed "the truth" about his sexual history. Up to this point, he had allowed her to believe that his dysfunction was the result of his previous marriage. Heidi became despondent, imagining that she and Peter would never have a normal sex life. She had believed that a few months of couples psychotherapy would cure him. The therapist explained that her expectations were unrealistic. He told her that she should think in terms of a year or more, and stressed that orgasm in her presence was a positive sign, as was his ability to sustain erections without injection. When they began to process Peter's revelation, Heidi was very understanding. She understood how Peter's abuse at the hands of a nanny and later humiliation in college might cause sexual problems. She herself revealed an adolescent molestation that had resulted in several years of promiscuous behavior, for which she had sought psychotherapy.

Their sexual accomplishments continued; occasionally Peter could have intercourse without injection, although he rarely ejaculated. They married and immediately became preoccupied with having a baby. The goals of therapy constantly shifted. Initially the goal was to have an erection with papaverine, then to have intercourse with injection, then to ejaculate, then to have intercourse and ejaculate without injection, and finally to conceive a child.

The therapist was unsuccessful in asking for a moratorium on "babymaking." Peter ejaculated into a syringe and Heidi inseminated herself; within 2 months, she was pregnant. Fear of hurting the baby then emerged as a sexual concern. Peter also feared he would not be aroused as Heidi's pregnancy advanced. For several weeks, both partners found themselves avoiding sexual play. Therapy focused on the adjustment to parenthood, fears of hurting the baby, and Peter's issues about loss of control. Though Peter's erections became more reliable, the couple generally still relied on injections to have intercourse.

Summary

Self-injection of papaverine and phentolamine is a relatively safe, reliable, and proven treatment for mixed and organic erectile dysfunction. Yet the low patient acceptance of this treatment alternative limits its usefulness. It will be necessary to develop a less objectionable delivery system and to search for new drug combinations that are efficacious and have fewer side effects than papaverine–phentolamine or prostaglandin E_1.

The role of this therapeutic option in the treatment of psychogenic erectile dysfunction is less clear. We continue to believe that psychotherapy remains the treatment of choice; nevertheless, we would like to see more research on the outcome of individual and conjoint psychotherapies supplemented with self-injection, in order to clarify the limitations and benefits of combined medical–psychological interventions.

EXTERNAL VACUUM DEVICES

Development

In 1917, Dr. Otto Lederer obtained a patent for a device that induced erection by creating a vacuum around the penis. This tumescent state was maintained by a constriction ring surrounding the base of the penis. No follow-up reports detailed the success of this venture.

Over half a century later, Gettings Osbon designed a device to cure his erectile dysfunction. In 1982, Osbon's system received FDA marketing approval and became commercially available by prescription; however, his product lay in obscurity while the company improved it. In 1986, Nadig, Ware, & Blumoff published the first scientific investigation describing the utility, efficacy, and safety of vacuum tumescence therapy. The concept seemed difficult for clinicians to accept, and our first response to this device was also skepticism. In an era of high technology, perhaps the low technology and simplicity of vacuum devices are disarming and provoke rejection.

Five vacuum devices are currently manufactured: (1) Osbon Medical System's ErecAid System (EAS) (see Figure 11.2); (2) Mission Pharmacal's Vacuum Erection Device (VED); (3) Smith Collins Pharmaceutical's Response System; (4) Performance Medical's Erection Inducer Device (EID); and (5) Dacomed's Catalyst System. They range in price from $200 to $400. All of the systems include a clear plastic cylinder, vacuum pump, lubricant, and tension rings. The systems differ in four ways: (1) use of a pressure-limiting device, (2) shape of the cylinder, (3) design of the tension rings, and (4) external versus attached pump.

The necessity for pressure-limiting systems is controversial. Those in favor of pressure limiting believe that it enhances safety; pain, bruising, and hematoma occur when pressure exceeds 225 mm Hg. Those opposed believe that pressure-limiting systems decrease efficacy without increasing safety, as some men require more vacuum pressure to create erection. The shape of the cylinders differs slightly from a tube of constant diameter to one that is more narrow at the base than the tip. The functional significance of these designs is not clear.

All tension rings are made of rubber and have handles or string to allow for easy application and removal; they differ in width. The narrower rings exert a more concentrated tension over a smaller area, while the wider band

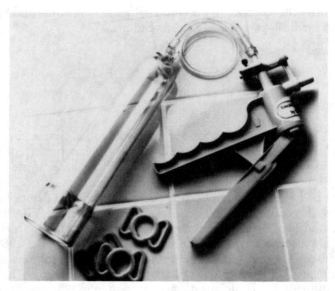

FIGURE 11.2.   Osbon Medical System's ErecAid System.

disperses the constriction over a larger area. The use of an external or attached pump is mainly a matter of patient preference.

Method of Action

The physiological changes produced in the penis by a vacuum pump and maintained by a tension ring differ significantly from naturally occurring and injection-induced erections. Active mechanisms, such as release of a neurotransmitter, relaxation of the smooth muscles, and alterations in venous return, occur with injection-produced or natural erection. The filling of the corpora cavernosa due to suction, and the venous stasis secondary to constriction, are both passive mechanisms.

These conclusions are based on Diederichs, Kaula, Lue, and Tanagho's (1989) work in *Macaca cynomolgus* monkeys. Suction caused the cross-sectional area of the penis to expand 150%, similar to the effect produced by papaverine injections. These erections differed from those produced by papaverine injections, however, in that the additional volume could only be maintained if a constriction device was placed at the base of the penis. Diederichs et al. discovered that the cross-sectional area of the corpora cavernosa during suction was only 50% of that induced by intracavernosal papaverine. They concluded that contracted smooth muscle limited the expansion of the corpora cavernosa.

Marmar, DeBenedictis, and Praiss (1988a) demonstrated the safety of vacuum devices by studying the penile plethysmographies of 51 men before, during, and after the use of this treatment. Continuous blood flow was maintained, although the men demonstrated a 70–75% decline in the amplitude of the pulse volume curve during tumescence. Within 1 minute after removal of the ring, the amplitude returned to baseline.

Procedure

We suggest that prior to deciding on this option and/or purchasing the device, a man and his partner should come in for a demonstration and teaching session. This meeting provides a better sense of whether and how the system will work. They are first shown a 20-minute video, and then spend 30 minutes with the nurse educator, who reviews the technical nuances of the system.

The man starts by stretching the elastic tension bands around the open end of the cylinder and connecting the neoprene tubing from the cylinder to the hand pump. Water-soluble lubricant is liberally applied to the penis and to the cylinder opening. The cylinder is then placed over the flaccid penis and pressed firmly against the body to create an airtight seal. The pump is used to remove air from the cylinder, thereby forming a vacuum that draws blood into the penis. An erection-like state is produced within 30 seconds to 7 minutes. Once the erection is achieved, the tension band is transferred from the cylinder to the base of the penis. After the band is in place, a vacuum release valve is then opened, allowing the cylinder to be removed from the penis. As the cylinder is removed, the tumescence band is slipped from the cylinder to the base of the penis. The patient should not keep the tension band on for more than 30 minutes. Upon removal of the band, the penis becomes flaccid, and penile blood pressure immediately returns to baseline levels.

The erection-like state produced by these external vacuum devices differs from a normal erection in several ways. Men with almost no spontaneous erectile capacity maintain tumescence only distally to the bands. The resultant penile pivoting can cause difficulty with penetration and intercourse. Also, the skin temperature of the penis falls an average of 0.96° C over 30 minutes, because of decreased arterial inflow.

Efficacy

Several studies have documented the efficacy of external vacuum devices. Ninety percent of men with organic, mixed, and psychogenic erectile dysfunctions were able to achieve erections sufficient for intercourse by utilizing this treatment alternative (Cooper, 1987; Koreman, Viosca, Kaiser, Mooradian, & Morley, 1990; Nadig et al., 1986; Nadig, 1989, 1990; Turner et al., 1990a; Witherington, 1989).

In addition, men who had failed to develop adequate erections with injection therapy achieved satisfactory erections with vacuum tumescence therapy. This treatment alternative was also successful in inducing erection in patients who had surgery to remove penile prostheses (Moul & McLeod, 1989).

Koreman et al. (1990) reported that the supine and exercising penile-brachial index increased significantly after 6 months of vacuum tumescence therapy. Also, one-third of their sample (all with abnormal nocturnal penile tumescence) were able to have intercourse occasionally without the device. Similarly, men in our study had statistically significant improvements in spontaneous erections after using the system for 12 months (Turner et al., 1990a). It was not clear whether these findings were attributable to "reconditioning of the penile vasculature" or to a reduction in the performance anxiety that coexisted with the organic erectile dysfunction. Further studies are needed.

By interviewing men and their partners at intervals of 1, 3, 6, and 12 months after receiving the device, we contrasted sexual functioning before and at various times after receiving the device (Turner et al., 1990a). During the year, men used the system in order to have intercourse four times monthly on average. Satisfactory erections resulted 78% of the time. Statistically significant improvements in quality of erection, frequency of intercourse, frequency of orgasm, and sexual satisfaction were initially apparent and persisted over the course of the year.

Follow-up interviews also included repeat psychological assessment. When baseline SCL-90-Rs (Derogatis et al., 1976) were contrasted with those at follow-up, 11 of 12 scales manifested statistically significant improvement. Also in contrast to their baseline status, the men demonstrated statistically significant positive changes in anxiety as measured by the STAI (Spielberger et al., 1970). There were however, no measurable differences in relationship satisfaction or self-esteem.

Side Effects

The primary side effects associated with vacuum tumescence therapy are (1) hematoma, ecchymosis, and petechiae; (2) pain; (3) numbness of the penis; (4) pulling of scrotal tissue into the cylinder; and (5) blocked and painful ejaculation.

Hematoma, ecchymosis, and petechiae are the most common side effects of vacuum tumescence therapy and have been seen in 8–50% of men (Turner et al., 1990b; Nadig et al., 1986). These symptoms occur with greater frequency in the initial phases of the process as the men are learning how to operate the systems. These side effects are generally not serious and disappear without medical intervention. Nadig (1990) believes that a safety valve limiting the maximum degree of vacuum pressure minimizes the occurrence of these side effects.

Patients' early experiences with external vacuum devices are often characterized as mildly uncomfortable to somewhat painful. This discomfort diminishes as men gain more experience. Men also report discomfort from wearing the tension rings; this, too, lessens with time. Sustained pain appears to be a major problem in about 10% of patients. Numbness of the penis has been occasionally reported, although fewer than 9% of patients describe it as a problem (Nadig, 1990). It was not clear why this occurs.

Scrotal tissue may be pulled into the cylinder as the vacuum is created. From 5% to 15% of patients experience this difficulty (Turner et al., 1990b; Koreman et al., 1990). To remedy this problem, cylinders now come with inserts of different sizes that prevent the scrotal tissue from being drawn into the cylinder. In addition to the use of inserts, this problem is often overcome by modifying the manner in which the man creates the vaccum (i.e., by repositioning the cylinder). As a last resort, we would also recommend that the man be given a trial on another system.

Compression of the urethra leads to blocked ejaculation in 39% of patients (Turner et al., 1990b) and painful ejaculation in 10–15% of patients (Nadig, 1990; Witherington, 1989). This can be remedied by loosening the rings just prior to orgasm.

A small percentage of men faint during their first encounter with the device, probably as a result of anxiety. To avoid injury from falls, clinicians should be alert to this possibility.

Finally, patients with tight foreskins may develop paraphimosis as suction is applied to the penis. Nadig (1990) recommends that such patients undergo circumcision before using a vacuum tumescence device.

Patient Acceptance

The patient acceptance rate for vacuum tumescence therapy hovers between 80% and 95% (Nadig, 1990; Turner et al., 1990b). The principal reasons for declining or rejecting this treatment option include mechanical difficulty, failure of the system to induce an adequate erection, complaints that the device is cumbersome, and objections to the artificiality of the erection. The majority of the mechanical difficulties can be overcome with practice. Those who decline or drop out do so early; these men are generally not sufficiently motivated to surmount the mechanical obstacles or psychological barriers. In those instances where the mechanical problem cannot be overcome, a combination of injection therapy and vacuum treatment may be considered (Marmar, DeBenedictis, & Praiss, 1988b).

The following vignette illustrates how vacuum tumescense therapy was helpful in reversing erectile dysfunction in a man with multiple medical problems.

Case Vignette

John G., a 42-year-old married black man, had risen through the ranks to become a supervisor at a large manufacturing plant. Because of severe hypertension and a seizure disorder, he was forced to seek medical disability. While on disability, he was involved in two car accidents that necessitated disc surgery at the level of L_4 and L_5. As a side effect of the medications he was prescribed, he developed erectile problems.

It was not possible to reverse his dysfunction by manipulating the medications. He was offered several treatments but preferred self-injection therapy. Trial dosing ensued; eight injections later, the ceiling dose of 60 mg of papaverine and 2 mg of phentolamine was reached without the patient's having had a good response.

We suggested that John consider a vacuum pump device. During the teaching session, he developed a good erection and was quite pleased. In the first month he used the device for intercourse twice weekly. He did, however, complain of discomfort around the tension rings. We suggested he use the wider bands; this alleviated the discomfort. At the 1-year follow-up, he was continuing to use the system in lovemaking twice weekly with 100% success. During the interview, he described a more optimistic outlook on life and noted that restoration of potency had "solved a lot of mental anguish." His wife confirmed these positive changes, and both expressed their gratitude by offering to speak with other patients about their experience.

Another vignette illustrates how the success of the external vacuum therapy in producing erection helped illuminate a couple's marital conflicts.

Case Vignette

George and Susan R. had been married 14 years; George was 46 and Susan was 52. Two years prior to seeking help, George began to experience erectile problems and a concomitant decrease in sexual desire.

After practicing with the system four times, George was able to achieve a good erection. When he planned to make love to Susan, she asked that he try it without the device. George again lost his desire. In individual treatment, George recognized his wish to avoid being sexual with his wife.

For a brief period of time, George considered divorce and then dropped out of therapy. When he attempted to use the vacuum system, Susan complained that it was artificial and his penis felt cold and clammy. He felt angry and turned off because she criticized his love-making and refused to make love the way he wanted (i.e., any place but in the bedroom). George then convinced Susan to participate in conjoint therapy. In the second session, he told Susan how he felt, and she walked out. In a follow-up meeting, George declared that the price for keeping the marriage together was his asexuality.

Contraindications for Use

Men with significant penile bends, such as those seen in Peyronie's disease, are unable to utilize vacuuum devices. Tumescence forces the penis into the side of the cylinder, which results in pain and limited tumescence.

Men with blood dyscrasia and those taking anticoagulants are at some risk for superficial penile bleeding because of capillary fragility. These men should be considered for other therapeutic options.

Finally, men with poor dexterity cannot operate these systems; their partners can, however, be trained to work the systems. Manufacturers are overcoming this limitation by developing battery-operated, rather than hand-operated, pumping systems.

Psychotherapy and Vacuum Systems

Although the studies cited above include a small number of men with psychogenic eretile dysfunction, no report has carefully examined how these devices can best be utilized with this population. Our preliminary analysis of vacuum tumescence therapy with psychogenically dysfunctional patients (most of whom were in concomitant psychotherapy) indicated that these devices helped to restore sexual confidence and moderate performance anxiety in approximately one-third of the sample. Patients felt that they "had insurance" if an erection was unreliable. The men seemed less dependent upon this alternative and were more willing than those on self-injection to attempt intercourse without an adjunct. Finally, a greater percentage of patients recovered their potency with a combination of psychotherapy and vacuum tumescence therapy than with a combinaton of self-injection and psychotherapy. We believe that vacuum tumescence therapy is viewed as a less radical alternative and mobilizes less resistance than self-injection therapy. A case illustration follows.

Case Vignette

Todd J., a 40-year-old physician, had induced a 9-hour erection by self-prescribing treatment with papaverine and phentolamine. At the time of evaluation, he had just been divorced from his wife of 10 years. The divorce had estranged Todd from his son, and he had lost a substantial portion of his savings. He was now dating a younger woman named Susan, and was experiencing erectile problems.

Todd had a number of concerns about his relationship with Susan. He feared being "trapped" into another marriage. Part of him looked down on Susan because she had had a child out of wedlock. Also, he was angry with her because she occasionally dated the child's father.

Agreeing that his dysfunction was psychogenic, Todd agreed to weekly psychotherapy. The initial approach was to point out the adaptive nature of his symptom (i.e., the ways in which it was his friend). The dysfunction was a means of not committing to Susan. It protected him from jumping into another relationship, with the attendant risks of "being used," while it also reflected some of his ambivalent feelings toward her.

Within three sessions, Todd's erections were somewhat improved but not reliable. He believed that a vacuum system would help him regain his sexual confidence. Over the next 3 months, he used the device several times a week. On occasion he was also able to have intercourse without the device. When he felt that Susan was unresponsive, he lost his erection and used the pump as a backup.

Todd and Susan settled into a monogamous relationship while maintaining separate residences. Although he felt increasingly comfortable with her, he did not wish to increase his commitment. He eventually terminated treatment because he was no longer experiencing any erectile dysfunction.

COMPARISON OF VACUUM PUMP THERAPY AND SELF-INJECTION

Self-injection and vacuum pump therapy appear to be equally effective in improving sexual functioning. Both methods have a positive impact on psychological well-being. The critical discriminations need to be made on the basis of cost, potential side effects, patient acceptance, and aesthetic preferences of the man or couple (Table 11.1).

Vacuum systems range in price from $200 to $400. Self-injection costs about $75 a month. Although the vacuum devices require a greater initial outlay of money, savings are evident after 3 to 6 months of use.

Side effects are less severe with vacuum systems. Also, they enjoy higher patient acceptance, as evidenced by the significantly lower dropout rate.

In terms of aesthetic preferences, some men object to making love while wearing the vacuum system's tension ring, because it serves as a reminder of

TABLE 11.1.   Comparison of Self-Injection and External Vacuum Devices

Factor	Self-injection	External vacuum devices
Efficacy		
Neurogenic	Good response	Good response
Vasculogenic	Poor–good response	Good response
Idiopathic	Good response	Good response
Psychogenic	Adequate response	Adequate–good response
Psychological benefits	Positive effect	Positive effect
Patient acceptance	40–50%	80–95%
Cost	$75/monthly; $900/yearly	$200–400 total outlay
Side effects	Prolonged erection	Hematoma, bruising
	Fibrotic nodules	Numbness
	Hepatotoxicity	Blocked/painful ejaculation
	Bruising	Pulling in scrotal tissue
	Pain	Fainting
	Vasovagal episodes	
	Infection	
Concealability	Easily concealed	Not easily concealed
Prolonged intercourse	Possible	Limited to 30 minutes
Frequency of intercourse	Limited to twice weekly	No limitation
Conception	No limitation	Possible blocked ejaculation

their perceived inadequacy. There are no such reminders after an injection is given. Couples trying to conceive prefer self-injection because the tension ring may block ejaculation. A few men also report that the blocked ejaculation diminishes their sensual experience.

The vacuum system's 30-minute time limitation concerns some men. In order to have sufficient time for relaxed intercourse, many men prefer to take time between foreplay and intercourse to use the device, rather than using the system prior to foreplay. Couples report that this breaks the mood and highlights the artificial nature of the treatment. Conversely, this can also be an advantage for a man with psychogenic erectile difficulty: He can begin to make love without performance anxiety, because he knows that he can use the vacuum device if he fails to achieve or maintain an erection.

The twice-weekly limitation on self-injection poses difficulties for couples who prefer a greater frequency of intercourse. Although there are no empirical data available to support this restriction, its intent is to reduce the possibility of nodule development. Such couples prefer the vacuum device because the frequency of its use is not limited. Similarly, should an injection fail to induce erection, the man will not be able to try again that day. Should he ignore the limitation, he places himself at substantial risk for inducing a prolonged erection. If the vacuum system should fail, one would simply try again.

Men who are single and trying to make love with new partners often prefer self-injection. Since injections can be given in privacy, it is easier for men to keep their erectile difficulty a secret from their partners. Married men who are having extramarital affairs also prefer self-injection because "a hypodermic needle is more portable." Or, as a couple who planned to travel overseas with a vacuum device remarked, "What do we say when this thing shows up on the X-ray baggage detector at the airport?" Men who are in steady relationships do not have this difficulty and may integrate a vacuum device into foreplay (e.g., "We do it together. I hold the cylinder and she works the pump. It works great that way.").

At our clinic, most patients select the vacuum device because it is less invasive, less costly, and freer of potentially worrisome side effects than self-injection. A minority of patients continue to choose self-injection, and a few patients employ both alternatives simultaneously.

CONCLUSION

Self-injection and vaccum pump therapy provide clinicians with two innovative technologies that temporarily reverse erectile dyfunction. These treatment alternatives are reliable and relatively safe, and tend to enhance the psychological well-being of patients who utilize them. These developments should be considered as "steps along the way," however. Both options need to be further refined while strategies for how to utilize them most effectively are developed.

This is an exciting time in the field of human sexuality as research gradually uncovers the pathophysiology of erection. This work will ultimately lead to the next generation of treatment alternatives.

Acknowledgments. We wish to acknowledge the help of our colleagues, Stephen B. Levine, M.D., Candace Risen, L.I.S.W., Donald Bodner, M.D., Elroy Kursh, M.D., Martin Resnick, M.D., and Larianne Jacob, R.N. We are also grateful to Doris Kurit for her research assistance and Barbara Juknialis for her editorial acumen.

REFERENCES

Althof, S. E., Turner, L. A., Levine, S. B., Risen, C., Kursh, E., Bodner, D., & Resnick, M. (1987). Intracavernosal injection in the treatment of impotence: A prospective study of sexual, psychological, and marital functioning. *Journal of Sex and Marital Therapy, 13*(3), 155–167.

Althof, S. R., Turner, L. A., Levine, S. B., Risen, C., Kursh, E., Bodner, D., & Resnick, M. (1989a). Why do so many people drop out from autoinjection therapy for impotence? *Journal of Sex and Marital Therapy, 15*(2), 121–129.

Althof, S. E., Turner, L. A., Levine, S. B., Risen, C., Kursh, E., Bodner, D., & Resnick, M. (1989b). *How do women respond to their partners' use of injection therapy for erectile dysfunction? A prospective study.* Paper presented at the meeting of the Society for Sex Therapy and Research, Toronto.

Althof, S. E., Turner, L. A., Levine, S. B., Risen, C., Kursh, E., Bodner, D., & Resnick, M. (1991). Long-term use of self-injection therapy of papaverine and phentolamine. *Journal of Sex and Marital Therapy, 17*(2), 101–112.

Bauer, B., & Capek, R. (1972). Studies on the neuropharmacology of papaverine. *Neuropharmacology, 11*, 697.

Bodner, D., Lindan, R., Leffler, E., Kursh, E., & Resnick, M. (1987). The application of intracavernous injection of vasoactive medications for erection in men with spinal cord injury. *Journal of Urology, 138*, 310–311.

Brindley, G. S. (1983). Cavernosal alpha-blockade: A new technique for investigating and treating erectile impotence. *British Journal of Psychiatry, 143*, 332–337.

Brindley, G. S. (1986). Maintenance treatment of erectile impotence by cavernosal unstriated muscle relaxant injection. *British Journal of Psychiatry, 149*, 210–215.

Buvat, J., Lemaire, A., Buvat-Herbaut, M., & Marcolin, G. (1989). Safety of intracavernous injection using an alpha-blocking agent. *Journal of Urology, 141*, 1364–1367.

Cooper, A. (1987). Preliminary experience with a vacuum tumescence device (VCD) as a treatment for impotence. *Journal of Psychosomatic Research, 31*(3), 413–418.

Derogatis, L., Rickels, K., & Rock, A. (1976). The SCL-90-R and the MMPI: A step in the validation of a new self-report scale. *British Journal of Psychiatry, 128*, 280–289.

Diedrichs, W., Kaula, N., Lue, T., & Tanagho, E. (1989). The effect of subatmospheric pressure on the simian penis. *Journal of Urology, 142*, 1087–1089.

Domer, F., Wessler, G., Brown, R., & Charles, H. (1978). Involvement of the sympathetic nervous system in the urinary bladder internal sphincter and in penile erection in the anesthetized cat. *Journal of Urology, 15*, 404–407.

Drieman, P. (1973). Papaverine—hepatotoxic or not? *Journal of the American Geriatrics Society, 21*(5) 202–205.

Girdley, F., Bruskewitz, R., Feyzi, J., Graversen, P., & Gassner, T. (1988). Intracavernous self-injection for impotence: A long-term therapeutic option? Experience in 78 patients. *Journal of Urology, 140*, 972–974.

Hashmat, A., & Abraham, J. (1987). Papaverine induced priapism: A lethal complication. *Journal of Urology, 137*, 829–836.

Ishii, N., Watanabe, H., Irisawa, C., Kikuchi, Y., Kubota, Y., Kawamura, S., Suzuki, K., Chiba, R., Tokiwa, M., & Shirai, M. (1989). Intracavernous injection of prostaglandin E_1 for the treatment of erectile impotence. *Journal of Urology, 141*, 323–325.

Koreman, S., Viosca, S., Kaiser, F., Mooradian, A., & Morley, J. (1990). Use of a vacuum tumescence device in the management of impotence. *Journal of the American Geriatric Society, 38*, 217–220.

Krane, R., Goldstein, I., & Saenz de Tejada, I. (1989). Impotence. *New England Journal of Medicine, 321*, 1648-1659.

Kursh, E., Bodner, D., Resnick, M., Althof, S. E., Turner, L. A., Risen, C., & Levine, S. B. (1988). Injection therapy for impotence. *Urologic Clinics of North America, 15*(4), 625-630.

Levine, S. B., Althof, S. E., Turner, L. A., Kursh, E., Bodner, D., & Resnick, M. (1989). Side effects of self-administration of intracavernosal papaverine and phentolamine for the treatment of impotence. *Journal of Urology, 141*, 54-57.

Lue, T., & Tanagho, E. (1987). Physiology of erection and pharmacological management of impotence. *Journal of Urology, 137*, 829-836.

Marmar, J., DeBenedictis, T., & Praiss, D. (1988a). Penile plethysmography on impotent men using vacuum tumescence devices. *Urology, 32*(3), 198-203.

Marmar, J., DeBenedictis, T., & Praiss, D. (1988b). The use of vacuum constrictor device to augment a partial erection following an intracavernous injection. *Journal of Urology, 140*, 975-979.

Moul, J., & McLeod, D. (1989). Negative pressure devices in the explanted penile prosthesis population. *Journal of Urology, 142*, 729-731.

Nadig, P. (1989). Six years experience with the vacuum tumescence device. *International Journal of Impotence Research, 1*, 55-58.

Nadig, P. (1990). *Vacuum erection devices: A review article.* Unpublished manuscript.

Nadig, P., Ware, J., & Blumoff, R. (1986). Noninvasive device to produce and maintain an erection-like state. *Urology, 27*(2), 126-131.

Nellans, R., Ellis, L, & Kramer-Levien, D. (1987). Pharmacological erection: Diagnosis and treatment applications in 69 patients. *Journal of Urology, 138*, 52-54.

Nelson, R. (1989). Injections of papaverine and Regitine into the corpora cavernosa for sexual dysfunction: Clinical results in 60 patients. *Southern Medical Journal, 82*(1), 26-28.

Padma-Nathan, H., Goldstein, I., & Krane, R. (1986). Treatment of prolonged or priapismic erections following intracavernosal papaverine therapy. *Seminars in Urology, 4*(4), 236-238.

Poch, G., & Kubovetz, W. (1971). Papaverine induced inhibition of phosphodiesterase activity in various mammalian tissues. *Life Sciences, 10*(3), 133-144.

Reiss, H. (1989). Use of prostaglandin E_1 for papaverine-failed erections. *Urology, 33*(1), 15-16.

Sidi, A. (1988). Vasoactive intracavernous pharmacotherapy. *Urologic Clinics of North America, 15*, 95-101.

Sidi, A., Cameron, J., Duffy, D., & Lange, P. (1986). Intracavernous drug-induced erections in the management of male erectile dysfunction: Experience with 100 patients. *Journal of Urology, 135*, 704-706.

Sidi, A., Cameron, J., Dykstra, D., Reinberg, Y., & Lange, P. (1987). Vasoactive intracavernous pharmacotherapy for the treatment of erectile impotence in men with spinal cord injury. *Journal of Urology, 138*, 539-542.

Sidi, A., Pratap, R., & Chen, K. (1988). Patient acceptance of and satisfaction with vasoactive intracavernous pharmacotherapy for impotence. *Journal of Urology, 140*, 293-294.

Sidi, A., & Reddy, P. (1990). Simplified tourniquet for intracavernous pharmacotherapy. *Urologic Clinics of North America, 17*(1), 19–21.

Spielberger, D., Gorsuch, R., & Lushene, R. (1970). *State-Trait Anxiety Inventory manual*. Palo Alto, CA: Consulting Psychologists Press.

Trapp, J. (1987). Pharmacologic erection program for the treatment of male impotence. *Southern Medical Journal, 80*(4), 426–427.

Turner, L., A., Althof, S. E., Levine, S. B., Kursh, E., Bodner, D., & Resnick, M. (1990a). Treating erectile dysfunction with external vacuum device: Impact upon sexual, psychological and marital functioning. *Journal of Urology, 144*(1), 79–82.

Turner, L., A., Althof, S. E., Levine, S. B., Kursh, E., Bodner, D., & Resnick, M. (1990b). *A comparison of the effectiveness of two treatments for impotence: Self-injection therapy versus external vacuum pump devices*. Unpublished manuscript.

Turner, L., A., Althof, S. E., Levine, S. B., Risen, C., Kursh, E., Bodner, D., & Resnick, M. (1989). Self-injection of papaverine and phentolamine in the treatment of psychogenic impotence. *Journal of Sex and Marital Therapy, 15*, 163–176.

Virag, R. (1985). Human penile erection: An extensive study of the effects of vasoactive compounds on the cavernous tissue and the penile arteries. *Journal of Urology, 133*(2), 191A. (Abstract 311)

Virag, R., & Adaikan, P. (1987). Effects of prostaglandin E_1 on penile erection and erectile failure [Letter]. *Journal of Urology, 137*, 1010.

Virag, R., Frydman, D., Legman, M., & Virag, H. (1984). Intracavernous injection of papaverine as a diagnostic and therapeutic method in erectile failure. *Angiology, 35*, 79–87.

Virag, R., & Virag, H. (1983). L'épreuve à la papaverine intracaverneuse dans l'étude de l'impuissance: Perspectives thérapeutiques. *Journal des Maladies Vasculaires, 8*, 293–295.

Waldhauser, M., & Schramek, P. (1988). Efficiency and side effects of prostaglandin E_1 in the treatment of erectile dysfunction. *Journal of Urology, 140*, 525–527.

Witherington, R. (1989). Vacuum tumescence device for management of erectile impotence. *Journal of Urology, 141*, 320–322.

Willis, E., Ottesen, B., Wagner, G., Sundler, G., & Fahrenkrug, J. (1981). Vasoactive intestinal polypeptide (VIP) as a possible neurotransmitter involved in penile erection. *Acta Physiology Scandanavica, 113*, 545.

Zentgraf, M., Ludwig, G., & Ziegler, M. (1989). How safe is the treatment of impotence with intracavernous autoinjection? *European Urology, 16*, 165–171.

Zorgniotti, A., & Lefleur, R. (1985). Auto-injection of the corpus cavernosum with a vasoactive drug combination for vasculogenic impotence. *Journal of Urology, 133*, 39–41.

Erectile Disorders
in Special Populations
IV

12

Treatment of Erectile Dysfunction with Single Men

BARRY W. McCARTHY

Treating the single man with erectile difficulties can present a major challenge. Quite often, the patient finds himself in a vicious cycle. On the one hand, he may believe that without adequate sexual performance, he will be unable to initiate or maintain a lasting relationship with a partner. However, these demands typically lead to increased performance anxiety and consequent erectile failure. It is clearly evident that in order for successful treatment to occur, the male's self-defeating belief system must be challenged at the same time that his sexual self-confidence is restored.

In this provocative chapter, McCarthy suggests a four-part approach to treatment of males without partners. He suggests that it is necessary for the patient's cognitive beliefs about sexuality to be changed; that sexual anxiety needs to be decreased while sexual comfort is developed; that building heterosocial and relationship skills is essential; and, finally, that sexual stimulation and arousal techniques often need to be expanded.

A central element in McCarthy's approach to treatment is encouraging the male to find a "sexual friend"—that is, a partner with whom he is sexually aroused and comfortable. The "sexual friend" can facilitate his learning of new skills, and at the same time may help the male to realize that such a relationship can be safe, mutually rewarding, and sexually exciting. McCarthy suggests that it is not as difficult for a single male to find such a partner as a client (or a clinician) may think, although he cautions that it may not be advantageous to include the "friend" in ongoing therapy, since it implies greater commitment than may be warranted.

McCarthy also addresses the special issues associated with primary erectile failure in single men, as well as with erectile difficulties in gay men. In the former case, he notes that a variety of factors may contribute to the erectile failure, from the establishment of an idiosyncratic masturbatory pattern to conflict over sexual orientation. Whatever the origin, primary erectile failure can be difficult to overcome once established, and may require extensive individual therapy. The single gay male *also presents a special therapeutic challenge, since many are intensely humiliated by their erectile difficulties, and adopt a sexually passive role that may put them at greater risk of human immunodeficiency virus (HIV) infection. McCarthy suggests that the gay male's homophobia may need to be confronted, as well as other maladaptive cognitive beliefs. Nevertheless, the concept of finding a "sexual friend" can be as helpful with the gay male as with the straight one.*

Finally, McCarthy notes that erectile difficulties in the single population may be difficult to treat, even under the best of circumstances. For the man without a stable partner, increased creativity is often demanded from the therapist. The use of imagery techniques, masturbation rehearsal, fantasy training, and other sensual exercises may be indicated. Even so, McCarthy admits that failures do occur, since many single men are reluctant to abandon the myth of achieving effortless and automatic erections with all partners. Nevertheless, he suggests that most single men with erectile dysfunction can profit from individual cognitive–behavioral sex therapy.

Barry W. McCarthy, Ph.D., is Professor of Psychology at American University in Washington, D.C. He is the author of numerous articles, chapters, and books on various aspects of sexuality, including Sexual Awareness *(1984, with E. McCarthy) and* Male Sexual Awareness *(1988).*

The classical sex therapy model developed by Masters and Johnson (1970) emphasizes that sexual problems are best conceptualized as couple problems, with the optimal treatment program being couples sex therapy. Although most sex therapists agree, in reality there are many males who are never-married, separated, or divorced, or whose spouses or partners resist entering sex therapy. Males without partners who have an erection problem (whether primary or secondary) are faced with a serious concern and need therapeutic help. This chapter describes a cognitive–behavioral treatment for males without partners, using an individual sex therapy approach.

In male sexual socialization, the man typically has his first experience with arousal and orgasm during masturbation, which begins in early adolescence. The masturbatory experience combines fantasy, visual, or reading material with active penile stimulation. The male has repeated experiences of masturbation in which he learns that arousal and erection occur in an intense, secretive, and very predictable sequence. The great majority of males masturbate in a rapid, goal-oriented manner. In adolescence or early adulthood, when the young man begins sex with a partner, intercourse follows the same scenario as masturbation—rapid and goal-oriented. The combination of novelty and illicitness adds to arousal. The most common sexual problem experienced by young males is early ejaculation (McCarthy, 1989), but this is not a major concern.

The male learns an approach to sexual expression that serves him well at that time, but often sabotages sexual satisfaction as he ages. He learns that sexual arousal is easy, automatic, and autonomous. In other words, he comes to believe that he needs nothing from the woman in order for erections and intercourse to work. This creates an unrealistic expectation about sexual performance, which interferes with the successful resolution of an erectile problem. The man's desire to return to the easy, automatic erections of adolescence (which sex therapy cannot deliver) is a prime motivation for seeking the medical remedies of surgical implants and papaverine injections. Even in cases where there is an organic impairment and a prosthesis or injection program is the treatment of choice, it is crucial to disabuse the male of the expectation that he will be returning to the ever-present erections of adolescent sexuality.

Another legacy from male sexual socialization that interferes with sex therapy is the belief that a "real man" can have sex with any woman, any time, and in any situation. In the therapeutic model proposed here, the man learns to view the woman as a "sexual friend." He is encouraged to choose a partner with whom he feels comfortable, to whom he is attracted, and whom he trusts; with this partner, he can discuss the sexual problem and work cooperatively to resolve it. For many males, thinking of a woman in this manner and talking directly about sexual concerns is a novel idea. Establishing positive conditions for a good sexual relationship is not in most men's repertoire.

PRIMARY ERECTILE DYSFUNCTION

The great majority of males seeking treatment have secondary erectile dysfunction. In other words, they have a history of successful erections and intercourse. Males with primary erectile dysfunction, by contrast, have never had successful intercourse. Contrary to clinical lore, my experience with treating primary erectile dysfunction has been positive and follows the cognitive–behavioral intervention model to be described later in the chapter.

There is no unitary profile for the male with primary erectile dysfunction: Frequent causes are (1) an idiosyncratic masturbation pattern, (2) paraphilic arousal, (3) conflict over sexual orientation, (4) a history of sexual trauma, and/or (5) guilt and anxiety concerning premarital sexuality. Regardless of which factors began the pattern, performance anxiety and a sense of stigma combine to maintain the erectile dysfunction once it is established. To that extent, it is similar to secondary erectile dysfunction, with similar treatment interventions.

Idiosyncratic masturbation habits make it difficult to transfer sexual arousal to partner sex. Examples of idiosyncratic patterns include not moving the penis, ejaculating with a flaccid penis, or rubbing against an object. Benign paraphilias include fetishes and cross-dressing, whereas noxious paraphilias include exhibitionism, voyeurism, and pedophilia. One way to conceptualize a "paraphilia" is as an intimacy disorder that blocks not only erections, but the development of a trusting, emotionally intimate relationship (Levine, Risen, & Althof, 1990). The male who is conflicted about sexual orientation or who is leading a double life is likely to experience erectile dysfunction during heterosexual relationships. The issue of sexual abuse of male children is only now being recognized. Males have a more difficult time coping with sexual trauma than females because, in addition to breaking the trust bond that adults should not use children to fulfill sexual needs, it also raises concerns about sexual orientation ("Why did this man pick me to abuse?"). Since males are supposed to be in control in sexual situations, an abused male frequently conceals the fact of sexual trauma. When the trauma is denied and kept secret, it becomes powerful and distorted, serving to victimize the male further. Finally, guilt and anxiety over prior sexual activity can interfere with sexual self-esteem and current sexual functioning. A religious or parental ban on premarital sexual activity may well backfire in causing adult sexual dysfunction.

Males with primary erectile dysfunction find this problem to be socially and emotionally crippling. It is more than a sexual problem; it defines their lives and their sense of masculinity. The stigma of being a "virgin" at 25 or 45 weighs heavily on self-esteem. Protecting the secret becomes more important than solving the problem.

The great majority of these males are able to masturbate to orgasm, usually with a full erection. However, rather than viewing this as positive evidence of ability to function sexually, they belittle it as a reminder that they cannot be successful with a partner. Most males have engaged in nongenital and genital stimulation, often getting erections and then losing them before or during intromission. It is not unusual for a male to have an unsuccessful first intercourse, whether caused by ejaculation before penetration or erectile failure. However, if intercourse continues to be unsuccessful, and especially if the lack of success is caused by erectile problems, the male becomes trapped in the cycle of anticipatory anxiety, performance anxiety, and sexual avoidance. The more partners it happens with and the longer it continues, the more he feels hopeless and helpless. The weight of the problem colors all aspects of his emotional and social life.

Althof (1989) has noted, and I agree, that the treatment of choice for males with primary erectile dysfunction is individual therapy. Some have suggested group treatment for single males with erectile dysfunction. Although it can be helpful, in clinical practice it has been extremely hard to organize and conduct these groups. The stigma against admitting sexual problems is very strong. Group programs for sexual problems work best if they are homogeneous (i.e., if they consist only of men with erection problems), rather than mixing males with inhibited sexual desire, early ejaculation, ejaculatory inhibition, paraphilic arousal, or problems with sexual identity. Programs using sexual surrogates have lost favor, since they raise complex legal and ethical issues. Moreover, few clinicians have access to a well-trained surrogate who would be open to professional supervision.

Many single males have inquired about the medical interventions of penile implants and injection therapy. Unless the male is unable to attain an erection through self- or partner stimulation, the use of these interventions (especially the implant, which is an irreversible procedure) is discouraged. If the single male is to learn to integrate sexuality into his life, he needs to directly address the anxiety, attitudinal, and behavioral problems that interfere with sexual interaction. Trying to bypass these issues by implants or injections can raise other problems and in some cases may be iatrogenic. An example is a male's desire for an implant so he can have intercourse with a woman and "cure" homosexuality.

Case Vignette

Paul was a 34-year-old single male who had a history of unsuccessful intercourse with seven partners. He was referred by an individual psychotherapist who had treated him for 3 years for depression and social isolation. This was Paul's fourth experience with psychotherapy; he had first sought therapy at age 16 because of his parents' concern over his lack of interest in dating and his social isolation. Although Paul's chief concern was sexual, he had never completed a detailed sexual history or received any direct sexual information from a therapist or physician. He was a bright, successful attorney who had achieved partner status in his firm.

In the course of providing a detailed sexual history, Paul revealed three major blocks to erectile functioning: (1) His masturbatory pattern was rubbing against the bed with a semierect penis (he had never manually stimulated his penis or achieved orgasm with an erect penis); (2) his sexual fantasies focused on a fetishistic arousal pattern of imagining a woman in high heels and long, painted fingernails; and (3) he was painfully shy with women. Interventions involved masturbation training; reducing fetishistic arousal and replacing it with a more involved, erotic, genital-oriented sexual scenario; and building social skills, including seeing a female partner as a sexual friend. (These interventions are described in greater detail later in the chapter.)

A chief issue for Paul was taking sexual risks and not feeling hopeless and humiliated by his prior failures. A helpful analogy was that he would have failed as a lawyer if he had had little understanding of law and minimal resources. Now that he had an increased understanding of erections and increased sexuality resources (attitudinal, behavioral, and emotional), he could learn to be a sexually successful person. Males with a long history of erectile failure need to implement realistic steps; there are few "miracle cures." Paul was pleased with his ability to gain full erections with his own and his partner's manual stimulation. As his sexual repertoire expanded in both fantasy and behavior, he felt more comfortable as a sexual male. He experienced his first successful intercourse with his third girlfriend after 8 months of individual sex therapy.

SECONDARY ERECTILE DYSFUNCTION

In secondary erectile dysfunction, performance anxiety almost always plays a major role. Young men experience easy, automatic, and autonomous erections, which lead to problem-free, predictable intercourse. There is little or no self-consciousness about erections and intercourse. However, once a sensitizing event (the inability to get or maintain an erection sufficient for intercourse) has occurred, the man does not return to automatic, un-self-conscious functioning. He can learn to be a pleasure-oriented and better lover, but will not return to the easy functioning of adolescence.

A common cause of erectile dysfunction is the breakup of a marriage or partner relationship. As the relationship deteriorates, sexuality often becomes problematic. The male arousal cycle is particularly vulnerable. A newly single male frequently attempts to prove his sexual prowess by "scoring" with new women. To build a false sense of confidence and lower inhibitions, he may also drink too much. Alcohol is a central nervous system depressant that inhibits erections.

Another common pattern involves the man who is an early ejaculator. Rather than talking to his partner and enlisting her cooperation, he decides to use a "do-it-yourself" technique to control ejaculation. He may bite his lip, think of how much money he owes, wear two or three condoms, or use a desensitizing cream. Rather than learning ejaculatory control, he becomes less sexually aroused and has difficulty maintaining his erection. The next step in this self-defeating cycle is that he becomes obsessed with performance anxiety and takes a "spectator" role, concentrating on and monitoring his penile response. The erectile difficulty initially occurs at the point of intromission, but then the male begins losing his erection during pleasuring/foreplay. As anticipatory sexual anxiety builds, functioning becomes more problematic; the male begins to fear that he will be unable to obtain an erection at all. The male becomes trapped in the syndrome of anticipatory anxiety, aversive experience, and sexual avoidance.

THE COGNITIVE-BEHAVIORAL ASSESSMENT
AND TREATMENT MODEL

Sexual function and dysfunction can be very complex. For treatment to be successful, with gains maintained and generalized, therapy must be approached with respect for this complexity. The treatment program for each client should be individualized and each component carefully considered. The treatment strategy my colleagues and I utilize has four components: (1) changing cognitions about sexuality, (2) decreasing sexual anxiety and increasing sexual comfort, (3) building heterosocial skills in choosing and developing a relationship, and (4) building sexual stimulation and arousal skills.

The most crucial assessment technique is taking a comprehensive, detailed sexual history. Of specific concern are the client's masturbatory pattern, sexual information (especially about penile functioning), any guilt-inducing or traumatic incidents, the parental model of sexuality, cognitions about male-female similarities and differences, social and sexual skills, first intercourse experience, most embarrassing or traumatic adult sexual experience, and desire for an intimate relationship. The clinician must take the sexual history with a sense of empathy and respect for the man and his experiences. Open-ended questions about masturbation, homosexual experiences, paraphilias, and trauma must convey the message that the clinician will listen in a nonjudgmental manner. In this therapeutic model, the assessment and treatment phases are linked and feed back to each other throughout the therapy. Sexual exercises do not just build comfort and skills; they serve diagnostically to identify inhibitions that require therapeutic attention. When therapy reaches an impasse, the clinician reviews the sexual history to generate hypotheses concerning past conflicts, ambivalence, or trauma.

Changing Cognitions about Sexuality

Annon's (1976) "P-LI-SS-IT" model serves as a useful framework for sequencing interventions. "P-LI-SS-IT" stands for "permission giving, limited information, specific suggestions, and intensive sex therapy." Especially important is giving permission for the male to be open and frank, to admit sexual problems, to raise questions about sexuality, and to ask for help. Males feel pressure to be sexual experts because of the myth that "real men" know all there is to know about sex. In addition, women seek therapy more frequently than men. The single male entering therapy for erectile dysfunction has to overcome cultural inhibitions and needs support and permission. For this reason, many such clients prefer a male therapist who can serve as a positive role model.

Males are more receptive, at least initially, to a cognitive, information-giving approach than to the nondirective, feeling-oriented strategy traditionally utilized in initial sessions. An example of information giving is describing the natural physiological process of waxing and waning of erections—a process of which most males are unaware. A diagram can be used to illustrate the process. Most males have the habit of striving for orgasm on their first erection. Accordingly, a client may well be unaware that penile stimulation when he is flaccid is counterproductive to sexual arousal, in that he becomes more self-conscious and tries to force or will an erection.

To increase information and awareness, an informational handout (Table 12.1) is given to each client at the first session. In addition to this handout, chapters from books on male sexuality are provided (McCarthy, 1988; Zilbergeld, 1978; Schover, 1984), depending on the client's motivation and reading ability. Because many males have distorted attitudes and beliefs concerning female sexuality, selected chapters from books on female sexuality (McCarthy & McCarthy, 1989; Heiman & LoPiccolo, 1988; Barbach & Levine, 1980) can be assigned at a later time. Cognitive changes alone will not alter sexual behavior, but knowledge is power. Positive attitudes toward male and female sexuality can and will help the client overcome erectile dysfunction.

Another area for cognitive restructuring is the male's attitude toward his penis. In our culture, sexuality plays an inordinately large role in the definition of masculinity (Tiefer, 1986). Because of erectile dysfunction, the client labels himself a "failure" as a person. The term "impotence" connotes lack of strength, competence, and masculinity, when in fact it is a specific problem in getting and maintaining an erection. Too much of the typical male's self-esteem depends on his penis. No wonder the penis buckles under such intense psychological pressure.

A cognitive restructuring strategy involves increasing the client's awareness of how stress and life transitions can affect both psychological and sexual functioning. Male mythology holds that men can go through difficult and traumatic life experiences (divorce, loss of a job, serious illness, death of a spouse) with no effect on their sexuality. The myth of the man and his penis as a perfectly functioning machine unaffected by stress or relationship factors is widely believed. In truth, occasional or temporary erectile dysfunction as a result of stress or transitions is a very common phenomenon.

An example of the effect of transitions is the "widower's syndrome." The male with a spouse who has suffered from an incapacitating illness and then died may not have had intercourse for a period of months or years. Males find the mourning process emotionally difficult and after a period of weeks or months are likely to try to establish a new relationship. The availability of women in the appropriate age group makes this all the more probable; especially after age 50, there are many more females without partners than males. A widower needs to realize that he probably will not have easy, automatic erections with the new partner. It will take time, communication, and the partner's cooperation to develop a comfortable and functional sexual relationship.

Another example of a life transition that can affect sexual functioning is the attainment of sobriety. Alcoholism and alcohol abuse constitute a major cause of erectile dysfunciton, but there are many men who remain sexually functional while drinking. Males use alcohol to build sexual feelings and lower inhibitions. Many alcoholics have seldom been sexual in a sober state. In essence, their sexuality has been a state-controlled learning process (i.e., sex occurs in conjunction with drinking). For these men, attaining sobriety is likely to be accompanied by transitory erectile dysfunction, because they have to learn a sexual arousal pattern focused on sensations and stimulation rather than on alcohol. The male who understands this transition can adopt a positive coping strategy instead of overreacting to the erectile problem. If the male (and his partner) realize that the difficulty is temporary—a natural result of the transition to sobriety—and continue to communicate and engage in sensual and sexual pleasuring, his sexual functioning will return.

Decreasing Sexual Anxiety and Increasing Sexual Comfort

The second major component of the model involves identifying and reducing sexual anxiety, especially anticipatory and performance anxiety. A variety of techniques, including relaxation, imagery, masturbatory rehearsal, and cognitive strategies, can be utilized. Deep muscle relaxation and cue-controlled relaxation are of considerable value. Many males have little awareness of their bodies or of the amount of tension and stress they experience in both sexual and nonsexual domains. Awareness of relaxation and body cues facilitates a comfortable and pleasure-oriented approach to touching and sexuality.

When there is phobic anxiety concerning sexual intercourse, a desensitization hierarchy can be utilized. Where anxiety is diffuse, variants such as guided imagery or cognitive coping strategies are more appropriate. Typical guided imagery scenarios include talking to the woman about the sexual problem, engaging in nondemand pleasuring, and rehearsing the transition from genital stimulation to intercourse. The imagery is repeated with variations until the man can see himself functioning comfortably. Cognitive coping strategies and cue-controlled relaxation together can teach the client to monitor and cope with sexual anxiety.

Another strategy is the use of masturbatory exercises. Detailed exercises are available in the book by Zilbergeld (1978) and on an audiotape by Reynolds (1990). An advantage of masturbatory practice sessions is that the

TABLE 12.1. Arousal and Erection Guidelines: A Handout for Clients

1. By age 40, 90% of males experience at least one erectile failure. This is a normal occurrence, not a sign of chronic erectile dysfunction.

2. The majority of erectile problems are caused by psychological or relationship factors, not by medical or physiological malfunctions. For an evaluation of medical factors, consult a urologist with special training in erectile function and dysfunction.

3. Erectile problems can be caused by a wide variety of factors, including alcohol, anxiety, depression, anger, side effects of medication, frustration, fatigue, and not feeling sexual at a particular time or with a particular partner.

4. The key is to accept the erectile difficulty as a situational problem, not to overreact and label yourself "impotent" or put yourself down as a "failure."

5. Don't believe the myth of the "male machine," ready to have an erection and intercourse at any time with any woman in any situation. You and your penis are human, not a performance machine.

6. One of the most pervasive myths is that if a man loses his initial erection, it means that he is sexually turned off and must work to regain it. In reality, it is a natural physiological process for erections to wax and wane during a prolonged pleasuring period.

7. In a typical 45-minute pleasuring session, the male's erection will come and go an average of three times. Subsequent erections, intercourse, and the ensuing orgasm can be more pleasurable.

8. You don't need an erect penis to satisfy a woman. An orgasm can be achieved through manual, oral, or rubbing stimulation and is sexually satisfying. If you have a problem getting or maintaining an erection, it is not necessary to stop the sexual interaction. Many women find it arousing to have a man use fingers, tongue, or penis (erect or flaccid) to stimulate the clitoral shaft or labia minora (inner lips).

9. Actively involve yourself in giving and receiving pleasurable touching. An erection is a natural result of sexual arousal.

10. You cannot will or force an erection. Avoid being a passive "spectator" who observes the state of his penis. Sex is not a spectator sport; it requires active involvement.

11. It makes sense for the woman both to initiate the moment of intercourse and to guide your penis into her vagina. It reduces pressure on you, and since the woman is the expert on her sexuality, it is the most practical procedure.

12. You can feel comfortable saying to your partner, "I want pleasuring and sex to be nondemanding. When I feel pressure to perform, I get uptight, and sex is not good. Let's make sexuality enjoyable by taking it at a comfortable pace."

13. Erectile problems do not affect the ability to ejaculate. A male can ejaculate with a flaccid penis. A male can also relearn to ejaculate to the cue of an erect penis.

14. One way to regain comfort and confidence with erections is masturbation. During masturbation you can practice gaining and losing erections, relearn ejaculating to the cue of an erect penis, and focus on fantasies and stimulation that can be transferred to sex with a partner.

15. Morning erections should not be used for intercourse initiation. The morning erection is associated with rapid eye movement (REM) sleep or may result from being close to your partner. Too many men vainly try to use their morning erection before they lose it. Remember, arousal and erections are regainable.

(continued)

TABLE 12.1. (continued)

16. Make clear, direct, assertive requests (not demands) for the sexual stimulation you find most arousing. Both verbally and nonverbally, guide your partner in how to pleasure and arouse you.

17. Stimulating a totally flaccid penis is counterproductive for sexual arousal, and can result in becoming obsessed about the state of your penis. Instead, engage in sensuous, nondemand stimulation until there is some arousal. Enjoy the stimulation rather than trying to "will an erection."

18. Your attitudes and self-thoughts influence arousal. The key is "sex and pleasure," not "sex and performance."

19. Feelings about a sexual experience are best measured by your sense of pleasure and satisfaction, not whether you got an erection, how hard it was, or whether your partner was orgasmic. Accept that some sexual experiences will be great for both of you; some will be better for one than the other; some will be mediocre; and some will be poor or will be downright failures. Do not put your sexual self-esteem on the line for each sexual experience.

20. Be aware that when sleeping, you get an erection every 90 minutes—three to five erections a night. Sex is a natural physiological function. Don't block it by developing anticipatory anxiety or performance anxiety, or by putting yourself down. Give yourself (and you partner) permission to enjoy the pleasures of sexuality.

male has a good deal of control: He can increase awareness, enjoy the arousal process, and practice waxing and waning of erections. Understanding that it is normal for erections to come and go helps to reduce feelings of panic. When a man is comfortable and confident with gaining an erection, letting it dissipate, and restimulating the penis to an erect state, he has established a base for regaining erectile functioning with a partner.

Still another technique is utilization of imagery during masturbation to desensitize anxiety and build sexual confidence. Imagery (fantasy) can serve as a rehearsal for partner sex. This proceeds along a graded hierarchy similar to the pleasuring/sensate focus exercises utilized in couples sex therapy. Finally, audio, video, or bibliotherapy materials can aid in the reduction of anxiety. We prefer educationally oriented materials rather than commercial erotic materials. The materials increase sexual comfort and focus on a positive, cooperative, non-performance-oriented view of sexuality.

Building Heterosocial Skills

The third component of the cognitive–behavioral model is increasing heterosocial skills, a crucial factor for males without partners. The central concept is that of viewing a woman as a "sexual friend." The male is encouraged to choose a partner—one with whom he feels comfortable, to whom he is attracted, and whom he trusts—to work with him in developing a satisfying sexual relationship. This requires changing assumptions regarding women and sexuality. In addition, he needs to develop behavioral skills, especially the skill of making assertive sexual requests.

Single males with sexual difficulties have self-defeating attitudes about relationships. They do not see women as friends, but rather as sex objects for whom they need to perform and who may embarrass and reject them. A man goes to a bar to "pick up" a woman, tries to impress and seduce her, drinks as a way to ward off anticipatory sexual anxiety, and is obsessed with proving himself. This results in a high likelihood of sexual failure. One strategy is to encourage the male to establish a nonsexual friendship with a woman. As the friendship develops and trust builds, he can communicate his feelings and concerns about sexual performance. Ideally, the female friend is emotionally supportive and can reassure him that women are not demanding and performance-oriented.

The male is encouraged to examine how he meets women and to choose a woman who will be a sexual friend. First, it is crucial for him to be comfortable with her; he cannot be sexual if he views his partner as demanding. The woman's sexual arousal can be accepted as a positive thing, not as a sexual demand that intimidates the man. Another important guideline is for the client to choose a woman to whom he is attracted. Some men deliberately date women they find unattractive, so that they have a rationale for their lack of erection. The client is encouraged to relate to his partner as an attractive, sexual woman, not as a sex object. In addition, firm cautions are provided against attempting intercourse on the first date and against drinking excessively or taking drugs before being sexual. The most important guideline is for the client to choose a woman he trusts. He needs to be comfortable discussing sexual feelings, hopes, and difficulties. Ideally, the woman is comfortable with her sexuality and has a positive attitude toward sex. She feels free to express herself; she is neither sexually inhibited nor sexually demanding. Especially important is that she not punish or embarrass the client. She needs to be viewed as someone to share pleasure with, not someone to perform for. Although selecting a sexual friend is not as easy as going to a pharmacy to fill a prescription, it is easier than most clients or clinicians may imagine, especially for men in their middle years. Most women do not expect men to be "studs." They are responsive to males who are involved, caring partners.

Through use of imagery, audiotapes, or behavioral rehearsal, the client learns to be clear and assertive in communication. This includes standing up for his rights and saying no; more importantly, it includes expressing emotions clearly and making direct sexual requests. The therapist should be as concerned with teaching the man to make clear and direct sexual requests as with teaching him to say "no" to sexual demands. He can learn to speak intimately, sharing feelings of desire as well as concerns. He can share sexual anxiety without putting himself down.

In preparing the man to talk about the erection problem to a new partner, modeling, behavioral rehearsal, imagery, and specific feedback are utilized. A typical script might go as follows:

> I care about you and your sexual feelings. I want us to develop a satisfying sexual relationship. I find you attractive and want the sex to be good for both of us. I can get aroused and have erections, but when I worry and view sex as a performance, it causes problems. You did not cause the problem and it's not your responsibility to cure it, but if you stay my sexual friend, I know erections and intercourse will be exciting and satisfying. It's likely to take time for me to gain sexual comfort and confidence. I need to know if I can trust you to be my friend in overcoming this problem. I want our emotional and sexual relationship to be satisfying.

One of the most difficult decisions is whether to involve the woman in therapy sessions. Putting a new, tenuous relationship under the scrutiny of therapy is a high-risk procedure. Unless the client and his sexual friend are committed to a long-term relationship, clinical judgment would argue against couples therapy. A not-so-funny joke among clinicians is that the best way to break up a badly suited couple is to put them in sex therapy; the intensity of the therapy and sexual exercises will underscore couple problems. A better strategy would be to see the woman on an as-needed basis, preferably in couple sessions. The client can be encouraged to share readings and exercises with her as a way to promote communication.

Building Sexual Stimulation and Arousal Skills

There are two major methods of improving sexual stimulation and arousal skills: fantasy rehearsal (especially during masturbation) and partner sexual exercises. As noted earlier, Zilbergeld (1978) has developed a detailed series of fantasy and masturbation exercises to teach the male focusing, stimulation, and fantasy rehearsal skills. Masturbation exercises give the male a sense of control, reduce performance anxiety, and allow for practice that is free from embarrassment or partner disapproval. Masturbation also permits the male to identify the types of touching and fantasy that result in arousal. With greater self-awareness, he is in a better position to guide his partner. The most important exercise is practice in the process of waxing and waning of erections. The client can develop confidence in his ability to regain an erection and proceed to orgasm with an erect penis. Understanding and gaining confidence in the coming and going of erections can reduce performance anxiety. Many men, as they experience erectile difficulties, develop a habit of ejaculating when the penis is semierect or flaccid. They find orgasm less satisfying, but ejaculate so that they can avoid further frustration and embarrassment. This short-term strategy causes a long-term problem: The erectile difficulty is compounded by a lack of fulfillment through orgasm. From this, it is a short step to sexual avoidance. The male is encouraged to put pleasure back into sexual stimulation and to enjoy ejaculation with an erect penis during masturbation. He can then generalize this to partner manual or oral stimulation.

The male is encouraged to develop arousing sexual fantasy scenarios, whether he is using imagery, video material, pictures, or written materials. He is also encouraged to utilize fantasy during partner sex. Fantasies block performance anxiety and heighten arousal. A client may need to be given permission to utilize fantasy; he may not realize that the majority of males use fantasy during partner sex.

If a client does not have a partner for *in vivo* sexual exercises, the therapist can use guided imagery or bibliotherapy (McCarthy & McCarthy, 1984). The client learns through reading, and then practices in imagery, the importance of nondemand pleasuring and multiple stimulation. Many males have the unrealistic hope that they can find a magical or esoteric sexual technique that will guarantee an erection. They need to understand and accept that erections are the natural result of sexual anticipation, genuine involvement in touching and sensuality, and response to genital stimulation and multiple stimulation scenarios. They also must learn not to allow anxiety or inhibitions to block the natural sexual response cycle.

The man with an erection problem often becomes so obsessed with the state of his penis that he does not attend to pleasurable sensations or to the woman's feelings and needs. He is preoccupied with failing to get a strong erection and satisfy the woman with his penis, so that the resulting emotions of frustration, anger, and guilt predominate. Negative motivation does not promote sexual arousal. Such a man needs to understand that a woman can receive pleasure from manual, oral, and/or rubbing stimulation. He can become more comfortable and skilled at giving stimulation. A great many males view nonintercourse sex as "second best," engaging in it mechanically without feeling; they "service" their partners instead of "giving" to them. A woman usually resents this and feels frustrated, not primarily because of the erection problem, but because of the obsession with failing and the negation of her emotional and sexual needs. A man needs to involve himself, enjoy giving stimulation, and share his partner's arousal. The woman's arousal is the most arousing sexual stimulus. For the male with an erection problem, female arousal is a cue for intimidation and performance anxiety. He needs to learn that he can give and receive touching; can be an active, involved participant in the sexual interaction; and can be responsive as her arousal builds instead of feeling threatened.

A suggested change in sexual technique is to allow the woman to take responsibility for initiating intercourse and guiding the man's penis into her vagina. This permits him to focus on pleasurable sensations instead of feeling burdened by anxieties and responsibilities. The woman is the expert on her vagina; moreover, her active involvement in intercourse can be arousing and can reduce pressure on the man to perform.

Many males with erection problems also have difficulty with early ejaculation. Such clients are assured that they can learn the skill of ejaculatory control, but at this point the focus needs to be on pleasure and arousal, not concern about ejaculating early. Once a client regains comfort and confidence with erections, he can focus on ejaculatory control.

A SUCCESSFUL CASE EXAMPLE: JAMES

James was a 47-year-old, twice-divorced journalist with a long history of psychotherapy. He was referred to sex therapy by his family physician after a comprehensive evaluation by a urologist indicated no specific hormonal, vascular, or neurological impairment. In the initial interview, James admitted he was disappointed that an organic cause was not found. He had taken massive doses of vitamin E and of yohimbine (a drug prescribed by the urologist), but without much impact. Not finding the hoped-for medical cause made James feel depressed and defective. Although James had not had a good erection in the past 4 years during intercourse, he did occasionally awake with morning erections. When he masturbated, between twice a week and once every 2 weeks, he ejaculated with a firm erection. He also had good erections when he engaged in manual or oral sex. In the sex therapist's opinion, the comprehensive medical evaluation was not warranted, given the behavioral history of masturbation and nonintercourse sex. The medical assessment reduced James's motivation for therapy because he felt that the promised medical cure had been denied him.

At the initial session, James was given information about the therapy process, agreed to a therapeutic contract of 10–20 sessions, received the arousal and erection guidelines (see Table 12.1), and was asked to read selected chapters from McCarthy (1988): "Erections," "Being Single Again," and "Pleasuring, Intercourse, and Afterplay." The second session involved taking a detailed sexual history. James had had minimal sex education from family, school, and religious sources. He viewed his parents' marriage as marginal in quality, and felt that most of the parenting was provided by his mother. James saw his mother as intrusive in many ways, but uninvolved in matters regarding relationships and sexuality. He had a younger sister who had married at 19 because of a pregnancy, divorced, and remarried. James was more professionally successful, but admired his sister's second marriage and was envious of the relationship with her three children. James had an 18-year-old son by his first marriage and a 9-year-old daughter by his second. He regretted having minimal contact with his son, although he had a better relationship with his daughter, seeing her every other weekend and occasional weekday nights.

James had begun masturbating at age 12 and experienced excitement mixed with anxiety about being discovered. His masturbatory pattern, which had continued to the present, was penis-oriented, rapid, and goal-oriented; he used *Playboy* pictures or fantasies of women he had seen in movies. He felt embarrassed that for the past 10 years masturbation had been his major sexual outlet. James felt he was a "late bloomer" sexually, having had his first orgasmic experience with a woman at 18 and first intercourse at 20. He recalled several emotionally painful adolescent experiences, especially taking an unattractive woman to the prom. James recalled college as somewhat more successful socially and sexually, but he continued to feel unsure of himself, believing that he did not measure up to peers.

At 23, James married the first woman who fell in love with him, and reveled in daily intercourse. A year after marriage his wife was complaining about their lack of communication, but James ignored these early warning signs and focused his energy on his career. He enjoyed journalism and felt rewarded and satisfied in his profession. Journalism is a very competitive field, and James felt it was one area where he was clearly a winner.

James had hoped that the birth of their son would placate his wife and improve the marriage, but, as often happens, it had the opposite effect. She was consumed with parenting, and James felt left out, sexually and otherwise. He had his first affair, with a reporter from a news magazine, 2 months after his son was born. James approached it as a harmless fling, but it turned into a complicated, time-consuming affair that ended bitterly after several months. His wife suspected that something was amiss, but ignored the cues until she receive an anonymous phone call. James tried to lie his way out of a confrontation, but the damage was done. They entered couples therapy and then individual therapy. The marital history of benign neglect, combined with the extramarital crisis, caused the marital bond to disintegrate. His wife began an affair to help in the transition out of the marriage, and James felt devastated and guilty. It was during this period that he experienced his first erectile difficulty, at age 31. His wife was not sympathetic. She complained about the poor quality of sex and his pattern of early ejaculation, and accused him of being a self-centered lover. James attempted to compensate by becoming overly concerned with her sexual satisfaction, which only compounded his sexual problems.

James was single from age 32 to age 37. Those 5 years were rocky, and he never regained his sexual self-confidence. He met women through the bar scene. James would attempt to impress the woman by "coming on" as if he were a "sexual star." From the first moment, however, he worried about whether he would be able to perform sexually. As the evening wore on, anticipatory anxiety increased. He attempted to reduce this anxiety by drinking—a self-defeating strategy, because alcohol interferes with sexual response, as noted above. The one-night stands were usually unsuccessful, and the cycle of embarrassment and performance anxiety was reinforced. James visited prostitutes on occasion and found that he had more success with fellatio than with intercourse. In partner contacts, James began avoiding intercourse, preferring oral sex.

When he met his second wife, their sexual relationship emphasized cunnilingus and fellatio. She was sexually experienced and uninhibited, and was multiorgasmic during cunnilingus. James was excited by her sexual responsivity and experienced good erections. Since she had never been orgasmic during intercourse, he rationalized that sex was perfect as it was. When they did attempt intercourse, James would lose his erection at the point of intromission or during thrusting. Increasingly, he avoided intercourse.

Unlike the son from his first marriage, his daughter from the second was planned and wanted. James was enthusiastically involved with parenting. He was sure that he had learned from the mistakes of the first marriage, and that this marriage was solid and the sex satisfactory. James was devastated when his wife revealed that she was leaving him for another man. This was the final blow to his sexual self-esteem. It was a bitter divorce proceeding, with much conflict about money and child visitation.

At the time he presented for therapy, James had been dating an emergency room nurse for 4 months. Virginia was a 34-year-old single woman who was interested in marriage and children; she was hesitant about James because of the age difference and his two previous divorces. James pursued Virginia because he found her attractive and her vivaciousness was very appealing. They had met on a group bicycling outing, and shared an interest in outdoor activities, dancing, and playing in a coed volleyball league. Virginia had had 2 years of therapy following the breakup of an engagement, and James thought she was a psychologically solid person.

Initially, their sexual relationship was exciting, and with use of manual and oral stimulation it was functional. However, James lost his erection the third time they tried intercourse. For the month prior to the consultation, they had avoided any sexual activity. James was feeling desperate, afraid Virginia was about to leave. The therapist suggested that James share information and reading materials with Virginia and ask how willing she was to be involved in the treatment. Virginia was enthusiastic about the reading and found it of value. James was surprised when she told him she interpreted his erection problem and subsequent sexual avoidance as an indication that he no longer found her attractive. Virginia had no interest in attending couples therapy sessions, because she felt that doing so would indicate a long-term commitment she did not have. She was willing to be his "sexual friend," a concept she found acceptable, but needed to understand what was expected.

James agreed to weekly individual sex therapy sessions. The sessions were usually focused on two or three major areas. The initial part of each session emphasized cognitive restructuring concerning his past sexual experiences and a present focus on enjoying an open, pleasure-oriented relationship with Virginia. James became aware of the self-defeating nature of his fearful, anxious approach to sexuality. Especially important was realizing that manual and oral stimulation could be pleasurable, were not "second-class" forms of sexuality, and need not be used simply to avoid intercourse. The second part of the session focused on relaxation and imagery to rehearse new sexual scenarios and stimulation techniques, especially making sexual requests before his erection began to wane. James only talked or made requests when he was feeling desperate. Between sessions, James was encouraged to continue bibliotherapy and, on nights when he was not with Virginia, to practice the exercise of waxing and waning of erections using masturbation.

After six sessions, James reported noncoital sexual activity two to three times a week, with erections over 80% of the time and almost always firm erections during orgasm. He reported better communication about touching and sexuality. The therapist was surprised to receive a phone call from Virginia the day before James's next scheduled session. She asked for an individual session, which the therapist scheduled with the understanding that James would be informed. At his session, James reported increased comfort and confidence with erections, but was understandably concerned about what Virginia would share with the therapist. James wanted to attempt intercourse that week, since he had met the agreed-upon criterion of having regained erections three times in nonintercourse sex and was feeling high levels of subjective arousal. The therapist believed that James would use intercourse to prove himself or win over Virginia, and advised keeping the intercourse prohibition in force. He did suggest trying a scenario involving being sexual outside the bedroom. Virginia indeed had something to reveal: She had accepted another job and was returning to her home state in 5 weeks. She felt that James was a warmer and freer sexual person than he had been 2 months before, and she did not want her leaving to be interpreted as a rejection or abandonment. Virginia agreed to attend the next session and share her feelings and perceptions with James.

James accepted Virginia's leaving as a reality, not a personal rejection or a negation of his sexual learning. Virginia clearly valued him and their sexual experiences, and wished him well in future relationships. It was a draining session for all three participants. At his next session, James reported that he and Virginia had attempted intercourse, but he was anxious and ejaculated as she was guiding intromission. At James's suggestion, the next sexual experience did not include intercourse. Their last sexual experience included successful intercourse. James said he now understood what he had read (McCarthy, 1988) and practiced during masturbation imagery: "Intercourse is a natural extension of the pleasuring process." James regretted Virginia's leaving and was grateful to her for being an excellent sexual friend. They decided to keep in touch, but not to attempt a long-distance romance. James was relieved because, although he very much liked and valued Virginia, there were such differences in age, life approach, and political views that he doubted they would have been able to have a successful long-term relationship.

After Virginia's departure, James reduced his therapy sessions to every other week and continued with the masturbation/imagery exercises. In therapy, he discussed his pattern of choosing women on the basis of physical attraction and romantic love. James was instructed to engage in a number of cognitive and writing exercises based on the concept of choosing a partner he was comfortable with, was attracted to, and trusted, and who was open to an intimate relationship. James became aware that it was crucial to choose a woman who had social and political views similar to his own and who did not want a child. Although this made perfect sense to the therapist, for James it was a stunning insight. He desired a woman with a positive attitude toward sex—one who was open to a range of pleasuring scenarios and techniques, and could be orgasmic with nonintercourse sex.

Two months later, James disclosed that he had begun a serious relationship with Barbara, a 43-year-old nurse he had met through friends of Virginia. He discussed the sexual problem and shared books with Barbara. She expressed a wish to attend therapy sessions with him. From the beginning, it was clear that Barbara was interested in having a serious, intimate relationship as well as in being a sexual friend. If this were a Hollywood movie, they would have had great sex, but sex therapy with erectile dysfunction is much more complex. James and Barbara were told that it typically takes a couple 6 months to develop a sexual style that is functional and satisfying. The advantage of dealing with a sexual problem for a new couple is that it focuses the partners on communicating about sexual issues and working together as an intimate team. If they are successful, it will inoculate them against sexual problems as they grow older. The concepts of nondemand pleasuring, multiple stimulation, and emotional and sexual intimacy reach fruition with the aging couple.

James and Barbara started couples sex therapy on a weekly basis, cut back to every other week after 2 months, and terminated regular sessions

3 months later. At the last session, a 6-month follow-up was scheduled. They agreed that they would focus in the intervening time on developing alternative sexual scenarios when one partner was anxious or not desirous of intercourse, on developing comfort with an additional intercourse position, and on expanding multiple stimulation techniques during intercourse. At least once a month, they would schedule a pleasuring session with the clear understanding that it would not proceed to intercourse. They would also discuss integrating children into a blended family, since they planned to marry within 4 months. James and Barbara realized that marriage and keeping marital sex satisfying requires time and energy, and were committed to making theirs a successful and stable marriage.

CLINICAL OBSERVATIONS CONCERNING SUCCESSFUL CASES

In our cultural myth of romantic love, the woman rescues the man, and love is enough to sustain the relationship and make sexual problems magically disappear. In truth, the process of regaining erectile comfort and confidence is complex, gradual, and seldom without setbacks. Love is neither necessary nor sufficient to overcome an erectile dysfunction. The male hopes that an external source will magically give him a perfect penis—a prosthesis, an injection, a perfect woman, a fail-proof sexual technique. He is in search of the easy, automatic, autonomous erections of his youth. Once there has been a sensitizing event, however, the male cannot return to the un-self-conscious time of guaranteed erections. Most males view this as a devastating loss. In my opinion, it is a long-term benefit in terms of a male's awareness of his body and the complexity of sexuality. Sex is more than his penis, intercourse, and orgasm. A man cannot really own his sexuality until he stops treating his penis as an automatic performance machine. His penis is connected to his thoughts, his feelings, and the relationship. Owning his sexuality means accepting variability. The overemphasis on medical interventions to create erections is a way of bypassing the complexity of male sexuality. Even if such an intervention is a technical success, it can be a psychological and interpersonal failure. The male who is aware of the complexity and variability of sexuality, both for himself and for his partner, is more likely to integrate a prosthesis or injection program successfully into his sex life.

In the case described above, James needed a number of cognitive, behavioral, and emotional interventions before his erectile comfort and confidence could be restored. The sexual relationship with Virginia, and an understanding of the limits of that relationship, were important. Developing realistic expectations allowed James to experience the loss without negating his sexual gains, feeling abandoned, or regressing. Even a steady, intimate relationship with Barbara did not restore perfect sexual functioning. A key concept in successful treatment of males with erection problems is to accept the natural variability of the penis and sexual responsiveness. Occasional instances of not having an erection are normal, not indications of a dysfunction. The female sexual script is healthier and more realistic. The woman does not demand desire, arousal, and orgasm at each sexual opportunity. The male has to learn a new sexual script that is pleasure-oriented, that includes a variety of sexual scenarios in addition to intercourse, that involves the woman actively as a sexual friend, and that is based on variability in sexual expression. A crucial lesson for James was that he could alter the sexual script when he was anxious or not aroused. Rather than trying to force intercourse, he could focus on giving pleasure to his partner. He could also accept a sexual interaction that was mediocre or that failed altogether without overreacting; if possible, he laughed it off. He was encouraged to initiate being sexual in the next day or two, when he was feeling more comfortable and aroused. This type of cognitive set allows a male to maintain sexual gains and erectile functioning.

AN UNSUCCESSFUL CASE EXAMPLE: KARL

Karl was a 49-year-old divorced real estate developer who sought therapy at the insistence of his present female companion. He was referred by a former client who had been successfully treated for inhibited sexual desire. Karl had been single for 4 years and was a very skeptical client. During his marriage he had been in family therapy, with his adolescent daughter the identified patient. He had participated in 2 years of individual and couples therapy before his wife decided to leave. Since separating, he had seen a therapist for seven sessions regarding difficulties with another woman. His present companion, Dorothy, was willing to attend sessions, but Karl insisted on being seen alone.

Karl presented himself as a hard-driving, successful businessman who could not understand why his personal life was in such disarray. He was the oldest and only surviving son of a family of five. His next younger brother had been killed in Vietnam, and his youngest brother had been killed in an alcohol-related car accident. His two sisters were married and continued to live in Oklahoma close to their widowed mother. Karl had grown up poor in rural Oklahoma, and felt more successful than anyone he knew from his small town. He reported no sex education from parents, Sunday school, or regular school. He was a business major in college, but did not complete his degree; he married at 22 following a very active social and sexual life, and moved to the Washington, D.C., area to take a job with a hotel chain. Karl was ambitious and willing to take risks. Most of his energy went into his career, and by age 30 he had his own development company, four children, and over 20 affairs. He viewed himself as a sexually oriented man who knew how to have fun, but was dedicated to his wife and children. Karl reported himself as "macho," envied by business colleagues and sought after by women. The women he had affairs with were all younger and less successful than he.

After the fourth child, his wife asked Karl to get a vasectomy, but he refused. She eventually obtained a tubal ligation. Although he had four children and described himself as a dedicated parent, Karl was a marginally involved father and viewed conception, contraception, and children as a woman's domain.

Most of Karl's sexual energy went into affairs. The frequency of marital sex decreased to once or twice per month, and he found it increasingly difficult to become aroused with his wife. Karl found affairs, especially with women in the real estate field, most arousing. Sex was his reward after closing a deal. He was particularly "turned on" at conventions or meetings, held at lavish hotels with expense account evenings.

As this chapter has emphasized throughout, men experience a transition in their 30s or 40s from easy, automatic, autonomous erections to erections that come from interaction and stimulation. The majority of males make this transition comfortably, but for a significant proportion (including Karl), sex becomes a major problem. Karl did not want to need anything from a woman; he merely wanted to impress her with his sexual prowess. Three things occurring in conjunction disrupted his erectile security—the stress of financial problems; his daughter's emotional problems and the ensuing therapy; and his inability to accept partner stimulation. If Karl was aroused, he enjoyed penile stimulation, but he rebelled against the notion that he needed a woman's stimulation to help him become erect.

Karl reacted very badly to his first erectile failure, blaming the woman and immediately terminating the relationship. When an erectile problem occurred with a woman he had had a 6-year casual sexual realtionship with, he panicked. Karl consulted a physician, who recommended that he eat less, stop smoking, and exercise more—good advice that Karl ignored. He went through a complete assessment at a medically oriented male sexual dysfunction clinic, where a penile prosthesis was recommended, even though he still had successful intercourse 75% of the time. Interestingly, neither his wife nor his present companion was part of the assessment process.

Six years later, Karl was a more cynical and less self-assured man, although he continued to display a good deal of bravado. He was not enjoying being single and felt alienated from his adult and adolescent children. He now had a grandchild, but had only seen her once. Karl was angry at his wife for leaving him and blamed her for his sexual and financial problems. He was stuck in a vicious cycle: anxious anticipation, sexual experiences consisting of hurried and usually unsuccessful intercourse, and increasing periods of sexual avoidance thereafter. The women he dated were in their 30s, involved with real estate deals that made them financially dependent on him. The woman who insisted he seek therapy, Dorothy, was a real estate agent hired to sell houses in his recently completed development. Unbeknownst to her, he was dating two other women. Karl's major sexual outlets were a prostitute and weekly appointments at a sexual massage parlor. In both cases, he would be totally passive while the woman "worked on him" and brought him to orgasm orally or manually.

It was difficult to establish a therapeutic alliance with Karl because he was so guarded about being in a "one-down" position. He emphasized his net worth and made it clear that his past therapists had disappointed him. Karl was resistant to bibliotherapy ("That's pop psychology, I'm paying money for a professional"), relaxation ("I need to be in control"), and guided imagery ("I want to face you, see you, and talk with you"). Karl did agree to masturbation exercises; he was pleased to discover that his erections would wax and wane, and that he could stimulate himself to orgasm with an erection. This convinced him that his penis was intact and that he did not need an implant. Karl also stopped visits to the massage parlor. The therapist's rationale was that impersonal sex and his passivity would not transfer to partner sex; Karl disagreed and said he would have more contacts with the prostitute and be more active with her. What transpired was an unusual hierarchy of implementing techniques. When the therapist encouraged Karl to request teasing, nongenital stimulation until he got a beginning erection, he did this first in masturbation, then with the prostitute, next with one of his two girlfriends besides Dorothy, and finally with Dorothy. The level of success was better with masturbation and the prostitute than with the girlfriend or Dorothy. The therapist interpreted this as indicating an intimacy problem. Karl was unable to view women as sexual friends, and did not find Dorothy sexually attractive.

Next session, Karl reported with great smugness that he had had intercourse twice with Dorothy, thus "proving" that there was no intimacy problem. During the week, Dorothy called the therapist and insisted that she come to the next session; Karl agreed. When the therapist met them in the waiting room, he was surprised how different Dorothy was from Karl's description of her. She was 40 pounds overweight, but elegantly dressed and very aggressive in her presentation. The session focused on her financial demands, since she had stayed with a housing project that wasn't selling and a man who couldn't get an erection unless she put on special gloves (which she had done the last two times). Karl's response was to brag about the progress he had made and assure her that if she stood by him he would make her rich. At the next session, Karl was making jokes about how obnoxious Dorothy had been, at the same time reporting continued erectile progress. When the therapist brought up the issue of a fetishistic arousal pattern, Karl denied it and said it was similar to the intimacy issue. Karl claimed that the therapist was raising additional problems to keep therapy going instead of realizing he was cured. The therapist tried to make a distinction between requests for special turn-ons and fetishistic arousal, but Karl remained defensive and denying. The therapist then switched tactics and discussed Karl's attraction to Dorothy. Karl's task was to make two requests of her that would increase his attraction to her. A few days after this session, however, Karl left a message on the tape machine saying that he would not attend further therapy sessions because he felt he had learned all he needed. Attempts to elicit a follow-up were not successful.

CLINICAL OBSERVATIONS CONCERNING UNSUCCESSFUL CASES

Sex therapy is a difficult and complex field, especially with male sexual dysfunction. Permission giving, sexual information, nondemand pleasuring, viewing sexuality broadly, and seeing the partner as an intimate and giving friend are concepts more acceptable to females than to males. This is particularly true for erection problems, since traditional male socialization puts such a high premium on the penis, erection, and intercourse as measures of masculinity. The single male with an erection problem yearns to go back to easy, automatic, autonomous erections so that he can perform any time with any woman. A crucial therapeutic task is to develop realistic expectations not only about erections, but about the male sexual role. The concept that sexuality works better when the male's attitudes, behavior, and emotions are congruent is not accepted by many males. They view erections and intercourse as independent of other elements of life and a relationship.

A crucial concept is that of viewing the woman as a sexual friend rather than as someone to perform for. In the case described above, this concept was not acceptable to Karl. He had a "secret" arousal pattern that helped erections in the short run, but that further alienated him from partner sex. The problem with fetishistic and other paraphilic arousal patterns is that they serve to wall off the man from erotic sensations, partner stimulation, and emotional intimacy. A man's use of fantasy during partner sex can serve as a bridge to increase arousal; however, Karl's use of fantasy and fetish material would eventually lead him to a sexual dead end. Erectile confidence is based on responsiveness to a variety of sexually arousing stimuli, not dependence on a paraphilia.

Dealing with the erection problems of a man without a regular (or a cooperative) partner can be frustrating for both client and therapist. There is a tendency to engage in "if-only" thinking—if only a spouse would be cooperative, if only a partner would be receptive to oral stimulation, if only the client himself had not wasted 10 years drinking, if only he had known this in his 30s rather than his 60s. The therapeutic focus needs to be on clarifying the present and planning for the future, not on engaging in "if-only" thinking about the past. The reality of the situation needs to be acknowledged and dealt with, instead of wishing that a relationship could be revived or that the man had sought therapy earlier.

By the time most men enter sex therapy for erection problems, they have a long history of sexual failures and embarrassment. Many males adopt a pattern of sexual avoidance, leading to inhibited sexual desire. They no longer own their sexuality or feel anticipation about being sexual. Rebuilding anticipation and sexual desire needs to be directly dealt with. One technique is ask a client to recall periods when he did anticipate sex and found it satisfying. Imagery techniques can then be used to project sexual anticipation and satisfaction into the future.

A particularly difficult issue is how to deal with the pattern of repeated or intermittent erectile dysfunction. No intervention guarantees that each sexual experience will be successful. If the man has difficulty 25% or more of the time, he will not establish erectile confidence. A threefold strategy can be used to address establishing positive, realistic expectations for the male with a chronic erectile problem. The first is to increase comfort, awareness, and responsivity to sexual stimulation. The male needs to be aware and to communicate which sexual scenarios and techniques build arousal. Second, he needs to understand that when he is anxious or not feeling sexual, attempts at intercourse are likely to be unsuccessful. Instead, he can suggest alternate pleasuring scenarios that are enjoyable for both partners. Sexual satisfaction has to be defined more broadly than intercourse. Third, there will still be unsuccessful sexual experiences, whether these occur once a month or once a year. The man needs to be able to shrug or laugh such an experience off and to initiate a pleasure-oriented sexual interaction within the next day or two. The essence of sexuality is giving and receiving pleasurable touching. When the male fails to achieve an erection or it fades during intercourse, he is likely to feel disappointed and frustrated; however, he need not overreact with a sense of failure and/or avoidance. He needs to accept and to communicate with his partner about the normal variability of erections and intercourse, as well as to enjoy the intimacy of sharing pleasure.

There is a dearth of well-controlled outcome studies in this area. Clinical lore and my own experience indicate that success rates for therapy with single men are lower than for couples sex therapy. However, over 60% of males with erectile dysfunction profit from individual cognitive–behavioral sex therapy. The male with the best prognosis is one who is open to adopting a broader-based approach to women, sexuality, and erections. Specifically, he is able to view the woman as a sexual friend; to be receptive to her stimulation; and to view intercourse as part of the pleasuring process, not as a pass–fail performance test.

SPECIAL ISSUES WITH GAY MEN

A few points must be made about gay men without regular partners. The most common pattern is to be embarrassed and try to hide the dysfunction by servicing the partner manually or orally or by being passive in anal intercourse (a high-risk behavior for contracting human immunodeficiency virus, or HIV). A second self-defeating strategy is to rely on "telephone sex," in which the dysfunction is hidden.

The man's negative attitudes toward homosexuality need to be confronted and cognitively restructured so that, emotionally and sexually, he accepts homosexuality as optimal for him. The concept of interacting with a "sexual friend" he is comfortable with, is attracted to, and trusts needs to be discussed. Use of behavioral rehearsal provides practice in disclosing the problem to a new partner. Especially important is his right to request stimulation that is arousing for him. Integrating emotional intimacy with sexual expression not only will increase erectile functioning, but can add to a more complete experience of gay sexuality. Although many of the strategies and techniques discussed in this chapter are transferable to gay men, sensitivity to special issues and good clinical judgment are crucial.

INCREASING MALE CONSCIOUSNESS
AND PREVENTING ERECTILE DYSFUNCTION

Clinically oriented books focus on diagnosis and treatment of dysfunctional behavior. This chapter has presented an integrated assessment–treatment model using cognitive–behavioral strategies and techniques for single males who have erectile problems. The model emphasizes (1) changing cognitions about sexuality; (2) decreasing sexual anxiety and increasing sexual comfort; (3) developing heterosocial skills, especially choosing a woman as a sexual friend; and (4) building sexual stimulation and arousal skills.

In the public health field, it is axiomatic that the best intervention program is one that emphasizes prevention. How can we as a culture prevent erection problems? Elsewhere, we (McCarthy & McCarthy, 1990) have emphasized that intellectually, emotionally, behaviorally, and sexually, there are many more similarities than differences between men and women. We have advocated an equity-based model of male–female relationships to replace the traditional double standard. Theorists have emphasized the negative impact of the double standard on female sexuality, but in the long run it has an even stronger negative impact on male sexuality, especially as the male ages. Adolescent and young adult males are capable of autonomous sexual functioning. However, in the 30s, 40s, and beyond, not only is sex more pleasurable as an intimate and interactive experience, but partner stimulation is necessary for male arousal. If males in their 20s could come to view sexuality as a cooperative, giving, pleasure-oriented experience, and their partners as sexual persons and sexual equals, this would help to prevent unwanted pregnancy, sexually transmitted diseases, and sexual trauma. Just as importantly, it would set the stage for lifelong sexual desire, arousal, orgasm, and satisfaction. Ideally, these attitudes and experiences would inoculate males against sexual dysfunction as they age.

A crucial element in preventing erectile problems is establishing reasonable expectations about penile functioning and sexual satisfaction. The "male machine" myth, and the view that the penis must always be functional regardless of stress, anxiety, relationship problems, anger, illness, or depression, must be confronted. Sex is a positive dimension of life, an integral part of a man's personality; it needs to be expressed in a way that increases self-esteem, pleasure, and intimacy. Males can be aware of and own their sexuality, instead of falling into the macho role of asking no questions and pretending to be sexual experts who can go it alone. Women make up the vast majority of those who attend sex and communication classes, read books about sexuality and relationships, and consult physicians and therapists with sexual concerns. Men need to accept that it is healthy and masculine to ask questions and to seek help for sexual problems.

Another crucial aspect of prevention is making it widely known that the hitherto dreaded experience of failing to achieve or maintain an erection sufficient for intercourse is in fact an almost universal phenomenon. Rather than overreacting and building anticipatory and performance anxiety, men can learn to accept occasional erectile problems. In subsequent sexual experiences they can focus on increasing comfort, making sexual requests, and increasing involvement and arousal.

The greater the extent to which men, therapists, educators, and the culture at large adopt a broader view of male sexuality—one that emphasizes pleasure rather than performance, and celebrates the similarities between men and women—the less erectile dysfunction there will be. Adopting these attitudes toward sexuality will serve males well as they age. With less efficient hormonal, vascular, and neurological functioning with aging, psychological factors, sexual stimulation, and partner emotional and sexual giving become central in preventing erectile dysfunction.

REFERENCES

Althof, S. E. (1989). Psychogenic impotence: Treatment of men and couples. In S. R. Leiblum & R. C. Rosen (Eds.), *Principles and practice of sex therapy* (2nd ed.): *Update for the 1990s* (pp. 237–265). New York: Guilford Press.

Annon, J. (1976). *The behavioral treatment of sexual problems.* New York: Harper & Row.

Barbach, L., & Levine, L. (1980). *Shared intimacies.* New York: Bantam.

Heiman, J. R., & LoPiccolo, J. (1988). *Becoming orgasmic: A sexual and personal growth program for women.* Prentice-Hall.

Levine, S. B., Risen, C., & Althof, S. E. (1990). The diagnosis and nature of paraphilia. *Journal of Sex and Marital Therapy, 16,* 89–102.

Masters, W., & Johnson, V. (1970). *Human sexual inadequacy.* Boston: Little, Brown.

McCarthy, B. W. (1988). *Male sexual awareness.* New York: Carroll & Graf.

McCarthy, B. W. (1989). Cognitive–behavioral strategies and techniques in the treatment of early ejaculation. In S. R. Leiblum & R. C. Rosen (Eds.), *Principles and practice of sex therapy* (2nd ed.): *Update for the 1990s* (pp. 141–167). New York: Guilford Press.

McCarthy, B. W., & McCarthy, E. (1984). *Sexual awareness.* New York: Carroll & Graf.

McCarthy, B. W., & McCarthy, E. (1989). *Female sexual awareness.* New York: Carroll & Graf.

McCarthy, B. W., & McCarthy, E. (1990). *Couple sexual awareness.* New York: Carroll & Graf.

Reynolds, B. (1990). *Personal potential* [Audiotape]. (Available from Barry Reynolds, 12304 Santa Monica Blvd., Suite 211, Los Angeles, CA 90025; 213-207-3157)

Schover, L. R. (1984). *Prime time: Sexual health for men over fifty.* New York: Holt, Rinehart & Winston.

Tiefer, L. (1986). In pursuit of the perfect penis: The medicalization of male sexuality. *American Behavioral Scientist, 29,* 579–599.

Zilbergeld, B. (1978). *Male sexuality.* Boston: Little, Brown.

13

Erectile Failure and Chronic Illness

LESLIE R. SCHOVER

Men with chronic illnesses are no different from healthy men in desiring an active, satisfying sexual life. Yet it is often the case that sexual difficulties accompany acute or long-standing illness, as a consequence of either the illness itself, the prescribed treatment, or the psychological and interpersonal concomitants. Sex therapists who are called upon to consult or treat chronically ill men experiencing erectile failure need to be conversant with a wide variety of specialized issues in assessment and treatment. Unfortunately, most therapists are relatively uninformed about the subtleties and particular problems associated with erectile dysfunction in men with chronic illness.

No one in the field is better able to address these issues than Leslie Schover, author of several books and many articles and chapters dealing with the sexual needs and concerns of the chronically ill. In this chapter, Schover begins by reminding the reader that several psychological sequelae to chronic illness may impede erectile function, apart from the impairment attributable to the illness itself. For example, some men are concerned about changes in their physical appearance, such as hair loss from chemotherapy, paralysis from spinal cord injury, or amputation. Many patients will react to these insults to their physical appearance or sense of self with emotional withdrawal and sexual avoidance, as well as profound feelings of depression, anxiety, or fear. Single men are at special risk for serious health problems, and may subsequently be unable to develop a satisfactory sexual life. For example, young single men who are ill with juvenile-onset diabetes, severe asthma, or congenital heart disease may not have experienced the developmental milestones associated with building sexual confidence, and may require social skills training prior to treatment for erectile failure itself.

In reviewing current assessment approaches, Schover cautions us regarding limitations of the usual diagnostic screening procedures when dealing with individuals with chronic illness. For example, nocturnal penile tumescence (NPT) testing may not be diagnostic in young diabetic men, since some of these patients are able to achieve satisfactory erections during sex, despite impaired sleep erections. Similarly, some men with diabetes, chemical dependency, or multiple sclerosis may experience *reversible episodes of erectile failure, suggesting that tissue-destroying surgical interventions may be contraindicated in these cases.*

Obviously, the approach to treatment—whether surgical, pharmacological, or psychological—must be tailored to the specialized needs of the individual patient. Often, the initial evaluation occurs in a hospital setting, where privacy is at a premium. Outpatient visits are often difficult to schedule. Patient support groups may be utilized as helpful adjuncts to therapy. Several issues arise in counseling chronically ill patients that are not characteristic of healthy men. For example, fatigue and shortness of breath during sex is not uncommon in patients with cardiac disease, chronic obstructive pulmonary disease, or other illnesses that reduce energy levels. Patients with spinal cord lesions, or individuals with limited movement because of severe arthritis or low back pain, may require advice about comfortable sexual positions. Men recovering from stroke or cardiac surgery may have erroneous fears about the risks associated with sexual exertion, and often need accurate information. Men who have lost control of bowel or bladder function will need assistance in dealing with concerns about body image and the aesthetics of sex. Safer sexual practices for men who are positive for human immunodeficiency virus (HIV) require special attention as well.

Treatment of erectile failure in men with chronic illness requires flexibility, specialized knowledge, and heightened sensitivity. Again, Schover reminds us that it is important to assess both the psychological and physiological impact of the disease and its treatment on sexuality. Partner involvement in the therapy process is critical, since partners often feel anxious, confused, and uncertain about how best to support their mates. Despite the special problems posed, results can be quite gratifying for patients and therapists alike.

Leslie R. Schover, Ph.D., is a member of the Center for Sexual Function at The Cleveland Clinic Foundation. She is the author of Prime Time *(1984), a book exploring male sexuality, as well as the coauthor (with Søren Buus Jensen) of a scholarly volume entitled* Sexuality and Chronic Illness: A Comprehensive Approach *(1988). Author of dozens of articles on sex and various diseases, Schover is regarded as an international authority on the sexual sequelae of chronic illness.*

Case Vignette
The gray-haired farmer leans close to his second wife of 3 years, a plump and cheerful woman, as if for reassurance. She holds his hand as they talk to the psychologist about options for sexual rehabilitation after cancer surgery to remove his colon and rectum. He cannot meet the clinician's eyes when she inquires about his colostomy care and about the occurrence of any embarrassing odors or leaks. Discussing his sexual desire and degree of erection since the operation is even more difficult.

He blushes and stammers, calling the psychologist "ma'am." His wife answers many of the questions for him. At the end of the interview, when the couple has decided to try a home program of intracavernosal injections, he says, "You know, you people have made me feel it was worth it to go through all this. Until now, I had my doubts. When the surgeon said that this operation would end my sex life, I told Jeannie, 'Honey, it looks like you made a bad mistake hooking up with me. Maybe you should go and find someone who's still a man.'"

Jeannie playfully punches her husband's arm to indicate her opinion of this advice.

"Really, that was the thing I was most afraid of, that she would leave me, even though I couldn't blame her if she did." The patient looks at the floor as his wife rolls her eyes and mouths the word "Men." "But now I think we just may be able to get back somewhere near normal. I can live with the bag and the dry climax, if I can just get it hard again."

A large percentage of men seeking help for erectile failure have a chronic illness. As previous chapters of this book have noted, medical conditions such as hypertension, diabetes, or cardiovascular disease can disrupt the hemodynamics of erection. Neurological damage to the erectile response is common in men with diabetes, multiple sclerosis (MS), other progressive neurological diseases, radical pelvic cancer surgery, and spinal cord trauma. Hormonal abnormalities that interfere with erectile function are seen in end-stage renal disease and cirrhosis of the liver, and also as a side effect of treating metastatic prostate cancer. In addition, chronic illness can contribute to sexual dysfunction through its psychological impact on mood, body image, and relationship satisfaction. This chapter focuses on the special issues in assessment and treatment of erectile failure for men who have serious and debilitating medical illnesses.

CHRONIC ILLNESS AND CAUSES OF ERECTILE FAILURE

This section highlights the psychological and medical concomitants of chronic illness that may cause erectile failure.

Psychological Causes

Many illnesses create changes in a man's physical appearance. Some changes are public, such as hair loss from chemotherapy or paralysis from a spinal cord injury. Others are private but visible to a sexual partner—for example, an ostomy, a surgical scar, or the loss of a testicle. Some illnesses do not change outward appearance, but nevertheless leave a man feeling stigmatized. Men may report such a reaction to needing to start injecting insulin or having a myocardial infarction.

Women in our society are given permission to grieve over lost attractiveness. The American Cancer Society designs programs to help women adjust to mastectomy or chemotherapy, and to help them use cosmetics, wigs, and breast prostheses to look as attractive and normal as possible. Men who want to wear a wig or have a testicular prosthesis implanted after cancer surgery have no special support programs, however. Instead, they are often ridiculed for being oversensitive and counseled to "tough it out." Faced with the fear of rejection by their mates or potential dating partners, plus the shame of admitting their distress, many men use our society's approved masculine coping strategy: withdrawal from intimacy. A man may invent excuses to avoid sex, such as fatigue or pain. He may avoid revealing his fears to a sexual partner, even if she is a wife of 30 years. This type of anxiety and emotional distance can contribute to erectile failure.

A similar but broader issue is the general way in which men handle their emotional reactions to an illness that is life-threatening or curtails normal activities. Traditional gender roles equate masculinity with strength and stoicism. A man takes care of his mate, sexually and financially. A threatened or real loss of sexual function is thus seen as a loss of manhood, especially if it is coupled with a loss of ability to work (Liss-Levinson, 1982). Again, it seems that emotional withdrawal is a strategy men often use to cope with their emotional distress. If a man anticipates that he will not be able to "perform" sexually, he stops initiating affectionate touch and may even avoid sexual situations by staying up later than his partner or avoiding private time together. Anxiety over loss of masculinity can result from an episode of erectile failure, and then contributes to future difficulties by the means of distracting cognitions about sexual failure during lovemaking (Abrahamson, Barlow, & Abrahamson, 1989).

Mood disturbance is common in chronic illness, especially in more debilitated patients (Bukberg, Penman, & Holland, 1984). In men, depression can be a reversible cause of erectile failure, affecting both nocturnal penile tumescence (NPT) and erections during sex (Howell et al., 1987; Thase et al., 1988). Increasingly, psychoses such as schizophrenia and bipolar affective disorder are regarded as chronic medical illnesses. Men with these disorders present a challenge to clinicians: Even if their condition is currently stable, their medications may contribute to sexual problems. It is difficult to judge whether the erectile failure under such circumstances is reversible. Psychotic episodes are very alienating to a spouse; their impact is similar to that of recurrent substance abuse. In an altered state, a patient may seem to be a "different person." The spouse may not be eager to resume sex or may fear that sexual arousal will somehow precipitate another psychotic episode.

Some illnesses bring specific anxieties regarding sex. Examples include myths that heart attacks and strokes commonly occur during sexual activity; that cancer can be sexually transmitted; or that sex is dangerous for diabetics because it often triggers hypoglycemic episodes. Other common misconceptions center around the idea that sex is sinful and unhealthy. Thus a man with a serious illness may believe that he can "bargain," giving up sex in order to live longer. A spouse can also avoid sex, feeling that it saps a man's strength or will interfere with his recovery from an illness. Even if the couple stays sexually active, cognitions like these promote severe anxiety during sex and can thus decrease arousal.

Men who are not married are more at risk for many serious health problems. They may have less healthy lifestyle habits than married men, or may lack the emotional buffering of an intimate relationship (Verbrugge, 1979). In clinical practice, it seems that men who are not married or are in newer relationships are more likely to seek help for an erection problem related to an illness than are those in long-term marriages. A man often fears that a new partner will leave or that he will not be able to attract dates if he cannot function sexually. It is as if erections were the currency of relationships. It is very difficult to convince such men that women, especially in older age groups, are often unconcerned about erections if men provide companionship, tenderness, and noncoital sexual activity.

Young single men who become ill as children (e.g., those with juvenile-onset diabetes, severe asthma, or congenital heart disease) may never have experienced common developmental milestones in relationships, such as casual dating in high school, exploratory sexual experiences, or a committed relationship. They may need training in social skills, or at least in sexual communication.

Case Vignette

Johnny was born to a working-class, first-generation Slavic immigrant family. He had severe hypospadias, so that his urethral opening was at the base of his penis and his erection curved downward. He was acutely aware of his difference from other boys, and was teased at school because he could not urinate standing up. His family never sought medical advice, and Johnny was 22 when he discovered that surgical correction was available.

Although his condition was corrected so that he had straight erections and his uretha opened just somewhat off-center on the glans penis, he remained convinced that his penis was abnormally small. He came in at age 30 requesting surgery to enlarge his penis. He had never exchanged more than a few kisses with a woman and denied homosexual fantasies or experience.

His girlfriend was alcoholic and highly critical of his ineptness on the few occasions that he coaxed her into trying some sexual touch. He would then always lose his erection. She had had several other partners in the past, but currently led an isolated life, drinking and taking care of her elderly parents. She only had an interest in sex when she was drinking.

Treatment for Johnny centered first on education about normal male anatomy and sexual function. His concept of penile size was derived from viewing X-rated videos. He estimated that the average man's erection was 15 inches long and was stunned to hear that at 7 inches, his erect penis was above the mean size. He also learned about women's genitals and the sexual response cycle.

As his girlfriend continued to refuse to come to therapy with him, or even to engage in sensate focus exercises at home, Johnny agreed that he needed to seek a new partner. He began to attend singles dances and met an older woman who was eager to try sexual activity with him. Although at first he was taken aback by her assertiveness, he gradually did try sexual activity and was eventually able to have intercourse. He continued to be anxious about penis size, however, and preferred to wear his shirts untucked at work so that nobody could see the outlines of his genital area.

Younger men with sexual dysfunction who have survived cancer treatment, renal transplant, spinal cord injury, or other chronic illnesses may also be worried about infertility. If their illness has impaired their fertility, sex may bring up feelings of grief or anger. Again, issues of lost "manhood" may be involved. If normal sperm count and motility are found, but erectile failure is interfering with intercourse, a primary motive for getting treatment may be to enable the husband to get his wife pregnant. When fertility itself is impaired, the options for treatment are limited in men (Tanagho, Lue, & McClure, 1988). A few men may be candidates for repair of a varicocele (varicose vein in the scrotal sac) or microsurgery to reconnect a blocked vas deferens. Another small group may respond to hormonal stimulation or to drug or mechanical therapy for retrograde ejaculation. Many couples, however, must choose among artificial insemination by donor, adoption, or childlessness. Counseling can often be helpful during the decision-making process.

Medical Causes

Medical illnesses, as well as their treatments, can interfere with the physiology of erectile function. Since previous chapters have covered much of this material, only a brief summary is presented here. These topics are also addressed more fully in Schover and Jensen (1988, Ch. 5).

Hormonal abnormalities are rare causes of erectile failure, but are seen with antiandrogenic treatment for metastatic prostate cancer; prolactin-secreting tumors of the pituitary gland; end-stage renal disease during uremia or dialysis; and perhaps in severe chronic obstructive pulmonary disease (COPD). Medications may block testosterone action (cimetidine), elevate prolactin (phenothiazines), or have estrogenic effects (digoxin, spironolactone).

Vascular pathology, including poor arterial filling or failure of the veno-occlusive mechanism in erection, is a more usual cause of erectile failure. Risk factors for vascular problems include the major risks for generalized arteriosclerosis: heavy smoking, elevated cholesterol or triglycerides, and diabetes. Men who have cardiovascular disease frequently have erectile failure as a result of vascular abnormalities in the hemodynamics of the penis. In addition, pelvic radiotherapy for cancer or use of pelvic arteries for multiple renal transplant surgeries can contribute.

Damage to the autonomic nerves that control blood flow to the penis may be seen in diabetics, men with COPD, chronic alcoholics, and men with end-stage renal disease. The prostatic nerve plexus can be damaged in pelvic cancer surgery. Injuries to the spinal cord or diseases such as MS are more rare and can attack not only the nerves that control penile blood flow, but the sensory pathways that mediate pleasure with touch on the genital skin as well as the sensation of orgasm. Sensory loss can obviously contribute to poor maintenance of erections. A number of medications, including the antihypertensives, beta blockers, antipsychotics, and antidepressants, can interfere with erections because of central or peripheral impact on the autonomic nervous system. Most anticonvulsant drugs appear to leave sexual function intact, however (Jensen et al., 1990).

Occasionally, men lose part of the penis through accident or as the result of a surgical treatment for penile or urethral cancer. Men can have erections after partial penectomy that are adequate for vaginal intromission and thrusting, however. Men often dread surgery involving the prostate, because they fear it will damage erectile capacity. Actually, the prostate gland itself is merely part of the semen-producing machinery of the body; it is the plexus of nerves that runs between the prostate and rectum that is crucial to erection. Although radical prostate removal for cancer indeed often damages these nerves, surgery through the penis to remove benign, overgrown tissues at the core of the prostate is rarely extensive enough to penetrate the capsule of the gland and thus to involve the nerve plexus. Unfortunately, this lesser surgery does damage the valve that prevents retrograde ejaculation, so that about 80% of men will have "dry orgasm" afterward. Although the muscular contractions and sensation of orgasm are intact, no semen is ejaculated. The semen instead flows backwards into the bladder, mingling with the urine stored there. If men are not clearly prepared for dry orgasms, many become angry and anxious after prostate surgery for benign disease; as a result, they may develop psychogenic erectile failure. Among other common side effects of prostate biopsy or surgery are episodes of blood appearing in semen or urine. Again, men should be warned of this possibility and reassured that it is rarely a serious problem.

Chronic pain can interfere with erection by distracting a man from sexual arousal. Men with low back pain or arthritis have high rates of sexual dysfunction. In a recent case series of 48 men with chronic, unexplained genital pain, about half complained of erectile failure (Schover, 1990). Pain occurred in a variety of sites, including the penis, testes, perineum, and bladder or urethra. In one-third of the men, pain was triggered by sexual arousal or orgasm. Like women with chronic pelvic pain, many of these men had psychopathology (particularly other chronic pain syndromes, somatizing disorder, depression, and chemical dependency).

SPECIAL ISSUES IN ASSESSMENT

The general principles of psychological and medical assessment of sexual function have been covered in previous chapters. Here the discussion is restricted to special issues relevant to the man with a chronic illness.

Adapting to a Hospital Setting

Most sexual dysfunction clinics are not located in a hospital environment and perform evaluations exclusively on an outpatient basis. Some have patients fill out a vast array of questionnaires, especially if the clinic is a research setting. Assessing chronically ill patients may require some modification of such a routine. Studies of patients with different diseases concur that most men or women prefer sexual counseling to come from their primary caregivers rather than from a sexuality specialist (Schover & Jensen, 1988, pp. 106–117). The reality, however, is that most physicians will not take the time to ask about sexual function, much less to acquire special knowledge in providing assessment or treatment. Erectile failure, with its often complex etiology and array of available treatments, is a problem usually delegated to specialists. Ideally, the assessment team should include a mental health professional expert in sex and marital therapy, as well as a physician who can perform the medical evaluation. Typically this would be a urologist, but in our center an internist guides the physiological assessment. His thorough evaluation is an asset, because in a tertiary referral hospital my colleagues and I see many patients with complex medical histories.

On some occasions, we visit the patient in the hospital for a psychological consultation. This interview is geared to building a relationship with the patient, assessing his individual psychological coping and reaction to his illness, getting a picture of the relationship issues, and taking a complete history of the sexual problem. The history should include causal factors present at onset; the situational versus global dimension; and dysfunctions that exist in the realms of desire, arousal, orgasm, pain, and sexual dissatisfaction for each partner (Schover & Jensen, 1988, Ch. 6). In addition to standard questions used to assess sexual function, the interviewer may ask the following:

> What did your doctor tell you about the impact of this illness or medical treatment on your sex life?
> Have you had a chance to try sexual activity since your recovery?
> What changes have you noticed?
> What concerns do you have about your sexual function?
> Have either of you had trouble communicating during lovemaking—for example, if your usual techniques are not working as well as usual?
> Do either of you have any worries about whether it is safe or healthy to be sexually active now?
> Are pain, fatigue, or other physical symptoms distracting to you during sex?

If the patient is recovering from surgery or an acute illness, the interview may need to be divided into two sessions to avoid fatigue. Although some men may be able to give a coherent history if they are taking opiate pain medication or benzodiazepines, their memories of the interview may be hazy afterward. We try to keep questionnaires to a minimum, again to avoid taxing patients' stamina. We use the Brief Symptom Inventory (Derogatis & Melisaratos, 1983) to gauge psychological distress. In medical patients, scores are often a standard deviation above the mean for a healthy community-based sample. Scores on subscales such as Depression, Anxiety, or Hostility are also helpful indicators of current problem areas. The Sex History Form (Schover & Jensen, 1988, pp. 131–135) provides a detailed picture of sexual function. The Dyadic Adjustment Inventory (Spanier, 1976) yields a global score for dyadic satisfaction as well as indicating areas of conflict in the relationship.

Hospital rooms afford little privacy. Often a roommate is in the next bed, so that even conducting the interview in a low voice or with the masking noise of a television in the background is a violation of confidentiality. If privacy is a problem and the hospital unit offers no alternative interviewing area, the first session may be restricted to an introduction to the assessment and treatment process, with the clinician giving information rather than taking the history. Arrangements for follow-up after hospital discharge can be made.

Even when interviews are conducted with outpatients, the medical chart in a large medical center presents a challenge to confidentiality.

Patients are justifiably upset to have details of their sexual practices or a history of homosexuality or extramarital affairs documented in a chart that is seen by all of their physicians, nurses, ward clerks, and so on. If possible, a sexuality program should keep chart notes brief, covering only what is ethically needed for good health care. More extensive notes can be kept in a private file that can be released in a legal case, but not on a casual basis. The patient should be told in the first interview about the program's charting system and about any exceptions (e.g., routine sharing of the complete assessment with the referring physician or psychologist).

If the patient is married or in a committed relationship, it is crucial to include the partner. In addition to the general reasons for bringing the partner into the evaluation of erectile failure, the presence of a chronic illness can create strains in the relationship. The man may either hide his fear and grief about his health from his partner or develop an unhealthy dependency, abdicating his usual roles in the relationship. It is easy to label the erection problem as an individual, medical issue, forgetting that any treatment chosen will also have an effect on the partner and will require her (or his) cooperation and support. The tendency to exclude the partner once an erection problem is seen as "organic" is unfortunate, because it ignores the fact that sex takes place between two people. Both will be affected by any treatment chosen, even a medical or surgical option. In an inpatient setting, the partner can often be easily contacted, since she will be visiting the patient frequently. When the evaluation is done on an outpatient basis, the clinician must often counter both the patient's resistance to a couple approach ("I'm the one with the problem; just fix it") and the partner's reluctance to come in ("I think sex is private and I don't want to discuss it"). Refusal to schedule a couple session is often a sign of underlying relationship tension.

In tertiary referral centers, such as major hospital or specialized institute, patients may live a long distance away. The limits on ongoing treatment and difficulty in finding trained sex therapists in rural areas or foreign countries can create pressure to find a medical solution to the problem, or to provide any sexual counseling in one or two sessions. Sometimes the clinician also must deal with different cultural values and with language barriers.

Case Vignette

Shlomo Jaakob, a wealthy 61-year-old Jewish businessman, came with his wife from Iran to have cardiac bypass surgery. The physician initiating the consultation told the psychologist that Shlomo had complained of intermittent erection problems over the past 2 years; these were especially severe with a 24-year-old extramarital partner, but also occurred frequently with Miriam, his wife. He still occasionally had firm erections in the morning, on waking from sleep.

When the female psychologist arrived at the patient's luxurious private room on the "VIP floor," he told her in broken English that his primary language was French, and that he would like to wait 30 minutes for the interview until his wife arrived and could interpret for him, since her English was more fluent. The psychologist happened to speak reasonably good French and explained to Shlomo that she wanted some individual time with him anyway, to ask about how the problem varied with his two partners. He was somewhat embarrassed that his physician had mentioned the affair, and explained that he loved his wife dearly and had tried another partner mainly to determine whether his erections would improve as a result of novelty. The psychologist reassured him that this was a common male strategy, and that her job was not to judge him but to find out as much as possible about what might be causing the sexual problem. She mentioned that sometimes men tried sexual practices with a new partner that they felt uncomfortable requesting from their wives, and gave the example of oral sex. Shlomo denied that his partner gave more stimulation than his wife did. He said that his wife was an excellent sexual partner, and that in fact he had better erections with her than he did on the few occasions that he was with his younger partner. The psychologist said that she was unsure how Shlomo would regard masturbation, given his cultural background, but that it would be normal for a man in his situation to try some self-stimulation or to look at erotic pictures or movies to see whether he could achieve an erection. The patient replied that he had not tried masturbation since his teenage years. He was not offended by the question, however, and noted that sex had simply never been discussed with his parents while he was growing up.

At this point, Miriam came in. The psychologist introduced herself and explained that, since she spoke French, she had been taking some time to get to know Shlomo. Miriam, an attractive, beautifully dressed, slim woman in her early 50s, switched the language to English. She asked the psychologist whether she was Jewish, and on finding that she was, wanted to know about her family background. A discussion of the stress of being Jewish and living in Iran ensued. The Jaakobs lived in fear that they would need to flee the country some day. Miriam saw her husband as holding in his anxiety and anger until he would explode. She also felt that he was disappointed that the couple had never had a son. One of their two daughters was helping run the family business, and Shlomo was extremely reluctant to delegate authority to her. He had a history of a panic disorder, treated in Europe with an antidepressant. It seemed that his beginning this medication had coincided with the onset of the erection problems.

As Miriam spoke in English to the psychologist, she would interpret the psychologist's answers in French for her husband. She often left things out, however. When the psychologist offered to continue the interview in French, Shlomo said that he preferred to use English and let his wife interpret. This was frustrating for the psychologist, who felt that Shlomo was distancing himself and receiving only partial input. The psychologist suggested that the erectile failure could result from an interaction among the antidepressant, performance anxiety, and possibly some underlying vascular disease. She suggested that a conservative first step in treatment would be for the couple to try a program of sensate focus exercises. It developed that Miriam had been reading some self-help books on sex and had already suggested this to her husband. "You see!" she told him triumphantly. "I told you we should try this!" Unfortunately, Shlomo's reception of the psychologist's suggestion was as lukewarm as it had been when his wife proposed the idea. He was more interested in the thought of changing his psychotropic medication and pursuing an evaluation of his penile hemodynamics.

When the psychologist asked about marital issues, Miriam focused again on her husband's poor coping with stress and his overly rigid standards for their daughters. As she talked, he became more agitated; they increasingly began to bicker in Farsi, leaving the psychologist totally in the dark. She pointed out that they had been talking for a long time, and carefully went over her treatment recommendation. Shlomo agreed to see his psychiatrist in Europe and to change or discontinue his antidepressant. He was scheduled to fly home the next day, and so put off any penile vascular examinations until some future visit to the hospital. He agreed that he would try the sensate focus exercises, but the psychologist was doubtful that he would follow through.

The psychologist subsequently received holiday cards from the couple, but no word on whether their problem improved.

This case illustrates the frustration of trying to intervene when the therapist is unsure of cultural values about sexuality and is also dependent on translation, missing the subtle nuances that are communicated when all parties speak the same language fluently. Advice or homework that is helpful within a Western value system may be too foreign to be useful to such a patient, especially for cultures in which gender roles are still very male-dominant.

Special Challenges in Physiological Assessment

Techniques of hormonal, vascular, and neurological assessment of erectile function have been addressed in other chapters. In our program at The Cleveland Clinic Foundation, commonly used modalities include outpatient two-night Rigiscan studies; penile infusion studies of the veno-occlusive mechanism (Padma-Nathan & Goldstein, 1987); duplex ultrasound studies of the penile arteries (Lue & Abber, 1988); sensory testing of the penis by electrical stimulation (Rowland, Greenleaf, Mas, Myers, & Davidson, 1989); screening hormonal assays for prolactin and free versus total testosterone; and a careful medical and urological workup. Even with these sophisticated tests available, some chronic illnesses present dilemmas for assessment and choice of treatment.

MS is a disease that frequently produces erectile failure because of damage to spinal cord centers. In our own clinical experience, symptoms may include preserved NPT but consistent failure of erections in sexual situations, reducing the value of Rigiscan monitoring in choosing treatments. Furthermore, the erectile problems may improve and then recur months or years later, just like other symptoms of MS. The possible reversibility of the problem makes both patient and treatment team reluctant at times to try a penile prosthesis or even intracavernosal injections, with their risk of penile fibrosis. MS can also affect penile sensation, causing numbness or paresthesias that continue to reduce sexual pleasure even if erections are restored. Orgasm and ejaculation can be impaired by MS in a whole spectrum of ways (Schover, Thomas, Lakin, Montague, & Fischer, 1988). Men need to understand that treatments producing penile rigidity do not directly enhance skin sensation or orgasmic pleasure.

Techniques have been developed to spare the autonomic nerves of the prostatic plexus in radical cancer surgeries, including prostatectomy, cystectomy, and abdominoperineal resection (Walsh & Schlegel, 1988). Although more men now regain functional erections after cancer surgery, the recovery process is slow and may take over a year. Even when recovery is as complete as possible, a large group of men are left with erections that are not fully rigid and satisfactory for penetration and thrusting. Since penile sensation and the ability to have orgasm remain intact after such surgery (Schover, 1987), men are eager to resume sex once they have healed from the operation. With the advent of intracavernosal injection therapy and vacuum pump devices, many of these men prefer to take a chance that such therapy will slow or prevent the natural recovery of their erections, rather than waiting over a year to get treatment. Fewer men now choose to have a penile prosthesis. I should note anecdotally that we have followed two men who began using intracavernosal injections a number of months after radical prostatectomy, and both have reported improvement over time in their ability to achieve and maintain erections without using their medication. It is important to let men know that nerve-sparing surgery is an important advance, but does not provide recovery of rigid erections to everyone. Additional sexual rehabilitation may be needed.

Although physicians and patients assume that erectile failure is an irreversible side effect of diabetes, spontaneous remissions are not rare (Jensen, 1986). When poor control of blood sugar is improved, diabetologists sometimes observe that erections also normalize (Meisler, Carey, Lantinga, &

Krauss, 1989). Assessment of NPT again may be of limited value in treatment planning, because young diabetic men with good erections during sex have impaired erections during sleep (Schiavi, Fisher, Quadland, & Glover, 1985). The influence of psychological factors in causing erectile failure in diabetic men is often minimized, and the most drastic interventions are offered with no couple or individual psychological assessment. Since diabetics are more at risk for postsurgical infection and also may have neurological damage to penile or orgasmic sensation, they merit a thorough workup before a penile prosthesis, venous ligation surgery, or medical treatments are advised. Unfortunately, no effective therapy is available to enhance diminished pleasure with touch or orgasm, except to use sex therapy techniques to maximize mental arousal.

Men with a history of chemical dependency also present a dilemma. Those currently abusing drugs or alcohol should be treated and stabilized before any further sexual dysfunction workup is pursued, since many cases of erectile failure are reversible with sobriety (Schover & Jensen, 1988, pp. 274–285). Those who have remained drug- or alcohol-free for months or years, but who still have erection problems, should have a thorough medical evaluation. If any irreversible organic condition is found, treatment needs to be carefully chosen. We have a concern that some men have the potential to abuse intracavernosal injections—for example, injecting a larger dose than instructed or using injections more often than is advisable. A treatment such as the vacuum pump device, with fewer potential side effects, may be safer to prescribe. A penile prosthesis is another alternative that is not so dependent on patient compliance once healing has occurred. Sexual counseling or formal sex therapy is often a helpful adjunct to a medical or surgical treatment, particularly if one or both partners have trouble with intimacy.

Some men with psychiatric disorders have delusions about the penis—for example, that it is shrinking into the body (Fishbain, Barsky, & Goldberg, 1989). Others have chronic genital pain without any clear organic cause (Schover, 1990). A clinical should use extreme caution in prescribing even a mildly invasive test or procedure, such as an intracavernosal injection, for such a patient. The risk is that he will accuse the physician of contributing to penile pain or shrinkage, so that the presenting problem is exacerbated and even a court case could result.

Another group of patients who may not be candidates for invasive vascular evaluations are men with severe cardiac disease. The intracavernosal injection of papaverine and phentolamine can result in hypertension, especially if the veno-occlusive mechanism of the penis is abnormal. If the test injection results in priapism, the medications used for reversal (epinephrine, metaraminol bitartrate) can cause hypotension, cardiac arrhythmia, and pulmonary emboli. Although prostaglandin E_1 is believed to be safer, it has not been in use long enough for clinicians to be certain (Stackl, Hasun, &

Marberger, 1988). Avoiding these tests should not present a major handicap, however, since a home injection program would not be a safe treatment option for such men, nor would extensive surgery to ligate penile veins or perform microvascular arterial repair. Monitoring of NPT is a safe way to find out whether an organic deficit exists—for example, to determine whether a vacuum pump device or a simple penile prosthesis is an appropriate option.

SPECIAL ISSUES IN TREATMENT

Just as chronically ill men need individually tailored assessment of their erectile failure, their medical condition often necessitates modifications in typical treatment formats. This section defines "treatment" in an interdisciplinary fashion as the combination of techniques needed in each case. These may include brief sexual counseling or longer-term sex therapy (Schover & Jensen, 1988, Ch. 7), sometimes combined with the array of options for organic erectile failure: the vacuum pump device, home intracavernosal injections, penile venous ligation surgery, penile revascularization (in rare cases), implantation of a penile prosthesis, hormonal therapy (in rare cases), or adjustment of medication that is affecting erectile function.

The Format of Sex Therapy

Because patients with a chronic medical condition often come to a central, urban area for specialized health care, the sex therapist may see men who live beyond easy commuting distance. Thus, the typical once-a-week spacing of therapy sessions is impractical. One option is to use the original Masters and Johnson (1970) model of daily sessions over a week or two, letting the couple reside locally and do homework exercises between therapy hours during this period. Another format is to have the couple come in every 2–3 weeks, perhaps with a phone contact between sessions to make sure the homework is going smoothly. This second option is less expensive, but does not work well if a couple has severe marital conflict or individual psychopathology.

A mental health clinician who works with a particular group of patients (e.g., cancer patients, diabetics, or men with MS) needs to become expert on the impact of the illness and its treatments on sexual function. Such knowledge can be gained by spending time with a physician in a clinical setting; meeting with health care workers, such as physical therapists, enterostomal therapists, or respiratory therapists; reading textbooks and journal articles; and, perhaps most importantly, interviewing many patients in detail about their sexual problems and the ways they have found to solve them.

My own approach generally follows the format of giving homework between sessions and using the therapist–patient contact time to discuss how the exercises have progressed, as well as to work on marital communication, expression of caring, and conflict resolution. Emotional and cognitive coping with the illness for both partners is a topic I usually address. The framework for behavioral exercises is the typical one of sensate focus with gradually increasing genital touch and sexual communication. I may also have the man practice gaining and losing erections in self-stimulation as well as with his partner. Penetration is introduced in a stepwise fashion, first without a full erection, then with a firm one, and then with movement. Sexual fantasy enhancement, focus on sensation, relaxation training, and distraction from anxious thoughts are cognitive techniques I often use.

One largely untapped resource for sexual rehabilitation is that of patient support groups. Many organizations, such as the American Cancer Society, the Mended Hearts Clubs, the Multiple Sclerosis Society, and the National Kidney Foundation, sponsor local chapters and programs. A group of men or couples coping with the same disease could attend a workshop or a series of sessions on issues of sexuality or intimacy. The drawback is that men in particular are reluctant to share such private issues with others whom they know. Some of the self-help groups for men with erectile failure, such as Impotents Anonymous, may have more success, because men attending a session know that all their fellow attendees have a sexual dysfunction too. An alternative would be to create a special time-limited group—for example, a group for men on hemodialysis who want help with sexual and relationship issues.

Since the erectile failure of many men with chronic illness does have an organic component, treatment often includes a medical or surgical intervention. Ideally, some adjunctive sex therapy can help the partner to be supportive and feel included in the new treatment, and can remedy other sexual problems such as male low desire, premature ejaculation, or sexual dysfunction in the partner (Schover, 1989). In practice, however, men who seek a penile prosthesis, home injections, or a vacuum pump device are usually not receptive to sex therapy. They will attend a session or two, but often drop out and only give follow-up information if pressed. Combined treatment programs are a promising idea, but can only succeed with clear cooperation between the urologist and the mental health professional.

Treatment Issues Specific to Chronic Illness

A number of medical conditions interfere technically with sexual expression, so that specific advice or problem solving must be included in sex therapy for the erectile failure.

Fatigue or Shortness of Breath

Fatigue or shortness of breath during intercourse can be distracting and contribute to loss of erection. Patients with cardiac disease COPD, or other illnesses that reduce general energy level should plan lovemaking for a time of day when they feel rested. Studies of healthy young men (Bohlen, Held, Sanderson, & Patterson, 1984) suggested that respiration and metabolic consumption were lower for a man if the woman moved more actively during intercourse. Noncoital sex was also less strenuous than intercourse.

Men who have angina can use a nitroglycerin tablet prophylactically before sex to prevent chest pain with exertion. Some patients with COPD need to be on continuous oxygen. There are two pamphlets for COPD patients that illustrate how partners can position themselves to minimize interference from breathing apparatus (Eckert et al., 1984; Hossler & Cole, 1983). For example, a man with COPD can sit on a chair or prop himself against pillows. His wife can face him during intercourse while sitting astride his body and doing more of the thrusting.

Limited Range of Motion

Patients who are quadriplegic or paraplegic, or who have limited movement because of severe arthritis or low back pain, also need counseling on comfortable positions for intercourse. A woman with arthritis in her hips may be comfortable kneeling with her thighs fairly close together while her partner enters her from behind. A warm bath or a painkiller before sex can sometimes minimize pain. For men with spinal cord injuries, several films and self-help books are available (Bullard, 1988). A booklet on sexuality is also published by the Arthritis Foundation (1982). Although pictures or films can provide suggestions on how to modify a sexual routine, the most important factors are open communication between partners and a willingness to experiment. A sex therapist can guide this process, using techniques such as sensate focus exercises and communication training. A physical therapist can often give helpful advice.

Men with loss of fine motor hand coordination can use a vibrator to stimulate themselves or to provide extra stimulation to their partners. Some men with extreme disability may need a vibrator that straps onto a hand.

Special Concerns of Men with Cardiovascular Disease

After a heart attack or a stroke, men often fear that sex may bring on another such event (Schover & Jensen, 1988, pp. 203–216). Most men can have intercourse or other sexual activity safely, although the data on cardiac events or sudden death during sex are still minimal. A sex therapist should always make sure that the patient's physician has been consulted about the safety of resuming sex. General principles for such patients include avoiding sex after alcohol or a heavy meal; making sure the room is at a comfortable temperature; and realizing that signs of sexual arousal, such as rapid breathing and pulse, are normal and do not indicate an imminent heart attack or stroke. It is important that hypertension be controlled with medication, since blood pressure can rise to dangerous levels in unmedicated hypertensive men during sexual activity (Mann, Craig, Gould, Melville, & Raftery, 1982).

Bowel or Bladder Dysfunction

Some men have lost control of bowel or bladder function because of a medical condition. This becomes a concern in terms of aesthetics or body image during sex. Men with neurogenic bladder dysfunction resulting from spinal cord trauma or neurological disease may have indwelling urinary catheters, which can be taped down and covered with a condom during sexual activity. Using a condom during foreplay and intercourse can also be a reassuring to men who experience mild leakage of urine (e.g., after radical prostatectomy). Men who intermittently catheterize their own bladders should do so before starting sexual activity. Bowel incontinence is a less common problem. Spinal-cord-injured men who use aids to empty their bowels should again use that procedure before sex.

A number of men have urinary ostomies or colostomies after cancer surgery, or ileostomies after surgery to treat ulcerative colitis. With good ostomy care, the appliance does not have to interfere with sex (Schover, 1986). Men may wish to wear an undershirt or sash to conceal the appliance, or may tape the ostomy pouch to keep it out of the way. Pouch covers made of soft cloth can be bought or made at home. Some men with colostomies can wear just a stoma cap or safety pouch during sex. A small urinary ostomy pouch is also available for short-term use. Ostomy pouches should, of course, always be emptied before sex. Surgery to create continent urinary or bowel diversions is becoming more successful, so that some men do not need to wear an external collection device. Many men with ostomies have had cancer. A booklet, *Sexuality and Cancer: For the Man Who Has Cancer and His Partner*, is published by the American Cancer Society (Schover, 1988).

In my clinical experience, it is more common for the patient who has an ostomy or incontinence to avoid sex out of fear of rejection than it is for the partner actually to be turned off. An exception is the case in which a man has poor personal hygiene and comes to bed smelling of urine or feces. Some plain speaking and better self-care can often make a difference for such couples. Occasionally, a partner has a strong negative reaction to a change in bowel or bladder function. Desensitization to the sight of an ostomy or catheter can be accomplished through gradual exposure and cognitive restructuring.

Human Immunodeficiency Virus Infection and Safe Sex

Human immunodeficiency virus (HIV) infection is also a chronic illness. Although issues for gay men have been noted in Chapter 12, safe sex is of course also relevant to heterosexual patients. Those who learn that they are infected are often not yet experiencing any symptoms and have normal levels of sexual desire. The fear of transmitting the virus to a partner leads many to stop all sexual activity. Others (though not nearly as many) disregard the danger or deliberately set out to infect others as a kind of revenge for what they themsleves have experienced.

For the typical heterosexual HIV-positive person in a stable relationship with a partner who tests HIV-negative, the knowledge of this status brings a terrible dilemma. The partners want to continue to express love and closeness through sex, but they fear contagion and are unsure what is safe. It is not uncommon to see couples who have been having unprotected intercourse for several years without seroconversion of the uninfected partner (Burger et al., 1986). It is clear, however, that the more often vaginal–penile intercourse contacts take place, the more likely the partner is to become infected (Padian et al., 1987). Anal intercourse may slightly elevate the risk. Unfortunately, the use of condoms seems only moderately effective in preventing infection of the partner over the long run (Feldblum & Fortney, 1988; Frosner, 1989). It is unclear how risky oral sex is for women or for men (Haverkos & Edelman, 1988), although HIV is clearly present in high concentrations in semen and in vaginal secretions. Deep kissing seems less likely as a route of transmission, but cannot be ruled out.

As professionals, we must stay current in our knowledge about HIV transmission and give our patients the most unbiased information possible. Rather than telling a couple what "safe sex" means, we must help the partners openly discuss a range of sexual practices and arrive at an agreement of how much risk the uninfected partner is willing to take. When we know that one partner is at high risk for HIV or is in fact seropositive, and yet refuses to inform the other partner, a legal and ethical dilemma results (Girardi, Keese, Traver, & Cooksey, 1988; World Health Organization, 1989). Clearly, the best outcome is to persuade the patient to tell the partner, with active help from the therapist. Both partners must be offered education and counseling. If the patient continues to refuse, the therapist should seek ethical and legal consultation, rather than acting alone.

Case Vignette

Mr. Bob Abbott was an unskilled laborer aged 35 who told our infectious disease department that he became HIV-positive through handling dirty linen while working in a hospital laundry. He denied ever using intravenous drugs, but had a history of heavy alcohol and marijuana abuse. He denied any same-sex contacts. He sought HIV testing, he said, after watching a TV show on syphilis and wondering whether an old infection that had been treated 10 years before could still be present and causing the lumps he had under his arms.

Bob sought help for an erection problem that was making it impossible to use condoms for intercourse with his wife of 12 years, Mary. She tested negative for HIV. He reported that his penis had always had a downward curve, "like a banana." His sexual history was tragic. He had grown up with an alcoholic and physically abusive father. At the age of 9, Bob had been repeatedly molested by his 16-year-old stepbrother; when he told his stepmother, she refused to believe him. He said that this abuse never caused him to doubt his own heterosexual orientation, but he did disclose in the individual psychological assessment that he had contracted syphilis in a brief, drunken homosexual encounter in an adult bookstore. He steadfastly denied any other homosexual activity. Despite his penile curvature, he had had successful intercourse at age 21 and continued to function well during the earlier years of his marriage. It was unclear on questioning whether he had an abnormal curvature or whether his perception of a normal penile appearance was distorted.

Mary had also come from a background of turmoil, with abusive parents and brothers in constant trouble with the law. She had married for the first time at age 15 and already had three children when she met Bob. Bob reported that in recent years he was only able to have intercourse if he held the base of his penis with one hand and then thrust hard for 20–60 minutes to reach an orgasm. He said that because of this practice, his penis was constantly abraded and bleeding at the base. The therapist warned him that bleeding during intercourse increased the risk of infection to his wife. Bob also believed that the firmness of his erections had decreased since he learned about his HIV status. He and Mary were counseled on safe sex, but when he tried to use a condom it just "fell off." Mary was so attracted to him that she did not trust herself to live in the same house and have only safe sex. Therefore, she took their children and went to stay with her parents in a neighboring state until Mr. Abbott could get "fixed" and begin to use condoms.

On physical exam, Bob's penis appeared entirely normal. Ordinarily, the staff at our clinic would use an intracavernosal injection to evaluate penile curvature with erection; however, Bob's platelet count was quite low, making it unsafe to pursue such testing or even to consider the home injection program as a treatment. He was asked to bring in an instant-camera photo of his erection, but he did not do so. Dacomed snap gauges used on two consecutive nights suggested that erections were rigid, with three and two snaps broken. Testosterone and prolactin were normal. The physician told him that the psychologist needed to see him with his wife before proceeding with any treatment, but it took 3 months before the couple came in.

Mary was an overweight woman with tangled hair. She giggled as she confirmed that it was hard for her to stay away from her husband sexually, though she said that his erections were less firm than in the past. She also said that she had trouble believing her husband had HIV. "He's not sick!" she repeatedly exclaimed. "He worries more than I do." Just in the past week they had had intercourse without a condom, but had felt comfortable because Mary had douched afterwards. When the therapist explained that douching was no protection, and might even increase the risk of HIV transmission by causing minor vaginal trauma, both partners were surprised. Mary flatly refused to help her husband put on a condom; she believed that to be his job. She also would not consider using a vaginal spermicide (Feldblum & Fortney, 1988). Although the psychologist tried to interest the partners in another session or two of sexual counseling, they were only interested in a vacuum pump device. Bob's physician was concerned that the pump could create too much internal bleeding, given the low platelet count. The staff was also concerned that Bob was too disorganized to use the device correctly—for example, that he might leave the band on his penis for too long after sex, even if he proved not to have a significant chordee. Both partners agreed that Bob continued to have drinking binges on weekends. Penile prosthesis surgery was out of the question.

Our staff concluded, sadly, that our program had nothing more to offer to the Abbotts, since they declined to pursue sexual counseling. Bob continued to be followed up by our infectious disease department. The staff was concerned by Mary's denial, but saw no clear way to change her thinking or behavior.

Ethical issues are also raised when a seropositive man wants treatment for erectile failure. As HIV infection progresses, loss of sexual desire and erection problems become more common. Nevertheless, many men want to continue partner sex. Sex therapy automatically involves both partners, and their knowledge about risks can be assessed. Other treatments, such as the vacuum pump device, home intracavernosal injections, or a penile prosthesis, should not be offered without involving a partner and making sure that safe sex counseling has been provided.

The safest sex practice (i.e., manual stimulation to orgasm, using a condom or latex glove) can be accomplished without the man's having a firm erection. Should we help our patients to have unsafe sex? Certainly, involving the partner in consultation minimizes ethical concerns, if he or she is well informed and still chooses to have oral, vaginal, or anal penetration. Many women are financially and emotionally dependent on HIV-positive men, however; they may not be assertive enough to insist on safe sex. And what if a clinician suspects that a patient will have sex with other partners who are uninformed?

Other ethical considerations have to do with medical procedures. The penile injections cause some bleeding, further increasing a partner's exposure to infected body fluids. Many surgeons refuse to implant a penile prosthesis in an HIV-positive man; they feel it is an elective surgery and that it is wrong to expose the surgeon and operating room personnel to HIV for such a reason. Is this a tenable position? Easy answers do not exist.

The Terminal Patient

Men with a clearly limited lifespan sometimes request treatment for erectile failure. Most often their problems are organic. In the days when the penile prosthesis was the only good treatment option, the surgeon had to balance the trauma of the operation and healing period against the probable number of months the man had left. Now the vacuum pump device and home intracavernosal injections offer more immediate relief with far less health risk. Even when a cancer is being treated palliatively or a man has progressive cardiovascular or neurological disease, sex remains a way of feeling pleasure and closeness. Sometimes sex therapy can also help a couple resolve relationship tension and feel more at peace with one partner's dying.

CASE EXAMPLE

The case of Bill Johnson illustrates a number of the issues discussed in this chapter. Bill, a 41-year-old machinist, had had chronic back pain for 7 years; he had been injured in a motorcycle accident and had a lumbar laminectomy 1 year later. He also had irritable bowel syndrome and engaged in drinking binges on weekends once or twice a month. He had married his wife, Dottie, when both were age 16. Bill had been physically abused as a child by his alcoholic father. Bill and Dottie came in for help after a 1-year history of erectile dysfunction.

About 4 months before the onset of the sexual problem, Dottie had cranial surgery to repair an arteriovenous malformation. Bill became very frightened of losing his wife, but did have successful intercourse at first when the couple resumed sex. Another stress was that the couple's first grandchild was born with a heart defect at about this time. Basically, Bill and Dottie had a strong marriage, with open expression of caring. Bill was more apt to yell when angry, while Dottie was a pouter. Their main conflict centered on Bill's perception that Dottie was not strict enough with their two daughters. They enjoyed their mutual hobby of going to rural auctions. Neither partner had symptoms of depression, and both had normal scores on the Brief Symptom Inventory.

Sexually, Bill was always the one who had a stronger level of desire. In recent years, however, Dottie had become more interested in sex and more easily orgasmic. She remained somewhat inhibited, however, preferring sex with the lights out and refusing to try oral stimulation. It was Dottie who first commented that Bill was taking longer to get an erection with her hand caressing, and that his erections were not as firm as usual. Soon after that, Bill began to try to penetrate as soon as his erection was at all adequate. He would then ejaculate within a few seconds. Frustrated at the reduction in their foreplay and short duration of intercourse, Dottie withdrew and began staying up late to watch television instead of coming to bed. She believed her husband no longer found her attractive, especially since her surgery. Soon afterward, Bill had a flareup of his back pain and was temporarily disabled for work. Bill also began to focus on the sexual problem; he was concerned that one of his testes hung lower than the other, and he noticed a large vein on his penis.

Bill's medical evaluation was negative for organic causes of erectile failure. A glucose tolerance test, free and total serum testosterone, prolactin, and thyroid hormones were all normal, although one of his liver enzymes was mildly elevated (probably from alcohol abuse). A Rigiscan study revealed normal erections during sleep on both nights.

Bill and Dottie came in for three sessions of sex therapy. Sessions included education on male and female anatomy. Dottie told Bill for the first time that she had always wanted more foreplay and afterplay. The partners went through sensate focus exercises, with progression from no genital touch, to genital touch, to orgasm from manual stimulation. Bill immediately began to get firm erections during the exercises. He agreed to limit his drinking to two beers a day, but would not consider joining Alcoholics Anonymous. His fear of losing Dottie and then being rejected by others because of his sexual problem was discussed. Bill complained, however, that on most occasions he lost his erection as soon as Dottie stopped touching his penis. Reassurance that this was normal did not help, nor did use of an erotic movie or sexual fantasy. The couple continued to progress through penetration and intercourse, with variable success. They could not come in as often as would be optimal because they lived in a rural area, 3 hours away from the hospital. Bill's premature ejaculation resolved, but on about half of the couple's attempts at intercourse he lost his erection during thrusting and could not regain it. He would then sometimes be able to reach an orgasm with a semiflaccid penis.

The therapist and couple mutually decided that Bill could try a vacuum pump device, in the hopes that the assurance of a longer-lasting erection would reduce his remaining performance anxiety. Bill had a teaching session with the program's nurse clinician, and was able to achieve a very firm erection with the pump. At a 3-month follow-up, he and Dottie reported successful intercourse once a week. On most occasions Bill used the pump, but about one-fourth of the time he had a very firm erection in foreplay and elected to proceed to intercourse without using the device. Bill and Dottie were both satisfied with the outcome of treatment. Bill had more reliable erections, and Dottie enjoyed the improved foreplay and more open sexual communication. Bill was back at work, with only minimal complaints of chronic pain. Liver enzymes were normal, and Bill reported a large reduction in his alcohol use.

This case illustrates that a therapist must be flexible in a medical setting. If the therapist had insisted that Bill enter alcoholism treatment, or had refused to work with the vacuum pump device, the outcome might not have been as positive. She tried to work within Bill and Dottie's frame of reference, however. She reassured Bill that his penis, testes, and erection reflex were normal, but allowed him to try a medical solution that made him feel comfortable. She and her colleagues used Bill's liver enzyme results and his current sexual problem as evidence to urge him to cut down his alcohol use. Neither he nor Dottie was willing to use the label "alcoholic." As Bill regained confidence that he was in control as a man, his somatic symptoms decreased, so that he functioned better at home and at work.

CONCLUSIONS

Chronic illness is a common factor in causing erectile failure. When clinicians evaluate chronically ill men, it is important to assess both the psychological and physiological impacts of a disease and its treatment on sexuality. A man's partner, as always, should be involved in the evaluation process and treatment planning, unless the man does not have a committed relationship. Working in hospital settings sometimes necessitates flexibility in the format of brief sexual counseling or sex therapy. Even the structure of the assessment can be influenced by the patient's stamina and the availability of a private setting for talking. Specific advice may be given on how to minimize the interference of medical problems with enjoyment of sexual activity. The clinician must become familiar with specific issues relevant to each particular group of patients.

REFERENCES

Abrahamson, D. J., Barlow, D. H., & Abrahamson, L. S. (1989). Differential effects of performance demand and distraction on sexually functional and dysfunctional males. *Journal of Abnormal Psychology, 98*, 241–247.

Arthritis Foundation. (1982). *Arthritis: Living and loving. Information about sex* (Booklet No. 9190, 9197-9182). Atlanta: Author.

Bohlen, J. G., Held, J. P., Sanderson, M. O., & Patterson, R. P. (1984). Heart rate, rate-pressure product, and oxygen uptake during four sexual activities. *Archives of Internal Medicine, 144,* 1745–1748.

Bukberg, J., Penman, D., & Holland, S. C. (1984). Depression in hospitalized cancer patients. *Psychosomatic Medicine, 46,* 199–212.

Bullard, D. G. (1988). The treatment of desire disorders in the medically ill and physically disabled. In S. R. Leiblum & R. C. Rosen (Eds.), *Sexual desire disorders* (pp. 348–384). New York: Guilford Press.

Burger, H., Weiser, B., Robinson, W. S., Lifson, J., Engleman, E., Rouzioux, C., Brun-Vezinet, F., Barre-Sinoussi, F., Montagnier, L., & Chermann, J. (1986). Transmission of lymphadenopathy-associated virus/human T lymphotropic virus type III in sexual partners. *American Journal of Medicine, 81,* 5–10.

Derogatis, L. R., & Melisaratos, N. (1983). The Brief Symptom Inventory: An introductory report. *Psychological Medicine, 13,* 595–605.

Eckert, R. C., Bartsch, K., Dowell, D., Gutline, A., Davis, R., & Cochran, J. (1984). *Being close.* Denver: National Jewish Hospital and Research Center.

Feldblum, P. J., & Fortney, J. A. (1988). Condoms, spermicides, and the transmission of human immunodeficiency virus: A review of the literature. *American Journal of Public Health, 78,* 52–54.

Fishbain, D. A., Barsky, S., & Goldberg, M. (1989). "Koro" (genital retraction syndrome): Psychotherapeutic interventions. *American Journal of Psychotherapy, 43,* 87–91.

Frosner, G. G. (1989). How efficient is "safer sex" in preventing HIV infection? *Infection, 17,* 3–5.

Girardi, J. A., Keese, R. M., Traver, L. B., & Cooksey, D. R. (1988). Psychotherapist responsibility in notifying individuals at risk for exposure to HIV. *Journal of Sex Research, 25,* 1–27.

Haverkos, H. W., & Edelman, R. (1988). The epidemiology of Acquired Immunodeficiency Syndrome among heterosexuals. *Journal of the American Medical Association, 260,* 1922–1929.

Hossler, C. J., & Cole, S. S. (1983). *Intimacy and chronic lung disease.* Ann Arbor: Department of Physical Medicine and Rehabilitation, University of Michigan Hospitals.

Howell, J. R., Reynolds, C. F., III, Thase, M. E., Frank, E., Jennings, J. R., Houck, P. R., Berman, S., Jacobs, E., & Kupfer, D. J. (1987). Assessment of sexual function, interest, and activity in depressed men. *Journal of Affective Disorders, 13,* 61–66.

Jensen, P., Jensen, S. B., Sorensen, P. S., Bjerre, B. D., Rizzi, D. A., Sorenson, A. S., Klysner, R., Brinch, K., Jespersen, B., & Nielsen, H. (1990). Sexual dysfunction in male and female patients with epilepsy: A study of 86 outpatients. *Archives of Sexual Behavior, 19,* 1–14.

Jensen, S. B. (1986). Sexual dysfunction and diabetes mellitus: A six-year follow-up study. *Archives of Sexual Behavior, 15,* 271–284.

Liss-Levinson, W. S. (1982). Clinical observations on the emotional responses of males to cancer. *Psychotherapy: Theory, Research, and Practice, 19,* 325–330.

Lue, T. F., & Abber, J. C. (1988). Penodynamics: Diagnostic studies of vasculogenic impotence. In D. K. Montague, (Ed.). *Disorders of male sexual function* (pp. 95–104). Chicago: Year Book Medical.

Mann, S., Craig, M. W. M., Gould, B. A., Melville, D. E., & Raftery, E. B. (1982). Coital blood pressure in hypertensives: Cephaligia, syncope and effects of beta-blockade. *British Heart Journal, 47,* 84–89.

Masters, W. H., & Johnson, V. E. (1970). *Human sexual inadequacy.* Boston: Little, Brown.

Meisler, A. W., Carey, M. P., Lantinga, L. J., & Krauss, D. J. (1989). Erectile dysfunction in diabetes mellitus: A biopsychosocial approach to etiology and assessment. *Annals of Behavioral Medicine, 11,* 18–27.

Padian, N., Marquis, L., Francis, D. P., Anderson, R. E., Rutherford, G. W., O'Malley, P. M., & Winkelstein, W. (1987). Male-to-female transmission of human immunodeficiency virus. *Journal of American Medical Association, 258,* 788–790.

Padma-Nathan, H., & Goldstein, I. (1987). Corporal leakage syndrome: The role of dynamic infusion cavernosometry and cavernosography (DICC). *Journal of Urology, 137,* 184A.

Rowland, D. L., Greenleaf, W., Mas, M., Myers, L., & Davidson, D. M. (1989). Penile and finger sensory thresholds in young, aging, and diabetic males. *Archives of Sexual Behavior, 18,* 1–12.

Schiavi, R. C., Fisher, C., Quadland, M., & Glover, A. (1985). Nocturnal penile tumescent evaluation of erectile function in insulin-dependent men. *Diabetologia, 28,* 90–94.

Schover, L. R. (1986). Sexual rehabilitation of the ostomy patient. In D. B. Smith & D. E. Johnson (Eds.), *Ostomy care and the cancer patient: Surgical and clinical considerations* (pp. 103–120). Orlando, FL: Grune & Stratton.

Schover, L. R. (1987). Sexuality and fertility in urologic cancer patients. *Cancer, 60*(Suppl.), 553–558.

Schover, L. R. (1988). *Sexuality and cancer: For the man who has cancer and his partner.* Atlanta: American Cancer Society.

Schover, L. R. (1989). Sex therapy for the penile prosthesis recipient. *Urologic Clinics of North America, 16,* 91–98.

Schover, L. R. (1990). The psychological evaluation of men with atypical genital pain. *Cleveland Clinic Journal of Medicine, 57,* 697–700.

Schover, L. R., & Jensen, S. B. (1988). *Sexuality and chronic illness: A comprehensive approach.* New York: Guilford Press.

Schover, L. R., Thomas, A. J., Lakin, M. M., Montague, D. K., & Fischer, J. (1988). Orgasm phase dysfunctions in multiple sclerosis. *Journal of Sex Research, 25,* 548–554.

Spanier, G. B. (1976). Measuring dyadic adjustment: New scales for assessing the quality of marriage and similar dyads. *Journal of Marriage and the Family, 38,* 15–28.

Stackl, W., Hasun, R., & Marberger, M. (1988). Intracavernous injection of prostaglandin E1 in impotent men. *Journal of Urology, 140,* 66–68.

Tanagho, E. A., Lue, T. F., & McClure, R. D. (Eds.). (1988). *Contemporary management of impotence and infertility.* Baltimore: Williams & Wilkins.

Thase, M. E., Reynolds, C. F., III, Jennings, J. R., Berman, S. R., Houck, P. R., Howell, J. R., Frank, E., & Kupfer, D. J. (1988). Diagnostic performance of nocturnal penile tumescence studies in healthy, dysfunctional (impotent), and depressed men. *Psychiatry Research, 26,* 79–87.

Verbrugge, L. M. (1979). Marital status and health. *Journal of Marriage and the Family*, 42, 267–285.

Walsh, P. C., & Schlegel, P. N. (1988). Radical pelvic surgery with preservation of sexual function. *Annals of Surgery*, 208, 391–400.

World Health Organization. (1989). Consensus Statement: Sexually transmitted diseases as a risk factor for HIV transmission. *Journal of Sex Research*, 26, 272–275.

Index

368